What people are saying...

"This outstanding book offers new insights into the causes of the childhood obesity epidemic by a pioneer in the field. The emotional messages from the kids themselves are oftentimes heartbreaking. The book offers fresh ideas for stemming the problem and preventing it from worsening. A major contribution to the field."

--John Foreyt, Ph.D.
Professor in the Department of Pediatrics, the Department of Psychiatry, and the Department of Medicine at Baylor College of Medicine, Houston, TX. Dr. Foreyt is the Director of the Behavioral Medicine Research Center at Baylor and has published more than 240 articles and 17 books in the areas of obesity, eating disorders, and cardiovascular risk factor reduction.

"I must congratulate you on having the bravery to persist on this amazingly TRUE piece of work. It really resonates true because it is what they say."

-- Rose Marie Thomas, MD, FAAP
Dr. Thomas is a pediatrician and directs the Frontier Kids weight loss program on Trinidad-Tobago in the West Indies.

"Dr. Pretlow's book reveals the pain and struggle of obese children from *THEIR* point of view, thus providing unique and valuable information about the childhood obesity epidemic. Dr. Pretlow presents solutions – his take on what should be done to treat childhood obesity and to prevent it. A must-read for anyone seeking to hear the voice of obese children and the advice of a pediatrician who has been listening to these children for the past 9 years."

-- Barbara J. Moore, PhD

President and CEO of Shape Up America!
Founded in 1994 by C. Everett Koop, U.S. Surgeon General 1981-1989
www.shapeup.org

OVERWEIGHT

What Kids Say

What's Really Causing the Childhood Obesity Epidemic?

Dr. Robert A. Pretlow, MD, MSEE, FAAP

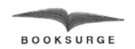

BOOKSURGE

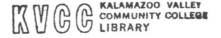

ISBN: 1-4392-4434-0 (trade paper)
ISBN 13: 9781439244340 (trade paper)

Library of Congress Control Number: 2009908469

Printed in the United States by
BookSurge
An Amazon.com Company
7290 B Investment Drive
Charleston, SC 29418

Visit us at www.booksurge.com

To order additional copies go to www.amazon.com

Manufactured in the United States of America

The information contained in this book is not a substitute for medical advice or care. All matters pertaining to your physical health or that of your child should be supervised by a health professional.

This book is dedicated...

To the millions of courageous kids from all over the world, who, on their own, seek help for their weight problem on the Internet and on our website. To those with the greatest measure of courage, who openly share their stories, struggles, and successes. And, to those with even a small degree of success, who become helpers to those just starting out.

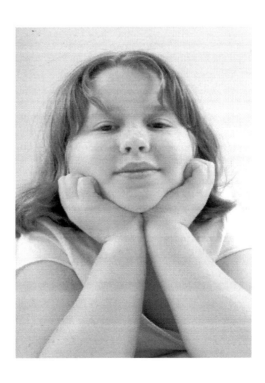

OVERWEIGHT: What Kids Say

Contents

FORWARD

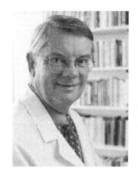

I first met Dr. Robert Pretlow in May of 2008 at a conference, where I spoke. At the end of my presentation he came up and told me about his unique website, where overweight kids have spontaneously posted over 130,000 messages over the last 9 years. After talking with Dr. Pretlow for only 5 minutes, I responded, "You should write a book!" He promised to send further information once he returned home.

Dr. Pretlow also shared his observation that these kids appear to be psychologically hooked on food, almost like an addiction. He expressed his frustration that healthcare professionals seem unwilling to consider this idea. I likewise have been perplexed by the rigidity of many healthcare professionals in this regard.

On returning home, Dr. Pretlow emailed me hundreds of posts from kids depicting their striking struggles to lose weight and many more describing using food to cope with stress, depression, and boredom. I wrote back: "I think that you have an enormous amount of information that would be lifesaving to many children and parents, and eye-opening to health care professionals. Your article on comfort eating is excellent and could serve as an outline for your book, focusing on what you know to be true, i.e., psychological food dependence is a major cause of childhood obesity, and how to break the dependence. The book, filled with examples from the posts demonstrating food dependence, followed by success stories to support your thesis, would make a significant contribution to the field."

Dr. Pretlow's book presents the heart wrenching stories of overweight kids, in their own words. These kids use food to cope with life. Unfortunately, they become hooked on this 'comfort eating' behavior and become overweight or obese because of it, which wrecks their lives. They hate being fat, yet they struggle to resist cravings for food, in spite of full awareness of the dreadful effects that further weight gain will have. Many state that their eating is 'out of control.' This is suggestive of an addictive quality or psychological food dependence. Displacement activity appears to be another factor in the kids' dependence on eating.

Dr. Pretlow shared a letter with me that he wrote to the editor of the journal, Pediatrics, in early 2008. In that letter he suggested that overweight and obesity in childhood be treated similarly to forms of substance abuse. Initially, his letter was rejected for publication, because none of the childhood obesity authorities would write a reply, and only letters with replies are published. Nevertheless, Dr. Pretlow persevered; his letter finally received a reply and was published in August 2008. The reply to his letter contended that a substance abuse approach would not work for childhood obesity, because "food is necessary for life *and kids cannot simply abstain from food." But, as Dr. Pretlow notes in this book, 'junk food,' which overweight kids say they have great difficulty resisting, is <u>not</u> necessary for life. The ideas of Dr. Pretlow's book are quite controversial, given our strong cultural dependence on food and belief by many that weight loss is only a matter of will power.*

I applaud Dr. Pretlow for his unwavering efforts, in the face of considerable opposition from mainstream medicine. As I once told him, "It's the pioneers that get the arrows." This book deserves a wide audience. It's a great book for the general public and for health care professionals and will make a significant contribution to the childhood obesity crisis in this country.

John P. Foreyt, Ph.D.
Professor, Departments of Medicine, Pediatrics, and Psychiatry
Director, Behavioral Medicine Research Center
Baylor College of Medicine
Houston, TX

Introduction

> The comedian, Jay Leno, recently joked: "What weighs 257 pounds and is made in America?" The answer: "An eighth grader."

The Facts

Jay Leno's joke is a bit reminiscent of the cruelty jokes of the 1950's, but it speaks grim truth. The United States, as well as much of the rest of the world, is in the midst of a childhood overweight and obesity epidemic. One third of America's kids are either overweight or obese, which is triple the rate of twenty five years ago. The rate in other countries isn't far behind.

Overweight and obes_____'s a serious health problem. Obese kids are devel_____ts, such as high blood pressure, high choles_____ 2 diabetes, poor sleep quality and sleep apn_____liver disease, and bone and joint problems. Most _____. Research studies are revealing that obese t_____vill have triple the rate of heart disease when th_____because of the current childhood obesity epic_____ids will not live as long as their parents.

So... what's this book _____nessages written by kids on an open access, interac_____ens, during the period from 2000 to 2009, with_____gg_____ ojjered by the author. This book presents what kids say about being overweight in their own words – their difficult lives, their striking struggles to lose weight, and their precious success stories.

This book contains information never before collected by academicians, researchers, or clinicians. The information was obtained from anonymous, amazingly outspoken, bulletin board messages from overweight kids, which is possible only on the Internet.

There are many ideas and tips from kids themselves, which are meant to offer help to kids struggling with their own weight issues, as well as to offer them hope. The more children and teens learn that they are not alone in their weight struggles, the more the stigma of overweight can be combated and genuine and meaningful dialogue can take place between those that suffer and struggle and those that wish to help.

What are the lives of overweight kids like? Why do overweight kids continue to overeat, knowing full well that staying overweight damages their lives? Why do they struggle to such a degree to lose weight? What's really causing the childhood obesity epidemic? What can be done about it? What overweight kids say concerning these questions is what this book is about. It's the author's hope that we can learn from their messages and offer strategies that are more in sync with what kids really need to succeed. If we risk new approaches, we can be better partners in helping them to combat the vicious cycles of being overweight.

The Chapters

This book first presents the lives of overweight kids, followed by the role that secrecy plays in their lives and the shame they feel. Then, what they say about their parents and healthcare professionals, what motivates them to try to lose weight, their extreme struggles to lose weight, and the reasons they struggle so much. "Comfort eating," "stress eating," and "boredom eating" are explained. Next, exercise posts are presented and the reasons overweight kids have such a problem with exercise. After that, the compelling "vicious cycles" overweight kids deal with are discussed, followed by their moving success stories. The final chapter is on 'Where do we go from here?' - what appears to be causing the childhood obesity epidemic, what should be done about it, how should we treat overweight and obesity in kids, and most important of all… what should be done to prevent it.

Science

This book is not a scientific work. It presents simply what kids type spontaneously on an interactive website for overweight teens and preteens. Results of multiple online polls are also included, which likewise are not scientific. Nonetheless, the polls do reveal trends, and the comments from kids about the polls are quite revealing. Steps were taken to render the polls as accurate as possible, such as use of browser "cookies" and logging of user IP numbers (user computer identifier numbers similar to phone numbers) to prevent duplicate responses. The polls are ongoing, so that as new kids come to the site they may also vote. Hence, results are stated in present tense.

The information in this book is obtained from a specific group, namely overweight kids who come to a web site seeking help, mostly on their own. It thus can't be assumed that overweight kids, who don't use this website or the Internet, have the same types of struggles and causes of their overweight.

Even so, overweight kids in healthcare or school groups referred to this site appear to have exactly the same struggles as the kids who come to the site on their own. For example, kids in the HealthyKids Weight Management Program at Children's Medicine Center, Charleston, WV, exhibit a high rate of 'comfort eating,' similar to the kids who use the site (see Chapter 9). Kids in supervised groups actually seem to struggle more, and are less motivated, than kids who come to the site on their own. Thus, the claim by some obesity professionals that kids who use this website may have a different cause for their overweight than kids who don't use the site, seems unlikely.

What Kids Say

In this book the original text of what kids have written in their messages is preserved as much as possible, for authenticity. For the sake of briefness, portions of messages are omitted. **Key points in messages are emphasized in bold by the author**. *A gold star beside a message indicates a success story. It was a daunting task to condense what thousands of kids say in nearly 133,000 messages into this small book. To help in this undertaking the messages are grouped according to the main issues raised, such as the struggle to lose weight, comfort eating, dealing with parents, etc. Every effort was made to include typical examples of messages in each category - a cross-section of what overweight kids say.*

Most messages were not posted by only a core group of a few kids, but rather by thousands of different overweight kids as they came and went on the site over the years. This is confirmed by varying IP numbers (computer Internet numbers). A few of the same kids have posted multiple messages over many years, and their individual stories may be followed by their sequential posts with the same name and/or IP number, but that may be the subject of another book.

Some of the information and ideas presented in this book may offend you. The information, nevertheless, is real. Therefore, if you decide to read this book, please keep an open mind. It's what kids say. Your responses and feedback are welcome!

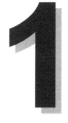

The Childhood Obesity Epidemic

Why do kids become overweight?

It is well accepted that overweight and obesity result from taking in more calories (food) by eating than are burned up by exercise. Food is your body's fuel. Your body can store fuel for later use, just like you can store fuel in your car's gas tank for when your car goes on a trip. Your body turns extra fuel into fat and stores the fat in your 'fat fuel tank' located all over your body.

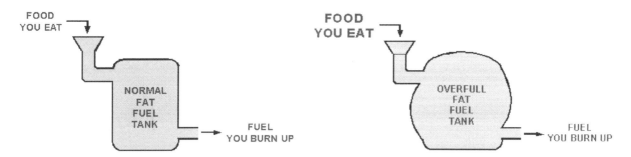

If the fuel that you burn up to run your body is equal to the fuel that you take in from food, then you don't gain weight, as shown in the left diagram above. Since there is no extra fuel, none of it is stored as fat. But if you take in more food than your body burns up, then the extra fuel is turned into fat, and your body gains weight. The extra fuel is stored in your fat fuel tank, which gets bigger and heavier as it overfills, as shown in the right diagram above. It's pretty simple.

But if it's that simple, why don't kids just eat less and exercise more to attain and maintain a healthy weight? Why do we have an epidemic of childhood obesity?

The Theories

There are at least five major theories on what's causing the childhood obesity epidemic: 1) genetics (the "thrifty gene"), 2) the weight "set point," 3) low metabolism, 4) the food rich environment, and 5) sedentary lifestyle. There are several minor theories, such as mothers are too busy to cook, poor people can't afford healthy food, and kids don't know how to make healthy choices.

Genetics - Thrifty Gene Theory

The so-called "thrifty gene," first proposed by Dr. James Neel [Neel 1962], supposedly drives humans to consume and store as many calories as possible in times of plenty in order to survive in times of famine (starvation). In ancient times, when food was scarce and famines were common, people with that gene would have survived better than those without it, so the gene would thus have been passed on to their children and eventually to modern day peoples.

But in modern times, with food in abundance and no famines, that gene may result in people becoming overweight. But is the thrifty gene really what's causing today's kids to overeat and become overweight and obese? There certainly is easily available, cheap, high-calorie food today. Although the thrifty gene theory is accepted by many health professionals as a main cause of the obesity epidemic, Dr. Neel eventually showed that his thrifty gene theory was actually untrue.

Dr. Neel found that populations, which have high rates of obesity, have no history of famine or starvation. For example, Pacific Islanders, who have a very high rate of obesity, have always lived on tropical islands, which had plentiful fruit and vegetation all year round and were surrounded by lukewarm waters full of fish. There were never any famines and thus no reason that Pacific Islanders with a thrifty gene would have survived better to pass on the gene.

Thus, the thrifty gene theory doesn't explain why we currently have a childhood obesity epidemic. Moreover, arguing that obesity is due to a gene that makes people consume as much food as possible in times of plenty to survive in times of famine is like arguing that alcoholism is due to a gene that makes people consume as much liquid as possible in times of rain in order to survive in times of dryness.

Weight Set-Point Theory

A theory presented at the 2007 American Academy of Pediatrics annual meeting, in regard to what's causing childhood obesity, is the "weight set point" theory [Fennoy 2007], [Bennett and Gurin 1982]. Each child or teen supposedly has a specific "natural" weight value set in his/her, brain, for example, 150 pounds, which actually may be medically 'overweight' for that individual. If that 150 pound child or teen tries to lose weight to 130 pounds, the weight set point would drive him/her to eat more in order to push the weight back up to the set point of 150 pounds, thus making weight loss or weight maintenance very difficult.

But what happens if the 150 pound child or teen gains weight to 180 pounds? Wouldn't the weight set point of 150 pounds cause him/her to eat less and push the weight back down to 150 pounds? That would seem logical, but according to the speaker, the individual's 'natural' weight set point would reset to the higher weight of 180 pounds, making weight loss again difficult. The weight set point resets up but not down? Does this make sense? No! Therefore, the weight set point theory doesn't account for the childhood obesity epidemic.

Low Metabolism Theory

"Low metabolism" has been proposed as a cause of childhood obesity. The "resting metabolic rate" is the rate at which food calories are burned up by a child or teen's body when he/she is not moving at all. Kids with a low metabolic rate or "low metabolism" would thus gain weight on less food eaten, compared to kids with a normal or high metabolic rate. Scientific evidence of this, however, has been mixed, with some research studies finding that individuals with low metabolic rates have higher rates of obesity, whereas other similar studies have failed to find such an effect [Hambly et al. 2005]. Therefore, thin kids, who supposedly can "eat anything they want and not gain a pound," simply eat fewer calories and/or exercise more than kids who gain weight.

Food -Rich Environment Theory

The food-rich environment is also claimed to be the cause of the childhood obesity epidemic [Swinburn 2009]. Kids are said to overeat simply "because the food is there." Presumably this theory refers to pleasurable foods like junk food and fast food. But if overweight kids don't see such foods in front of them, i.e. the food is no longer "there," do they stop overeating and lose weight? No, they still seek out such foods. This theory is a bit like saying that smoking and alcoholism are caused by a tobacco and alcohol rich environment, and teens become alcoholics or two pack-a-day smokers simply "because alcohol and tobacco are there?"

Sedentary Lifestyle Theory

Lack of playtime, little or no physical education at school, video games, and excessive TV viewing time are proposed as a major cause of the childhood obesity epidemic [Leatherdale and Wong 2008]. To treat childhood overweight and obesity the Expert Committee on Child and Adolescent Overweight and Obesity recommends "less than two hours of screen time" and "at least 60 minutes of physical activity per day." Low activity levels can certainly contribute to overweight, but this does not sufficiently account for the childhood obesity epidemic. For example, walking roughly a mile is required to burn up just 100 calories, the equivalent of one soda. There are about 3500 calories in each pound of fat, or 350,000 calories in 100 lb. A 257 pound eighth grader would thus have needed to exercise the equivalent of walking 3500 miles in order to be a healthy weight of 157 lb. Kids today aren't less active to that degree. Something else is going on. The sedentary lifestyle theory does not sufficiently explain the childhood obesity epidemic.

Other Proposed Causes of Childhood Obesity

Moms Today are Too Busy to Cook

Mothers tell me that kids become obese because parents are extremely busy and don't have time to cook at home, so they must purchase "fast food" in order to feed their family. But would a parent really allow his/her child to become obese with health risks, etc., just so the parent may save time? Also, a child can remain at a healthy weight on fast food if the type and amount is controlled. Something else seems to be occurring here. Does the mother herself simply prefer high calorie fast food or give it to the child in order to please the child?

Poor People Can't Afford Healthy Food

Obesity rates are higher among poorer peoples, for example minorities, such as Hispanics and Native Americans. A speaker at a recent childhood obesity conference argued that the inability to afford healthy food is the reason for higher obesity rates in those minorities, which is a popular theory [Drewnowski and Darmon 2005]. Also, food stores in poorer neighborhoods not offering healthy foods is given as a reason for higher obesity rates in poorer peoples [Black and Macinko 2008]. But if these theories are true, when poorer peoples become wealthy, wouldn't it be expected that they would then buy and eat healthy foods and attain healthy weights?

For example, what about Native American tribes, who become wealthy from casinos on their tribal lands? I visited two such tribes near Seattle, several years after they had begun reaping huge profits from their casinos. The tribal members still ate the same high-calorie native 'comfort foods,' such as 'fry bread,' and had just as much problem with obesity as before they became wealthy.

The above mentioned conference speaker, who proposed this economic cause of childhood obesity, confessed that poorer peoples typically do not eat healthier once they become wealthy. They still seem to prefer the high-calorie comfort foods, to which they are accustomed. Therefore, the theory that childhood obesity is due to parents' not being able to afford healthy foods seems questionable.

Kids Don't Know How to Eat Healthy

Many health professionals feel that if overweight kids (and their parents) would just learn to "eat healthy" that this would reverse the childhood obesity epidemic. For example, the U.S. Expert Committee on the Assessment, Prevention and Treatment of Child and Adolescent Overweight and Obesity released new recommendations in 2007 for the management of overweight and obese children and adolescents [https://secure.in.gov/isdh/files/51_resource_file1.pdf].

The Expert Committee's recommendations include the following:

- Consume at least 5 servings of fruits and vegetables daily
- No sugar-sweetened beverages
- Prepare more meals at home as a family (the goal is 5-6 times a week)
- Limit meals outside the home
- Eat a healthy breakfast daily

But is lack of knowledge on healthy eating really contributing to the childhood obesity epidemic? We asked kids about this in an online poll (http://www.blubberbuster.com/cgi/poll_new_85.cgi):

Do you think information on healthy eating helps you to lose weight?

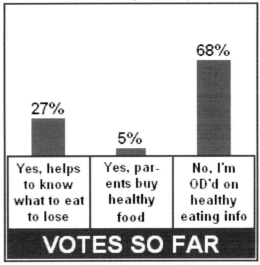

88 kids voted

Most kids responding say that they're overdosed with information on healthy eating and that what they need is information on how to resist cravings. Most also say they've learned about healthy eating in school.

Have you learned healthy eating info in school?

YES: 55 votes (62%)

NO: 33 votes (38%)

Thus, kids' lack of knowledge on healthy eating may not be a cause of the childhood obesity epidemic.

Below are some comments from kids about the preceding poll:

Age 14, female, 5'6, 185 lbs - **i know what i should eat but i eat bad food no matter what. Hate being fat :(**

Age 12, female, 4"10, 95 lbs - **The My Pyramid sucks!!**

Age 13, female, 5ft 4in, 240 lbs - I think we all know about it, more or less, but knowing isn't going to nreally help anyone unless they acttually do it. **I took a poll at my school. 95% knew a lot about eating healthy but 99% said that they really didn't do any of the stuff we learn about.**

From Lucee, Age 16 - 3/14/08 -
Ht. 5'8", Start: 147 lb, Current: 183 lb, Goal: 140 lb - OMG i cannot believe it. I have GAINED ... 37lbs since August. That is freakin crazy ...**i have a lot of knowledge about healthy eaing, calories etc. so i know how to eat to lose weight and i do eat like that 80% of the time but because the other 20% is just bingeing** i cannot lose weight..just gain it. ..

Treatment

How do we then treat childhood overweight and obesity? There are all kinds of weight management programs, which produce at least some weight loss in kids. But after leaving such programs kids typically gain the weight back [Assessment of Childhood Overweight and Obesity, Supplement to Pediatrics, Dec. 2008].

Gastric bypass surgery (stomach stapling) and gastric banding are currently the only treatments that have sustainable long term results. Gastric bypass is now being performed on morbidly obese teens, who fail multiple times in weight loss programs. Gastric bypass or banding makes the stomach very small, so that the teen feels full much, much faster and can therefore eat only small amounts of food. But gastric bypass doesn't work in some teens, who continually gorge gallons of milkshakes after surgery [Washington 2008]. Some take up drinking after bypass surgery, as food no longer comforts them. Moreover, such surgery poses significant risks for the remainder of the teen's life and may even be fatal. The real question is, "Why do teens eat so much that they become morbidly obese and need major surgery in order to stop overeating and restore their health?" What's going on here?

None of the above described theories on the cause of the childhood obesity epidemic adequately explains the dramatic rise in childhood obesity over the past 25 years, or why current treatments are only marginally successful, with poor long term results. What does explain it? Kids do! Read what they say...

2 | The Internet & the Website

The Internet

Most of us have had some experience with the Internet, such as email or search engines. For those who don't know what the Internet is, the Internet is a global electronic network of computers, somewhat like a television network. But instead of channels or TV programs, the Internet consists of things called "websites", made up of "webpages," similar to the pages of a magazine or book. One may "visit" websites with a computer. Websites may be "open-access" where anyone in the world may visit the pages, or they may be "closed access" where the pages are viewable only if you know the site's password. Websites may consist either of plain, static pages, which are simply viewed, or changing, interactive pages, where one types information and receives immediate responses on the page. Website polls, bulletin boards, and chat rooms are examples of interactive pages.

The website of this book

*The source of what kids say in this book is an open-access, interactive website for overweight kids and teens at **www.weigh2rock.com** and **www.blubberbuster.com** (identical sites). This website was created in the year 2000 to help overweight teens, preteens, and parents.*

The website contains several monitored bulletin boards and chat rooms, where overweight kids from all over the world may anonymously post messages and chat live about their weight problems and other issues. The kids tell their stories, ask for tips and support, or simply express their frustrations. Other overweight kids may read the messages and post replies. The website includes a school area, where kids learn about why they become overweight, what the health risks are, and what they may do to lose weight. A weight calculator tells them if they are healthy weight, overweight, or obese and what the healthy weight range is for their height, age, and sex, based on U.S. Center for Disease Control growth charts data files. The site has age appropriate areas for preteens, teens, young adults, and parents. There is a weekly tip and a Q&A Area where kids may post questions to the site's dietitian or nurse, which are answered in a format similar to a "Dear Abby" column. Lastly, the site has a monthly poll, where kids may vote and write comments on what they think about various overweight issues.

The website receives an average of 50,000-100,000 visitors per month, mostly children and teenagers. Typically, 5-15 messages per day are posted on the bulletin boards. As of this printing, more than 166,000 messages have been posted by kids, 133,000 of which have been archived in a user searchable database.

Bulletin Boards

A portion of a typical Teens Bulletin Board page is shown below. Kids post messages and other kids may reply to the messages.

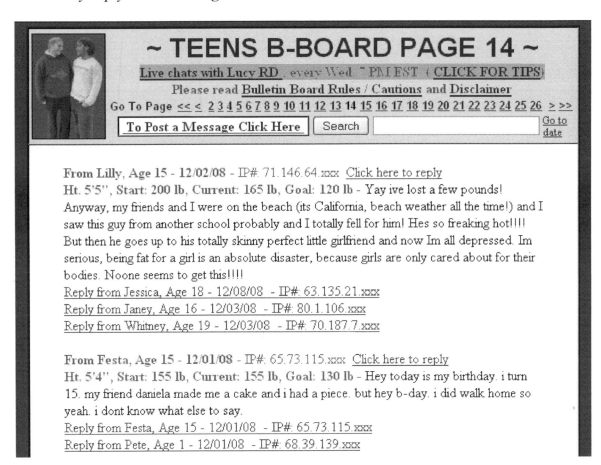

The bulletin boards are monitored by our staff, and offensive or hazardous posts are promptly removed. For security reasons, IP numbers of users are recorded and partially displayed (Internet addresses of users' computers, similar to phone numbers). Users who do not abide by the rules may be banned from further posting by blocking their IP numbers.

Kids are required to post their age, height, starting weight, current weight, and goal weight with their messages. In the initial years of the site, kids weren't required to post their weights, as it was felt that this would embarrass them. Hence, early kids' posts in this book do not show weights. However, a few kids would post their height, starting, current, and goal weights anyway, so we began requiring it. Once user stats were required with posts, use of the boards increased dramatically, as kids valued seeing how everyone else was doing.

Success Stories

The Success Stories Board is where overweight kids post their successes - how they've lost weight or how they've been able to keep the weight off. Kids gain inspiration from the stories, seeing that others have experienced their same problems, and that it is possible to overcome these problems. A portion of a typical success story page is shown below:

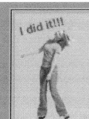 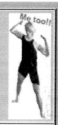

SUCCESS STORIES PAGE 1

Please read **Disclaimer**

Go To Page 1 2 3 4 5 6 7 8 9 10 11 12 13 14 15 16 17 18 19 20 21 22 23 > >>

To Share Your Success Click Here   Search

 From elle, Age 14, female - 10/25/08 - IP: 58.168.198.xxx

Dear anyone that struggles with their weight,

My name is Elle and just one year ago i decied to stop being in denial about my weight and change my life for the better. It was hard but looking back on all the hard times it was the best decision i have ever made and most likely will ever make in my life.

I never knew how big i was until i lost it all, the biggest shock came when my friend told me i used to be morbidley obese. The biggest girl in the entire school. I was so hurt, i knew i was big, but i had no idea. I don't know what made me finally decide to lose weight. I think it was a variety of things, there was no final click. I got sick of being looked at in disgust and not being able to fit into any fashionable clothes. I remember seeing myself in the mirror and not recognising myself. I had stretchmarks everywhere and a double chin. My thighs were so big that when i didn't wear bikeshorts underneath my clothing they would rub together so much they would bleed. I am ashamed of how big i let myself become. I was old enough then to make my own decisions and i couldn't blame my parents anymore.

I am fourteen now. I weigh fifty seven kilos (125 lb.) and am 166cm (5'6") tall. I lost about 35kg (77 lb.) maybe more in just one year. I thought i would be fat for the rest of my life, i wanted to die. I proved to myself that anything is possible.

I used to eat not only a lot of junk food but also large portions and just binge even when i wasn't hungry. Food was like a drug for me. Combine that with little education for whats good for you and little or no exercise and you have me.

One defining moment of my weightloss jorney was seeing this book called the diet for teenags only by Carrie wiatt and barbara schroeder. IT CHANGED MY LIFE.

i started running and walking and exercising and eating well. it was hard at first, and i didn't do it all at

Chat Rooms

Chatrooms are where kids may interact live with other kids having similar issues. Before interacting in the chatrooms or posting on the bulletin boards, the kids are referred to the rules and safety information on the website and asked to read the information and abide by

the rules. Kids are requested to give out only their first name and age on the site, in order to maintain privacy and keep identifiable information confidential.

Chatrooms work in the following manner. When you type a comment in the message box and click "Send," the message instantly appears on the chatroom screen area for others to see, as shown below for a typical chatroom. The names on the right are kids in the room, with their ages. On the left is the public conversation. The little red bug 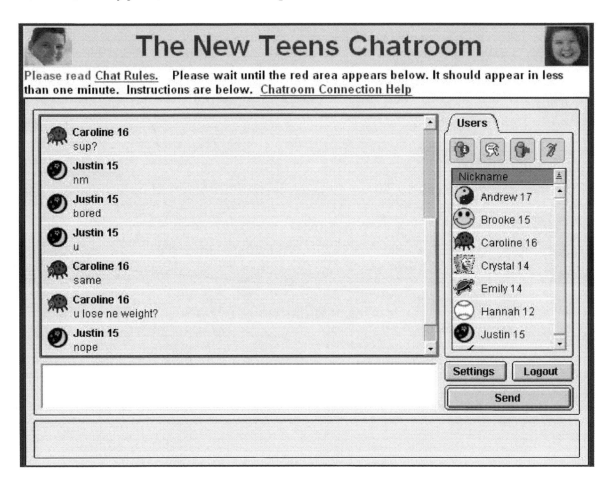*, baseball, half moon, turtle, smiley face, etc. are the kids' personal 'icons.'*

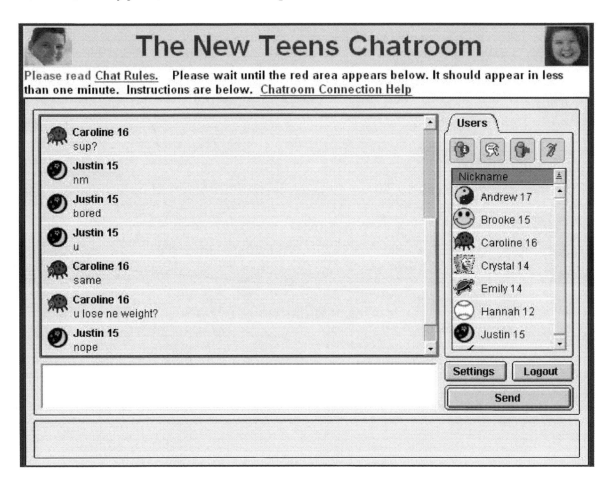

Anonymity

*In most cultures being overweight carries a social stigma and feelings of shame. Thus, overweight kids tend to be embarrassed to talk to anyone about their weight (see Chapter 4). A wonderful advantage of the Internet for overweight kids is that the Internet is **anonymous**. On the web, no one knows who you are or what you look like, so you can communicate about anything, without being embarrassed. Most kids do post their first name and age to personalize their messages, but no other identifying information is allowed.*

From Alice, Age 12 - 12/01/04
I just want to say, all of you are doing a great thing, and this is already boosting my self-esteem. I luv this website, cos its positive, and **we shouldn't have any trouble talking to each other. Especially since we will probably neva meet each other!!!!!!!!!!**

From Heather, Age 15 - 01/31/04
Hey guys Im heather, I have tried dieting but it has not worked for me. IT is to hard.. **Im glad my mom found this place for me to talk to ppl like me.....=)**

Graphical icons 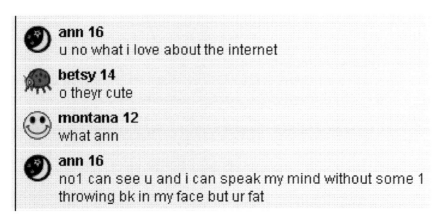 *further personalize interactions in the chatrooms, while still preserving anonymity.*

ann 16
u no what i love about the internet

betsy 14
o theyr cute

montana 12
what ann

ann 16
no1 can see u and i can speak my mind without some 1 throwing bk in my face but ur fat

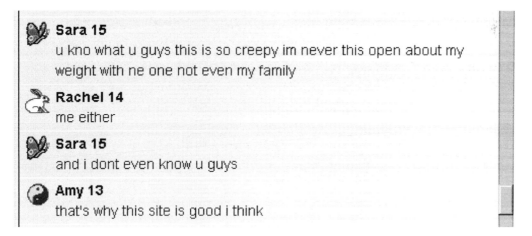

Sara 15
u kno what u guys this is so creepy im never this open about my weight with ne one not even my family

Rachel 14
me either

Sara 15
and i dont even know u guys

Amy 13
that's why this site is good i think

The information in this book

Because of the anonymity of the Internet, kids are stunningly honest in what they say on the bulletin boards and in the chatrooms. It would be nearly impossible to obtain this kind of information in the face-to-face world. Thus, the information in this book provides a new perspective on what it's like to be an overweight kid, what's really causing the childhood obesity epidemic, and what should be done about it.

Privacy

The website protects the identities and privacy of the kids by: 1) not allowing identifying information on posts on the boards or in the chat room, 2) logging user IP numbers to track any predators, and 3) monitoring postings to assure high standards and prevent hackers, predators, and individuals with eating disorders (anorexia and bulimia) from using the site.

Website Traffic

The chart below shows the number of monthly visitors to the site during a typical year:

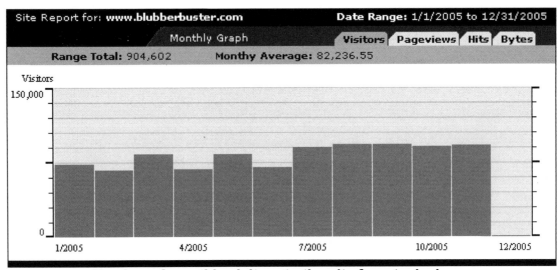

Number of monthly visitors to the site for a typical year

The next chart shows the number of daily visitors to the site during a typical week:

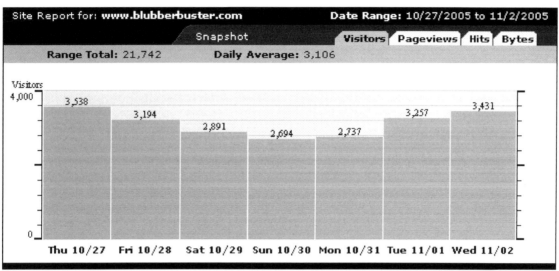

Number of daily visitors to the site during a typical week

Q & A Area

Two fictional characters host the site: the Wiz (below left), who in a story helps a teen baseball player lose weight and become a star; and Lucy (below right), who is overweight as a child, successfully loses weight, and grows up to become a registered dietitian in order to help other kids lose weight.

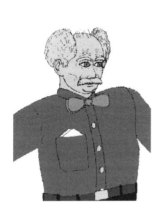
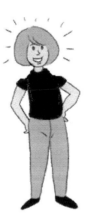

Thousands of kids have sent emails to the Wiz and to Lucy. Registered dietitians and nurses respond to these emails in the Q & A Area, with general suggestions and comments, as shown below:

Q: dear lucy i feel so bad about my self my friends say im not fat but i look in the mirror and all i see is this giant 5;7 180 pound elephant and i cant help it im bigger than my mom and my dad im having trouble i can walk good and its just when i run or jog do u have any advice on like a diet besides fruit please help me it really getting 2 me and i want a boyfriend in high school and if im fat im gonna be lonley and i dont want that do please help me   sincerly kristi   p.s (crying)

 Kids tell me that looking different can be hard and it can make them feel alone. Sounds like you feel frustrated and sad about your body. Consider talking with your parents, your school counselor, or another trusted adult about your feelings. In order to live healthier, you may need to feel better about yourself. Check out the chat room and bulletin board. Many other people are going through the same thing as you and may be able to give you support. Good Luck!

How do kids find the site?

Kids find the site mostly on their own, using Internet search engines, such as Google or Yahoo, as illustrated in the chatroom conversation below:

bill 16
so how di find the website

Sierra 14
i was looking up overweight-ness on google and found it about a year ago.

From Cassidy, Age 13 - 10/28/08
Ht. 4'10", Start: 142 lb, Current: 142 lb, Goal: 110 lb - Hey everyone.I am new to Blubberbuster, and **I found it on Google!** My wieght isn't AWEFUL. But I am so short, that it shows, A LOT. If any of you have any tips for me... PLEASE feel free to give them. I need help.

Some kids learn of the site by word of mouth, as shown on the following page.

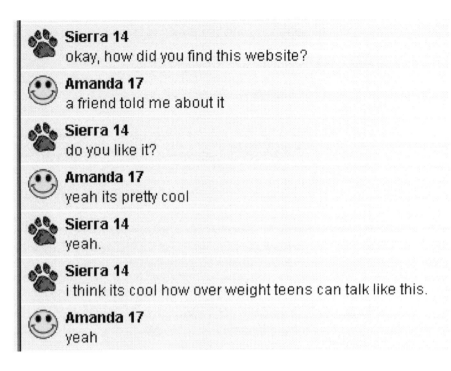

From Kelly, Age 16 - 01/05/06
Ht. 5"9, Wt. 377 - Hi guys. First post. iv recently decided to loose weight.**My dad introduced me to this site last night because hes really been trying to help me loose weight.** Well i guess im overweight thats why im here and i would like somebody to talk to about it.

The kids use search engines to search on key words such as "teen weight loss", "weight loss success stories", "weight calculator", or "self esteem quiz", as shown below:

Site Report for: www.blubberbuster.com		Date Range: 1/4/2005 to 1/4/2005	
Top Keywords		**Visitors** | **Pages/Visitor**	
Previous #Shown 10 ▼ GO	**Visitors**	**Percent**	0 .... 2.2%
1. teen weight loss	14	2.2%	████████████
2. weight loss success stories	13	2.1%	███████████
3. blubberbuster	12	1.9%	██████████
4. blubberbusters	9	1.4%	████████
5. dietsforpreteens	7	1.1%	███████
6. self esteem quiz	5	0.8%	█████
7. bmi calculator for teens	4	0.6%	████
8. blubberbusters.com	4	0.6%	████
9. what am i supposed to weigh	2	0.3%	██
10. weight percentile chart	2	0.3%	██
▼ Next			

Typical top keyword searches by kids who find our site

16

Some are referred via direct links to our website on 173 or more other sites, as the below link analysis report of our site indicates.

Inbound links (from other sites to yours):
29 Inbound links to orphaned URLs
173 Inbound Links
0 Broken Inbound Links

A few are referred by their teacher or healthcare provider,

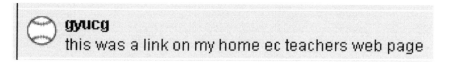

gyucg
this was a link on my home ec teachers web page

...or from listings of sites in books:

From Nicole, Age 16 - 7/19/06
Ht. 5'8'', Wt. 192??? - Hey Guys! I just joined. If you guys could tell me how to do things that would be great!! **I heard about this website through a book** I bought Calle **"The Diet for teenagers only" by Carrie Wiatt and Barbara Schroeder**. I highly recommend it!!!

Where do kids access the site?

Where are their computers located? We asked kids about this in a poll (http://www.blubberbuster.com/cgi/poll_new_48_percent.cgi).

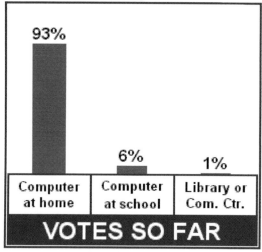

Where do you usually access this site?

93%		
Computer at home	Computer at school 6%	Library or Com. Ctr. 1%
VOTES SO FAR		

135 Kids voted

As you might expect, the vast majority access the site from their home computers, but a significant number access the site at school or at a library or community center.

Support Community

Kids say that it helps greatly to know that they are not alone in their weight struggles. Additionally, they say that it helps to be able to communicate with and receive support from other overweight kids.

Reply from Kathleen, Age 12 - 01/21/01
I know just how you feel. I am the same age and I weigh exactly the same weight. My friends are all really thin and I always feel huge compared to them. **I'm glad to know theres someone out there like me.**

From whitney, Age 15 - 06/11/07
Ht. 5'3", Start: 188 lb, Current: 188 lb, Goal: 150 lb - hey guys i love comin to this website at least **im know im not the only over weight teen** i need motivation so please email

From Brianna, Age 13 - 5/28/01
Hey everybody. I am 12 years old and 226 pounds. I want to loose weight by the next school year. Preferably 50 pounds... **I wished I had people to talk to about my problem, but talking to friends or family members would embarrass me. I guess talking to perect strangers and not having them see me is the best way for me.** Can anybody help me. Thanks a lot
Reply from Summer , Age 16 - 3/20/03
Reply from sally, Age 14 - 7/26/01
Reply from Amber, Age 16 - 6/8/01
Reply from Jeremy, Age 16 - 6/1/01
Reply from Erin, Age 17 - 5/31/07
Reply from Sarah , Age 14 - 5/31/01
Reply from Robert, Age 12 - 5/31/01
Reply from Courtney, Age 13 - 5/30/01
Reply from Katie, Age 14 - 5/29/01
Reply from Julie, Age 17 - 5/28/01

Note the many replies to the above post.

Kids from all over the world may access the site and the bulletin boards, for example the post below from a teen from the UK .

From anne, Age 16 - 11/27/03
happt thanksgiving to all americans out there! yay abe lincon!

The Website's Name

Initially, the site's name was "Blubberbusters." However, that name was offensive to a few parents, schools, and health professionals, thus in a poll we asked the kids who used the site what name they would suggest (http://www.blubberbuster.com/poll/comments_47.htm). Most did not want to change the name; therefore, we kept Blubberbusters.com and created a second "storefront" with the name "WeighCool" for schools and health professionals, but connecting to all the same areas of the Blubberbusters.com site. However, some kids then told us that the name WeighCool was "lame" and a name for young adults. Hence, we surveyed, via email, hundreds of kids who used the site, as well as health professionals and teachers, as to what name they would like. The result was"Weigh2Rock." "You rock" is a high compliment in today's kidspeak.

The next chapter presents what overweight kids say about their difficult lives.

3 | The Life of an Overweight Kid

What's it like being an overweight child or teen? The following are examples of what kids have written on the website bulletin boards. Their posts have been left in the original form, and the author has emphasized key points in bold. Here's what kids say:

This is ANGELICA's story:

i am **16, i really hate being this ffat**. my stomsch is so huge. a lot of **people assk me if i am pregnet**, its ok if i am alone but i want to die if my mom hears it or my brother or my best friend. **its real hard for me to find clothes that fit my belly**. alot of the time i shop in mens sections because they are bigger and they fit me. i really hate my size, i am so scared to find out what i weigh, i dont want to know how hevey i got!!!last time i was weighed, it was **208 ponds**. that is so sick. i get teased alot, but **i never ever talk about this at home** i never talk about my weight at home if i do, i will just cry, because i hate being fat, **i hate that i always want to eat**,hate that i dont have any nice clothes and the ones i do are ugly, **i hate ssneaking food**, i really hate how flabby and blubbery my stomach is, i hate that **my bf broke up with me beacuasw he said i was too fat, i hate that i broke up with my other bf when he liked me fat , because i was too ashamed of my bodysize**, and emabarrassed if he ever saw how blubbery i am. I just wish i could wake up skinny i would be so happy. i just wake up fat and overweight, with my belly so big I can pick it up, **and still I will be hungry. that is my story that none wlse knows, i never said it before to anyone. but it my story of what its like being FAT:(**

The last sentence of the post shows how the anonymity of the Internet can help bring out the feelings of kids to start a conversation.

Appearance

Overweight kids are distressed about how they look.

From Claire, Age 19 - 08/22/08
Ht. 5'4", Start: 210 lb, Current: 175 lb, Goal: 150 lb - **I hate looking in the mirror :(it's the saddest part of each of my days.** I hate myself.

From S.J., Age 17 - 07/08/06
Ht. 5"4, Wt. 245 - ... i'm considered "extremely obese"... I don't know what to do because in order to be healthy i would need to lose atleast 100 pounds. **I ruined my body and stretched out my skin and now have a lot of stretch marks.** Also, i'm extremely depressed. **I feel like even if i lost the weight my body couldn't be fixed.** This weight is **holding me back from being who i want to be.** It's at the point where i **hate to look in the mirror...**

From Tiff, Age 13 - 8/1/08
Ht. 5'6", Start: 216 lb, Current: 220 lb, Goal: 160 lb - ... **i think im soo ugly because of fat. When i go out and buy clothes its hard for me.** Also when **people underestimate me because of fat.** Like one time we were doing a relay race and no one wanted me on there team for the first round. But then i had my turn to run and I REALLY wanted to prove to them that i can run even thou my appearance doesn't like so. I ran as fast as i could and everyone was like OH TIFFANY UR REALLY FAST and i was happy but a boy said... "for a fat girl she can run fast" and my Best friend stood up for me and thats why im glad to have him. But ya **i don't want to be known as the fat girl. I wanted to be known as Tiffany because thats MY NAME.** and proud of it... I want to get into some nice clothes before the beginning of school! ...

~ ANDREA'S STORY ~
I an **13 and i am 185lbs..**I look so fat.What ever I where I look so bad in..So **when I take pichers of myself I only take them of my face most of the time.**It school I get called names like(fat,ugly,fat)..I live in a house with 4 other kids and my older sister calls herself fat all the time and she is not. She makes my fell bad abot myself all the time.!! My other brothers and sisters are not big at all. I am so big I am the only big kid in my house..!!This summer I whant to lost 60lbs.Becase **I want to look good at my 8th grade dance..!!!And also I whant to fell good about myself..!!!**

From Ki, Age 17 - 01/15/09
Ht. 5'4", Start: 165 lb, Current: 170 lb, Goal: 135 lb - ...I've been eating sucky foods. I'm just getting so discouraged because I'm graduating this year and prom is coming up. If I look the way I do now when prom comes around, I'm not going to go. **I even decided not to take senior pictures because I feel so unattractive and self conscious about my weight.** I love dressing up and wearing heels and getting my hair done and stuff, but because of my weight I always wear jeans and sweatshirts! **I have missed out on being a GIRL.** Prom is my last chance. I have to lose this weight...

From sad and depressed, Age 16 - 8/2/08
Ht. 5'9", Start: 320 lb, Current: 320 lb, Goal: 210 lb - **i really am sick of being fat. honestly i hate it.** ive been a big kid ever since i can remember and during all that

time **ive been teased and made fun of. i hate myself for being the size i am and i pretty much have no self esteem.**

Stretch marks

In over 331 different messages overweight kids ask what can be done about their embarrassing "stretch marks." Stretch marks are large, red, jagged areas on the skin of the abdomen, back, chest, legs, and arms, which occur when weight gain is rapid. The skin does not have time to stretch and literally breaks apart on the surface like ice on a pond. After losing weight, stretch marks tend to fade, but may not disappear completely.

From Katie, Age 15 - 5/13/07
Ht. 5'4", Start: 189 lb, Current: 174 lb, Goal: 130 lb - **I have stretch marks i hate them so much** any ideas how to get rid of them?

This is KAYLA's question:
Being overweight is hard. I am currently **235 pounds and 16 years old**. I am overweight by 100 pounds. Its hard when you go to school and all your friends are skinny and wearing belly shirts. The mall is the worst part because when my friends and I go to the mall, all this guys flirt with my friends, but ignore me. I get depressed and sad. **I eat when I am bored** and have nothing to do. I was diagnosed with depression a year ago and I think the reason is because I am overweight. Everyone tells me how they think I would be so beautiful if I was skinny. I agree with them. I have a cute face and beautiful eyes but my body is not so pretty. **The worst part is the stretch marks.** It looks like I am pregnant. I mean you dont know how much I wish I was skinny.

From Lexi, Age 14 - 8/26/07
Ht. 5'1", Start: 140 lb, Current: 180 lb, Goal: 100 lb - i try to lose weight but i just impossible **im addicted to food** i cant stick to a diet wen people pick on me i eat loads which is ever day i eat like 4000 calories a day **i'd got loads of stretch marks and i hate it.** i look huge and i hate it

From Jesso, Age 15 - 12/16/06
Ht. 5'5", Wt. 176 - Hey lovelies. I used to be really overweight, but I've recently lost a bit of weight, 25 kilos (not sure how many pounds that is) anyway, still have a bit of a way to go. So yes, my question is, well **I have these massive stretch marks all over me**, and I was wondering if anyone had any ideas of what I could do to prevent getting more or getting rid of the ones i have at the moment. **They make me feel really self conscious**

Saggy skin

Saggy skin is worrisome to kids when they lose a lot of weight.

From Tina, Age 16 - 06/23/08
Ht. 5'5", Start: 203.3 lb, Current: 184 lb, Goal: 125 lb -
hey people wasup? I've lost about 20 pounds so far. I can kind of notice a difference. **Im really worried about stuff like excess skin and stretch marks.** Im looking to lose about 50 more pounds any advice or comments?

Reply from jacquie, Age 18 - 06/23/08 -
1 that is a commen worry i am worried to **i have been over weight my entire life i'm afriad my body dosent know to go back**
2. **strech marks can be faded or completly removed** with fading cream or skin bleaching kind...
3. **toneing should help the skin tighten up** and go back. **lifting weights every few days is great...**
5.... **if the skin becomes a problem or the marks do we live in a world where those problmes can be fixed by a doctor.. if it comes to it......** however i highly doubt it..

Many overweight kids do not understand that physical problems associated with their weight gain and weight loss, such as stretch marks and saggy skin, are treatable. Thus, open dialogue about treatment options is an opportunity for healthcare providers to educate and alleviate fears among their overweight patients.

Disapproval from others

Overweight kids are quite distressed about how others think of them, even their family.

From michelle, Age 16 - 1/2/08 -
Ht. 5'6", Start: 213 lb, Current: 221 lb, Goal: 135 lb - ... i have a doctors app. tomorrow and **the one thing i dread is getting on that scale in front of my mom,** because i know i'm gonna get a lecture right after. **those lectures only make me feel worse.** i mean, it's not like i'm hearing anything new. this is the heaviest i've ever been in my life and it's the worst feeling. all of my friends are skinny and **when we go shopping, it's embarrassing that i can't fit into anything** that they shop for. **the worst thing about being overweight are the jokes. skinny people don't understand how hard it is for overweight people to be the way that they are. they dont understand how hard it is for us to change our eating habbits and our way of living...**

This is SARA's question:

I'm **270 pounds** and feel awful. Plus I have 2 familys on my dad's and mom's side that are so **critiSIZEing**. They always find a way to say im fat in different words to me.I feel left out in school b/c im different and nobody wants to be with me for appearence.I have heard that i should talk to a trusting adult,but when i do i see a little smirk on their face,which just shuts me down b/c nobody listens.

hi im morgan heres my story

im an over weight littile girl i weigh **250 pounds** and it emmberesing **i would like to have friend but im own best friend when i need some one to talk to i talk to my self** last weekend this girl was giving out invites to a slumber party and i wasnt invited. last year on **my birthday** nobody came **i invited 50 people no one showed up** and i started to cry all i want is friend if anyone can give me any tip

From jill, Age 16 - 6/27/08
Ht. 5'4", Start: 160 lb, Current: 160 lb, Goal: 130 lb - I have hit **an all time low.** I was visiting my grandmother and **she told me i looked to be about 4 months pregnant!** She was sitting next to me on the couch and I was so self consious, so I was sucking in my stomach. She took her hands and was still able to grasp 2 big handfuls of belly fat and said, "you need to be doing situps. once you put the weight on, its hards to take it off." then she started grabbing my arm and leg fat. i pretended not to care, but i did. later i saw her trying on my shorts and she said, " look at this. i am a grandmother and i can fit into these." i need to lose weight. HELP ME!

Physical challenges

The excess fat and extra weight is physically difficult to deal with.

From Amanda, Age 13 - 12/04/08
Ht. 4'11", Start: 260 lb, Current: 260 lb, Goal: 100 lb - **I hate being overweight because it's so UNcomfortable!** Who agrees with me?? I'm way too fat and I can't stand how it feels on my body. When I sit down my pants are TOO tight. My stomach is really fat and it rolls up and feels like someone's pushing on it when I'm sitting down. It's HARD to breathe like that. When I stand up it takes some pressure off my stomach but then it's SO heavy, my back HURTS and I get tired fast. This MOUNTAIN of fat is like torture because it's TOO heavy and it's ALWAYS there even when I NEED a break! I know I should lose weight but that takes a LONG time! What can I do to feel better until then???

~ LAURA'S STORY ~

Hello, my name is Laura. I am **17 years old and weigh 265 pounds. It's very tough being as big as I am. The world isn't built for bigger than average people...**

From Jaime, Age 19 - 01/12/09
Ht. 5'9", Start: 350 lb, Current: 350 lb, Goal: 180 lb - Hello everyone I am 19 years old weighing 350 pounds... I have a intern in Florida as an lifeguard for Disney in August and I will be very embarrassed to wall around in a swim suit looking the way I look at the moment. **Also being the size that I am I am unable to ride the rides at the amusement park...**

Many overweight kids have a problem with their thighs rubbing together and chafing.

From Ellie, Age 15 - 8/5/08
Ht. 5'4", Start: 164 lb, Current: 160 lb, Goal: 112 lb - even more than having a flat stomach i really really want a gap between **my thighs so they dont rub..**

From Rachel, Age 17 - 04/01/09 -
Ht. 5'2", Start: 10 stone 2, Current: 10 stone 2 (142 lb), Goal: 9 stone 0 - Ok, i've actually had enough of being my size... **I chafe. I said it!!! blimey..** anyone got any tips on that subject?

A parent in the Parents Chatroom talks about this problem in both herself and her teen daughter:

Sarah
just working out has been so hard for us because of the way our weight goes. right to our thighs and bottom so its so difficult to move them....i mean you proboly dont understand, but the both of us our legs just dont go past eachother. i just dont know what to do some times

Clothing is hard to find

Shopping for clothes is frustrating and embarrassing.

From sad and depressed, Age 16 - 8/2/08
Ht. 5'9", Start: 320 lb, Current: 320 lb, Goal: 210 lb -... school starts next week and my mom and **i went shopping for clothes and i havent found anything that fits correctly.** if it is my size then chances are its not something i would wear in public let alone to school. most of the clothes in my size are ugly old lady clothes and the fact of the

matter is i want to wear the latest fashions and feel good about myself just like everybody else...

From Kelsey, Age 10 - 04/04/09 -
Ht. 4'10", Start: 150 lb, Current: 150 lb, Goal: 120 lb - **No clothes every fit me!I can go to anystore in the free world clothes never fit me!** Sometimes I find the odd "cool" outfit that I can squeeze into but seriously!I always get stuck wearing lady clothes and grandma clothes.

From Jackie, Age 15 - 03/30/09 -
Ht. 5'8", Start: 240 lb, Current: 240 lb, Goal: 100 lb - **Nothing 'cool' fits me, it sucks!!!! :(**

Dating difficulty

Finding a romance with the opposite sex is difficult for overweight kids.

From Leah, Age 18 - 7/22/08
Ht. 5'4", Start: 228 lb, Current: 206 lb, Goal: 150 lb - ... **Being fat is horrible and im sick of it. for so many reasons im sick of it. and one of the most is romantically. i cant feel comfortable with someone, even if they are happy and comfortable with me. it just sucks...**

From Claire, Age 17 - 7/21/08
Ht. 5'2", Start: 200 lb, Current: 200 lb, Goal: 100 lb - Hey everyone, I'm here to let a little pain out... All i want is to be skinny, it's not much to ask. I know i'm the only one that can do it but it's just getting started ya know? But atm i'm more motivated than ever because **i've got a new boyfriend,** i've been with him a week today and **when we chill out and watch a dvd or something and he puts his hands on my leg of stomach or something i cringe and think he will break up with me because of my flab,** i would be sooo happy if i was skinny!

Not fitting into desks at school

Some obese kids must have special desks at school.

From BROOKE, Age 11 - 11/07/08
Ht. 5'7", Start: 245 lb, Current: 265 lb, Goal: 100 lb - IM FAT! I BROKE A CHIAR A COUPLE OF DAYS A GO! **I DO NOT FIT IN THE desk AT SCHOOL! SO I HAVE TO SIT ALONE AT A TABLE!**

From Justin, Age 15 - 10/18/07
Ht. 5'7", Start: 305 lb, Current: 305 lb, Goal: 175 lb - ok i was trying to lose weight at the beginning of this school year i was 295- now im up to 305 and **im sick of not being able to fit into the desks at school** or getting tired going up 1 flight of steps and as a guy its embarrasing to be fat

From patty, Age 12 - 07/21/03
i have 2 have a special desk i weigh 267 and want 2 loose fast but only gain weight fast my mum and dad say fat camp is 2 expensive and out of the question and do research on the net so i am but no help yet so please help **my nicnames r hipo,elephant,floor crusher,fatty patty,giant gut,massive,chubs and more names that depress me**

Frustration at failed weight loss

Most overweight kids have failed at trying to lose weight.

This is Francheska's Story
Help Me!!!!!!!!!! I am very obese. I currently weigh **171 pounds. I am 11 years old.** I want to lose weight but **I can't stop eating. I try many different things like eating less. I never works.** There is always good food in the house...

From Hollie, Age 11 - 7/28/08
Ht. 4'10", Start: 9 stone 1, Current: 10 stone 0, Goal: 6 stone 0 - Ok, **I have been giving in to my temptations** but I'm starting to give in. I'm eating a lot more fruit and veg and a lot less choccie and crisps. **I was jsut about to go out and ride my bike around but the it started raining! Honestly, I think someone up there wants me stay like a whale!** But I'm trying hard, really! (Note: 10 stone 0 is 140 lb.)

Special events

Many kids want to lose weight for an event, like a special dance or school starting back.

From Becky, Age 15 - 09/29/08
Ht. 5'5", Start: 180 lb, Current: 198 lb, Goal: 160 lb - hey everyone i am just so upset. today after school, me and some of my friends went **shopping for homecomming dresses** and they are all skinny and fit into every dress they wanted. **i tried on 14;s 16's and even 18's and none of them would fit** over my belly...do you know where i could get one??

From brittney, Age 16 - 8/9/08
Ht. 5'3", Start: 173 lb, Current: 164 lb, Goal: 125 lb - **junior prom** is in 279 days or something like that. do you think i can lose **30 pounds by may 15th**? i really hope i can.

This is RANDY's question (7/25/08)
hey im randy live in arkansas i am overweight i am **5'3** i think and weigh **160 i want to way 145 before school starts which is august 19** can u please help me im crying and begging for dis to happen!

Other countries

Kids from many countries struggle to lose weight.

From Sioned, Age 13 - 10/25/08
Ht. 5'5", Start: 18 stone 1, Current: 18 stone 1, Goal: 7 stone 0 - Hello,... **I Come From Scotland**, I Am Clinically Obese And All My Life I Have Been The 'Fat' One. The 'Ugly' One. I've Tried Loads Of Diets, But They Hardly Last A Day... I Know That I Am Disgustingly Obese And I Want To Change It, Please Help?. I Know Others In The World Are Going Through The Same As Me And I Was Just Wondering If Anyone Has An Any Tips Or Anything Else?
(: xx (Note: 18 stone 1 is 253 lb.)

From Steph, Age 18 - 8/4/08
Ht. 170 cm, Start: 100 kg, Current: 87 kg, Goal: 59 kg - Hey I'm Steph and **I'm from NZ**. I've struggled with being overweight since form 2 (12 years old) when I first started to get **bullied** by the girls in my class. It lasted 5yrs, and I finally got some closure after joining a church and youth group where I made alot of friends and had the chance to share what happened to me infront of 400 people. ... I feel disappointed with myself because I was meant to have lost twice as much weight as I have lost by now, because I wanted to get to 130 pounds after a year, but I am proud of myself for keeping the weight I have lost off... I lost 10kilo's in 2 months when I was doing everything properly, and the further three kilo's took 4 months because I wasn't really putting any effort in. We are currently in the middle of winter and getting outside is a real drag and we live a long way from town where **I have a gym membership, and with the price of petrol these days it nearly doesn't seem worth it**. Any pointers? ... **I no longer binge eat at night time**, but I don't feel like I've made any real progress in the last three months!
(Note: **170 cm, 87 kg is 5'8", 191 lb.**)

From hannah, Age 15 - 11/28/05
Ht. 5'3, Wt. 22 stone 0 - Hi, i'm 15 **i live in england** and i am 22 stone!!! thats **308 pounds.** I want to go to a fat camp but my parents cant afford it... I know that if i could

just lose the wieght at camp, i would enjoy being thin so much i would just not eat. .. **I have no friends, because people dont want to know anyone who is fat. I am so depressed that my school work is suffering**. People laugh and stare at me when i go out.**I am addicted to food**.I spend all my money on it-macdonalds,kfc,burgerking. I cant help myself. Even my old friends are begining to get embarrassed I **but i am disgusting**...

From Taryn, Age 18 - 12/28/08
Ht. 157cm, Start: 86 kg, Current: 86 kg, Goal: 65 kg (Note: **157 cm, 86 kg is 5'2", 189 lb.**) - I have always been fat. I have been on countless diets that work until i give up. I found one that worked for about 6 months.I was doing so well...I had lost 15kg and still going strong and then my family and I were hijacked when leaving my house. **I live i South Africa** so crime is well just one of those sucky things. A week after we were hijacked we were burgled. I just lost it completely. **When I was scared I ate chocolates or icing sugar, when I am angry or sad or depressed I also ate**. Food was one thing i had or rather have control over. I WANT TO LOSE WEIGHT. I want to look great in a dress for my only school dance in March and I do want a boyfriend although i tell everyone i don't because it is just easier that way. I don't want to be the victom anymore and I hate being teased because **I just eat more on the sly then**. I want to live and stop pretending...but how?

Gainers

The posts below are from obese kids who say they do not want to lose weight. Some even want to get fatter. These kids call themselves "gainers," and they attempt to recruit others. One also posted his photo. We remove such posts, as they sabotage kids' weight loss efforts. These gainers are very real, and one wonders about their psychological coping with the pain of being overweight. Are they trying to justify their health risks?

From Dylan, Age 16 - 11/12/07
Ht. 6'2", Start: 302 lb, Current: 302 lb, Goal: 180 lb - This may sound weird, but...**I like being fat, and wouldn't mind getting fatter, but i also wouldn't mind being normal**. being like everyone else. being able to fit into normal clothes, at least XXL or under. I'm a size 5XL, and its so hard having to find clothes that i like and are my age's look... Yea, i'm from **Australia**, and i only use this sight because there's nothing like it. **Australia has none of this sort of stuff.**

From Imi, Age 15 - 03/11/01

Ht. 1.68 meters, Wt. 152.7 kg - Hi everybody !!! You've got a vistor from **Germany** !!!... In my opinion, it doesn't matter if you're fat or not. **I like it to be fat. I'm trying to get bigger all the time,** I eat everything I want to eat. I've got many friends who are thin and some who are big, and they repect me like I am. Now, I try to get in contact with some other teens or kids, who like it also to be fat. So write me back Imi **(Note: 1.68 meters, 152.7 kg is 5'7", 336 lb.)**

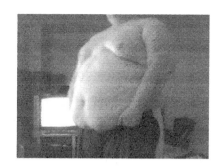

From James, Age 16 - 10/20/08

Ht. 5'6", Start: 180 lb, Current: 250 lb, Goal: 350 lb - This is for any **gainers** out their, if you wana chat send me an email. For those of you who don't what that is, **a gainer is someone who is actually comfortable with living in a fat body and might not mind growing a bit bigger.**

Some kids are bothered by their desire to get fatter and ask for help.

From dana, Age 12 - 08/27/09

Ht. 5'8", Start: 190 lb, Today: 225 lb, Goal: 110 lb - help me, i actualy want to get fatter,**what is wrong with me???**

Home schooling

Sometimes kids, who have become obese, are home schooled, in order to avoid teasing and other problems at school, such as not fitting into desks, difficulty climbing stairs, etc. Although home schooling has many benefits, obesity issues may become worse.

Kids chat about home schooling below:

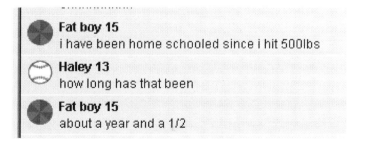

(Chat examples continued on following page)

30

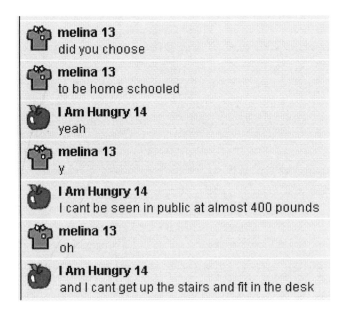

melina 13
did you choose

melina 13
to be home schooled

I Am Hungry 14
yeah

melina 13
y

I Am Hungry 14
I cant be seen in public at almost 400 pounds

melina 13
oh

I Am Hungry 14
and I cant get up the stairs and fit in the desk

From GG, Age 13 - 11/02/06
Ht. 5ft.5in, Wt. 245 - ...I'm ... overweight. **I even started being homeschooled so that i would not be teased in gym class.** I have tried two times already to go on a diet, and after about a month each time, I start eating unhealthy things little by little, and then constantly. I do not feel good in my body and everytime I go outside it seems like people look at me. Well, anyways I was just hoping that maybe someone could post some healthy foods that i should be eating and stuff and what type of exercise i should do. That would be great! Thank you VERY much!

From jill., Age 14 - 2/8/07
Ht. 5'2", Wt. 245 - ok guys i really need your advice! i know this is off subject but i am homeschooled. i started about a month late into the year. i have really been slacking off and they withdrew me from the online school.i dunno if they will let me back in.because i **stopped public school because im so fat.** anyways, will they MAKE me go back to public school or do you think my mom can just buy a few books like math reading and english and i could study them for the rest of the year! thank you so much if you took the time to read this. PLEASE PLEASE PLEASE tell me what you think about it. i would really appreciate it. it would be very helpful. i just needed someone to tell that to, so would you please reply with your thoughts? thank you!

This is ATIYA's question:
Im being home schooled right now because kids at my old school were making fun of me. I broke down one day and my mom and I talked. I want to loss as much weight as i can be for the school year start next year. I want to prove to the kids at school and myself I can change and I can do it. ... **(I am 198 pounds)**

From Fiona, Age 14 - 05/12/04
Every day i wake up with a sore body and after sleeping for 12 hours i am still soo tired i cant even stand up . i weight **240 pounds and i am only 14. i am taking homeschool cuz i am to embarrased and depressed to go to school.**

Further social isolation and less activity may result when home schooled, thus increasing the child's or teen's weight problem. Therefore, those who choose to home school should include regular physical activity and also social activities involving other kids.

Some kids say it's hard to lose weight and that they even gain weight when home schooled.

From Meg, Age 14 - 01/13/09
Ht. 5'5", Start: 210 lb, Current: 210 lb, Goal: 145 lb - I'm a homeschooled freshman and i really need to loose weight **its really hard when homeschooled cuz i dont have pe and stuff**... i would like a weight loss buddy... let me know asap if you wanna be mine!! thanks!!

From Ashley, Age 17 - 1/26/06
Ht. 5'6", Wt. 272 - I am new to this sight and would like some advice about starting to lose weight. I have tried losing weight before but could not stick with anything for long. I need something fun and interesting to do. Any suggestions? I am 272 pounds. I wasn't always this big, but **2 years ago I started getting homeschooled and since I wasn't doing as much as I used to the weight just poured on.** As you can see I need some help.

From Leah, Age 14 - 11/14/03
Hi, I'm 4'11 and 130 pounds! I'm so fat! I don't get teased that much by my friends, just my family. I've tried billions of diets but I crave and I give in, and **I'm homeschooled, so the food is there whenever I want it.** Someone pease help! I needto lose at least 30 pounds. That'swhat my mom says. Is anyone out there really short for their age and overwheight? If o, please reply!

From Krissy, Age 14 - 08/02/04
Hey Everyone!!! it's been a fast summer!! and all those diets I was suposed to go on didnt happen!!! **I dont want to go back to school to get made fun ofand teased again!!! so ... I have an alternative!!! homeschooling, yeah great idea!! but hows that gonna help me lose weight??** it probably wont i will probably just gain weight...

Suicide

Overweight kids sometimes reach the point of suicide, as the below posts illustrate. Our site has crisis prevention numbers posted for kids that feel suicidal.

From miserable, Age 14 - 04/16/01

hi everyone. im a **14 female who weighs 200 pounds and i am 5'2"**. i am so un happy, **i have no friends, im homeschooled,** i stay at home all day 5 days a week, and i sleep til noon. when im awake all i do is read and watch jerry springer.i am so lazy **i dont exercise at all. in the evenings i binge and then before i go to bed i cry my eyes out. i have even considered suciside.** someone please help me!!!

From Emily, Age 14 - 08/17/08

Ht. 5'5", Start: 118 lb, Current: 159 lb, Goal: 105 lb - i feel like just giving up...i gained about 12 more pounds in 2 weeks(vacation), and im really putting on weight too fast and i look horrible! even when i eat healthy, obesity runs in my family and its in my genes....so i guess im meant to be fat my entire life!!! **i just cant take it anymore!!! i cant stand all the people who make fun of me** and are always soo skinny and good looking...**it just makes wanna kill myself...**

From lisa, Age 12 - 12/20/08

Ht. 5'2", Start: 208 lb, Current: 214 lb, Goal: 160 lb - **i hate it i hate it i hate it** i was in the locker room changing the other day and this girl was stareing at me and i was all what? and she went oh nothing ..its just your stomach is really gross.. and those strech marks really dont help
i hate myself so much..
the her friends started laughing at me and one went its like jello! shes such a fat ass...
please just kill me you guys

From no name, Age 11 - 04/19/03

I'm really fat!! **I weigh 408 pounds** and I have to get clothes made for myself!!!! **I want to die**. People make fun of me and I just keep on eating and eating and eating!!!! HELP ME!

Thinner friends

Being upset by thinner friends or family members is a common feeling among overweight kids, particularly if the thin friends claim that they themselves are fat.

From meg, Age 13 - 6/26/08

Ht. 5'10", Start: 185 lb, Current: 172 lb, Goal: 155 lb - hey you guyss well i spent all week at my friends house i still did good with the eating but **i feel depressed when ever i hang out with my friends sometimes becuase they'll stand in front of the mirror and be like omg im so fat** and the people that i stayed with this week are size 0 and size 2 . it really makes me feeel bad about myself and i dont understand how they can actually think their fat. ugghhhh does anyone else feel this way?

This is ALEXIS's question:
HI THERE!!! **IM 11**... THIS MIGHT BE KIND OF A BIZARRE WAY OF SAYING IT BUT IM JUST "FAT" AND I KNOW IT. **I WEIGH 160!!!!!!!** WAY TO MUCH. IN SCHOOL ALL THE GIRLS ARE JUST BRAGGING HOW THEY ONLY WEIGH 60 POUNDS BUT **IM OVER THERE IN TEARS BESAUSE I AM SO OBESE.** PLEASE HELP ME I REALLY NEED HELP. P.S **I AM 5'1** BYE AND THANKS!!!

From Lisa, Age 17 - 10/25/08
Ht. 5'7", Start: 176 lb, Current: 176 lb, Goal: 140 lb - I don't understand why some people have to be fat for. its not fair. I just want to be skinny is that really impossible. Three of my closest friends are sooo tiny its like i dont even fit in the picture with them and i cant go shopping with them bc im not size 0 (or double zero for that matter)!!... :(and if i have to hear them talk about gaining weight one more time.. **its actually really instulting when they call themselves fat in front of me.. and how they need to go on a diet. it really upsets me**... i will do anything to be as skinny as my best friends .. so i can fit in and enjoy going out with them..

From Amanda, Age 19 - 7/21/08
Ht. 5'8", Start: 225 lb, Current: 170 lb, Goal: 150 lb - do any of you girls ever get **jealous of a skinny girl and automatically dont like them**? i know thats bad, but i do it all the time. llike when at a party, or whatever, if a girl is around and tries to talk to me im nice but automatically dont have an interest in being their friend because of my jealousy issues. its like unless the person has some kind of flaw i cant see myself hanging out with them. i think maybe once im thinner it wont be so bad, but ive been like this ever since i can remember. is there something wrong with me or what. cause like, i know no ones perfect but if they arent a little chubby, or **if theyre too pretty and skinny i want nothing to do with them.**

What kids say about healthy weight kids posting that they think they're overweight

We encourage everyone to check the weight calculator before posting, but healthy weight kids do sometimes post that they are fat. This is quite upsetting to the overweight kids on the site as the posts below indicate.

Here is a reply to a post by a teen claiming to be overweight at 5'10" 130 lb.

Reply from *Ray*Ray*, Age 13 , Ht. 5'7", Wt. 250 - 2/26/05
Actually 5'10" and 130 is healthy...maybe a little underweight actually. Either way, you're not overweight at all. And, honestly **I don't appreciate you calling yourself fat because**

if you're fat then what the hell am I -- or the other people on this board? Next time check the weight calculator and then post...

And a reply to all thin kids claiming to be fat.

Reply from anne, Age 19, Ht. 5'6", Wt. 191 - 3/29/06
youguys need to work on your mental state- ... **it hurts when thin people who don't think they 're thin come on here and call themselves fat, because if you're fat- what the &*^(&%^ are we?**

Healthy weight posts claiming to be overweight produce outright anger from kids who are truly overweight, as they feel this is mocking them. We therefore do not allow healthy weight posts. All kids posting on the bulletin boards must enter their current weight. We designed the bulletin board and chatroom software so that it checks the child's weight against growth chart tables for kids issued by the U.S. Centers for Disease Control. If the child's weight is in the healthy weight range, the software blocks the posting. Only kids, whose weight is in the overweight or obese range, or kids at a healthy weight, whose starting weight was in the overweight or obese range, are allowed to post.

Is there a sex difference in perspectives on weight loss?

Girls vs. guys poll

Most of the users of the bulletin boards are girls. It seems that girls may care more about losing weight than guys. We asked kids about this in a poll (http://www.blubberbuster.com/cgi/poll_new_23.cgi):

Why do you think more girls want to lose weight than guys?

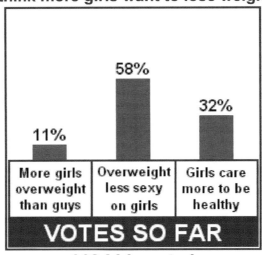

113 kids voted

Nearly 80% of the 113 kids responding to this poll are female. But of the 58% of kids choosing "Overweight is less sexy on girls," 80% of those are female, as well. Thus, it appears that girls want to lose weight more than guys, because the girls believe that overweight is less sexy on girls than on guys. Or the girls may be anticipating what guys would say, that overweight girls are undesirable from a boy's perspective. By contrast only 46% of the guys feel that overweight is less sexy on girls than on guys. Interestingly, only 4 (16%) of the 24 guys in the poll chose, "There are more overweight girls than overweight guys," and only 8 (9%) out of 89 girls chose that same answer. Thus, both feel that overweight guys outnumber overweight girls or they are equal numbers. One reason for the perception that less girls are overweight than guys (whether true or not) may be what weights guys and girls believe are acceptable to the other sex.

Comments from kids on this poll

Age 12, female, Ht: 5ft 3, Wt: 80 kg (176 lb)
boys like fit girls, but **girls dont mind** too much

Age 16, female Ht: 5'5", Wt: 151 lbs
guys are allowed comforting clothes. Baggy stuff can make them look thinner. **Girls are expected to wear form fitting clothes** and that causes alot of pressure =/

Age 16, male, Ht: 6'3, Wt: 235 lbs
Because **there is more expected of girls** ...**But girls DO care if men are overweight**, and actually it IS a big thing because you see great looking built, or muscular men all over the place, and there ARE some guys on this site, so I'd say it's about even except girls have been expected to stay "looking good for their man" longer!

Age 19, female, Ht: 5'6'',Wt: 250 lb
i think that girls think the **guys have the power because grls are more worried about being in a relationship thatn guys are and it is easier for a not good looking guy to get a hot grl than it is visa versa** and also grls care more about personality in a guy than most guys care about in a grl many guys are concerned about looks more so it puts more pressure on grls im jsut glad that my boyfriend is a true hot sweetheart and sees me for me i just got lucky.:) also **many guys are concerned about their looks they just dont show it as much**. they may not be worried about their weight as much but they are usually worried about muscles or their build

Age 17, female, Ht: 5'3", Wt: 101 lb
Society has simply placed all the attention on women in the media. Women have to be this "perfect" shape and figure. Less emphasis is placed on men simply because the media chooses to do so. Despite this, **guys who are over weight still think about it just as much as women who are overweight do.**

Age, 12, female, Ht: 5'1, Wt: 170 lbs
girls do care about guys being overweight but they dont say anything cause usually they are desperate and need someone to be there boyfriend and talk about

Kids' misperceptions

Many overweight kids have the misperception that normal weight kids can eat the same thing as they do and not gain weight.

Reply from ellie, Age 15 - - 08/18/08
i know exactly how you feel like you wanna be thin but you know youll be fighting your whole life to be it and **its so unfair how ppl are just lucky and can eat the same as you but not gain weight...**

From Nicole, Age 12 - 07/12/05
Ht. 5"0", Wt. 155 - HI! my name is Nicole.. **All my friends are really skinny! and we eat the same food!...**

This has to do with the belief by many overweight kids that they have 'low metabolisms' compared to normal weight kids. But this has never been conclusively proven in medical research studies. Some studies show this to be the case, whereas other studies do not. Therefore, overweight kids simply have eaten more calories or exercised less than kids who are healthy weight.

Kids' questions

How do I lose weight?

The most common message on the bulletin boards and in the Q & A Area is, "How do I lose weight?" and similarly, "Please give me weight loss tips."

This is BRI's question:
How do i lose weight. Im **187.5 and im 12** and I want to lose it because every time I go out side i get teases about mi stuipd weight

This is CHELSEA's question:
Please help me! **I have to lose weight and I don't know how.** I am **14 and 194 pounds** about. please help me or I will loose hope. I need help.

From courtney, Age 14 - 12/27/08
Ht. 5'4", Start: 220 lb, Current: 220 lb, Goal: 130 lb - well, **i want to loose weight i need to loose weight...i just don't know how** to..well i do but **i don't know were to start at all** do i start big small? do i count cals or what? i really need some help...

From anahi, Age 17 - 06/04/06
Ht. 5'2, Wt. 210 - hey guys, i'm new to this and would like some help gettin started. **i honestly have no clue what to do but i feel it's time to lose weight.** i don't even know what a reasonalble goal would be so if you can help i'd really appreciate it...thanx

From kimberly, Age 12 - 07/21/05
Ht. 5'4 , Wt. 166 - **i just need tips for losing weight**

More than a year and a half later the same child in the post above (same IP#) still asks for tips on how to lose weight (see below post), and she has gained 55 pounds.

From kim, Age 13 - 04/13/07
Ht. 5'5", Start: 220 lb, Current: 221 lb, Goal: 150 lb - can some one **please give me weight loss tips........**

From Lauren, Age 12 - 05/29/07
Ht. 5'1", Start: 144 lb, Current: 144 lb, Goal: 120 lb - Hi I just started and this and i would like to know what you do to lose weight and **how do you lose weight** if you have any ideas please!!!!!!!!!!!!!! tell me!!!!!!!!

From Jill, Age 16 - 03/31/07
Ht. 5'5", Start: 220 lb, Current: 220 lb, Goal: 175 lb - Hey,Im jill i weigh like 220 pounds,i was wondering **how to lose weight????** any info would be helpful! How much exercise should i get a day?? Has anyone ever tried slimfast?? im unsure about my goAL WEIGHT! thanks!

The many postings like the ones above suggest that kids are interested in losing weight but don't know how and don't know where or whom to turn to in order to find the help they need. Are we as parents, healthcare providers, and others missing the opportunity to help kids with their weight loss issues? Why are we missing this conversation? Is it lack of time, lack of money for payment for weight counseling, or something else?

How long will weight loss take?

A very common question from the kids is, "How long will it take for me to lose weight?"

From shannon - 07/30/06
Ht. ..., Wt. big - **I dont want to put my weight.** But if i eat very healthy and exercise

alot **how much weight could i lose by september 7th?** and **How long will it take to lose 25 pounds?**

From Kaitlyn, Age 14 - 02/21/08
Ht. 5'7", Start: 175 lb, Current: 160 lb, Goal: 130 lb - heyy. **How long will it take to loose like... idk 15 pounds?**

From lucky, Age 17 - 6/27/08
Ht. 5'4", Start: 138 lb, Current: 180 lb, Goal: 120 lb - **IS IT POSSIBLE TO LOSE 20 POUNDS IN 2 MONTHS AND 3 DAYS? IF I WORK REALLY HARD?**

From Motivated, Age 19 - 7/9/08
Ht. 5'7", Start: 215 lb, Current: 203 lb, Goal: 150 lb - **what was the most weight you've lost in a month?** i have a wedding i'm in next month and need to lose as much as possible!

The typical posts above show how little kids really know about the mechanism of losing weight in a healthy way. It's therefore important for parents, doctors, and other health professionals to talk to overweight kids about what's really involved in losing weight and all the other issues (psychological and physical) that go along with healthy weight loss. Websites, such as ours, can provide information and peer support.

Nutritional information?

The kids who use the site seldom ask, "How do I eat healthy?" Information on nutrition doesn't seem to really help them.

From sara, Age 13 - 06/04/06
Ht. 5'7, Wt. 175 - **i know alot about food and nutrion i just keep binging** though ugggggggggggggg......;/
any ideas

Reply from *.:Teresa:.*, Age 14 - 04/02/06
the usual stuff. **people are always asking HOW to lose weight. everyone knows HOW.** stop eating junk, and starting drinking a whole lot of water. add in excersize. eat smaller portions.

Once kids are provided the information on how to lose weight, most seem unable to follow it, even though they desperately wanted the information.

From ann, Age 17 - 11/02/04
does any 1 else notice **how desperate we r to find out how to lose weight and ask how and then dnt follow it.** we all no how to lose weight. anywayz bye

From Lauren, Age 17 - 6/14/06

Ht. 5'4, Wt. 155 - Hey guys; I just wanted to add a little bit of a rant here. Sorry if it is a bit on the offensive side, but I just wanted to get it out. **whenever someone gets on here and is excited about losing a few pounds, I hardly see any congratulations. Instead, I see "How'd you do it?!!!! Tell me!!! How did you do it?!!!"** It looks so **desperate;**

The above two posts show how desperate overweight kids are to find some other way to lose weight that doesn't require giving up any of the food they love. Why is this food so important to these kids, even though they are desperate to lose weight? What's really occurring here?

Poll – why is "How do I lose weight?" so often asked?

The question, "How do I lose weight?" is so common on the boards and in the chat rooms that we asked kids in a poll why they think that question is asked so much. Do the kids not want to take the time to read the weight loss information on the website, or are they just looking for support from other kids? (http://www.blubberbuster.com/cgi/poll_new_24.cgi)

Why do kids on the bulletin boards mainly say, "How do I lose weight?"

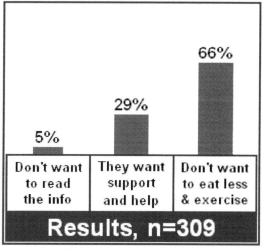

309 Kids voted

Most kids voted that the reason kids on the boards ask "How do I lose weight?" is that they don't want to eat less and exercise more. They are looking for some other way to lose weight. Here are comments from the kids who responded to this poll:

➔ "most kids and teenages are suffering from been overweight. **adults don't realise the depression and hullimation that teens suffer at school and at home**"

➔ "They might have **no one to show them in the right direction** to lose weight."

➜ "Many kids know they want to lose weight but **don't know how**. They need information and support."

➜ **"every 1 is looking for a way to loose wayt"**

➜ "They probably know that they have to cut down on food, and increase exercise, but **they are looking for some other FASTER way**, because Americans today are How can I have what *I* want **FAST WITHOUT having to work so hard**, and wait so long to get it???". And the bad part is, the answer to that question continues to be answered EVERYDAY - ways you can lose weight fast without having to work for it, and unfortunately, **that is what American kids today are born into…"**

➜ "I t hink they do it because they want to lose weight and **everything they do it fails** so they are asking for help or tips"

➜ "I'm Overweight and most kids like myself **just want smiple steps** to lsoe weight with out alot of work. "

➜ "probably they have tried to lose weight by excercising more and eating less,however **it hasnt worked and they are trying to find something that will"**

➜ "by saying this, people are looking for attention. **they are just fishing for people to take care of them** in any way."

➜ "i mean if they are over weight they are not going to want to get up and excirse… because they think that there is more to what people are saying than what is on the site. **They just dont want the way that they are going to have to slim down come to a reality."**

➜ "take me for an example i'm overweight and **i know i have to cut down on sugar sweets and junk foods but it is very hard to give it up"**

➜ "It's not so much that they are lazy, its that **people make them the butt of insulting and humiliating jokes**, that shouldnt be made about anyone ever and they feel like **they just can't leave the feeling of hoplessness and worthlessness** behing fast enough."

➜ "Kids will always want the easy way out.....but **healthy weightloss is hard and long process."**

➜ "well yeah or at least me!i love fatty foods and in huge portions!**its hard to let it go!**no wonder i am so fat!"

→ "**we love food so much we cant let it go** or at least me cause im so fat!! 153lbswhat a pig!! besids exersizing hard and boring."

→ "**I think they probably want support**, or some tips on how to make it easier."

→ "**Teens are not stupid!** They know what they need to do, but **they need encouragement!**"

In other words, even though these kids ask how to lose weight, they actually realize that they must eat less and exercise more. But eating less, as well as exercising more, is just too hard for them. Why is it so hard? The next three chapters reveal why losing weight is so hard for these kids.

Weight loss camps

Weight loss camps are a method used by many kids to lose weight. What do kids say about them?

Age 13, female, Ht: 5`9", Wt: 200 lb
I Have been to one and **it has really paid off**. I go to one at least every summer. They are really fun. It is just like a regular camp. Except you loose weight. I was so happy. I was at the camp for three months. Now i am old enough to be a canslour. I was one and i loved seeing **how happy the kids got when they saw they were loosing weigt and having fun at the same time.**

Age 11, female, Ht: 5`3", Wt: 160 lb
i would go, but i would tell me dad **NOT TO TELL ANYONE IM GOING... itl be so embarssing...** like, tell them i went to calif. or something.+...

Age 16, female, Ht: 5`8", Wt: 178 lb
it is great i can meet new people and nobody is gonna laugh at me cause i'm nat ganna be the fat kid. i think is gonna be fun because i need to leave home for a while, i haven't been out for six years i usually go home, sholl, and church, and then home,school and home again, and is boring. **with a camp i think i'll have lots of experiences, and learn alot of things, and will keep my mind of food, because i eat when i'm bored.**

From Charlotte, Age 11, female - 11/7/05
I has always been chuby until 3rd grade then I went up to 150 pounds in 3rd grade.When I went in fourth grade I was still that same weight.My mom let me do Weight Watchers with her because it was safe but I cheated so badly. **That summer i went to a weight loss camp wher i lost 20 pounds and was at 156 when i first started and went down to 136. In 5th grade i gained it all back, I think it was because it was impossible not**

lose weight in weight loss camp because they choose what you eat and make you exercise(it doesn't prepare you for real life at all). I gained up till I was 169 pounds....

Below is a "live" conversation in the chatroom, where two girls and others talk about the experience of going to a weight loss camp:

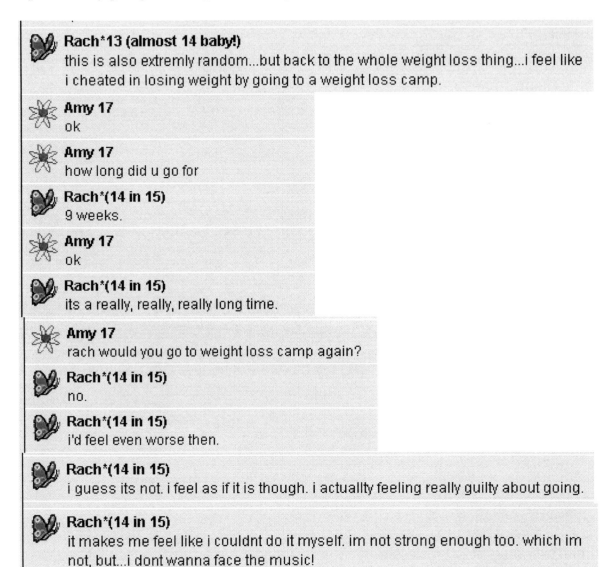

Rach*13 (almost 14 baby!)
this is also extremly random...but back to the whole weight loss thing...i feel like i cheated in losing weight by going to a weight loss camp.

Amy 17
ok

Amy 17
how long did u go for

Rach*(14 in 15)
9 weeks.

Amy 17
ok

Rach*(14 in 15)
its a really, really, really long time.

Amy 17
rach would you go to weight loss camp again?

Rach*(14 in 15)
no.

Rach*(14 in 15)
i'd feel even worse then.

Rach*(14 in 15)
i guess its not. i feel as if it is though. i actuallty feeling really guilty about going.

Rach*(14 in 15)
it makes me feel like i couldnt do it myself. im not strong enough too. which im not, but...i dont wanna face the music!

And a bulletin board post:

From Rachael, Age 14 - 4/7/05
Hey guys...I've been hearing some people talk about **fat camps** on this board, and **I don't think it's the best way to lose weight.** I mean, you'll definetely lose weight there, but **what happens when you come home and go back to your old habits?** You'll have to deal with passing on the candy and stuff, and at fat camps they only serve healthy stuff, so you won't be used to resisting things, and it will be much harder to keep the weight off. I

think the best way is to just develop healthy eating habits and exercise, **not take the easy way out and go to a fat camp where there's no temptation.**

Another chat conversation:

 Chewy 13
165 lbs., 5'6, female

 Chewy 13
i actually went to fat camp last summer

 Chewy 13
it was great- i lost 20 pounds

 Chewy 13
i gained it back now, but i am determined to loose it back

 Scar Face 14
idk... i wouldnt go to fat camp

 Michelle 14
k

 Scar Face 14
its sort of degrading

And still another:

 Sierra 14
have you ever been to one of those camps?

 Amanda 17
no

 Amanda 17
my cousin has

 Sierra 14
did he lose alot of weight?

 Amanda 17
not really. she didnt lose much at all

Amanda 17
and then she gained it all back and more

(Continued on the following page)

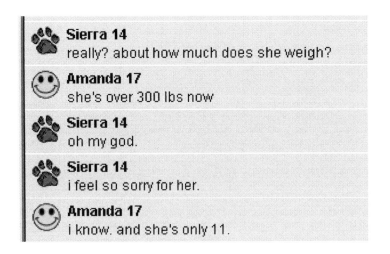

Sierra 14
really? about how much does she weigh?

Amanda 17
she's over 300 lbs now

Sierra 14
oh my god.

Sierra 14
i feel so sorry for her.

Amanda 17
i know. and she's only 11.

As these chats and posts suggest, weight loss camps didn't work for these kids. When they returned to the home environment (out of the controlled food and exercise environment of the weight loss camp) they often gained the weight back.

We ask kids about weight loss camps in a poll (http://www.blubberbuster.com/cgi/poll_new_36.cgi):

What do you think about a weight loss camp, if you could afford it?

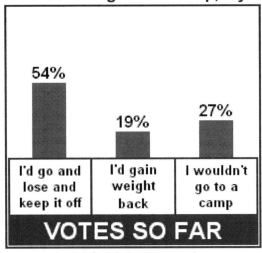

149 kids voted

More than half of 149 kids voting say they'd go to camp, lose weight, and keep it off. About a fifth of the kids believe they'd gain the weight back, and about a fourth wouldn't go to a weight loss camp. Comments from kids who responded to this poll are below. Several say that they would be embarrassed to go to a weight loss camp.

Would go:

➜ I weihg 210 pounds and i am 11 i am obese and hate it if i went to a weight loss camp i **would lose weight there and put it all back and more when i got back home**

➜ i would atleast try to keep the weight off but **at camp they have you running and playing all day and thats just not how it is at home**

➜ I would go and keep it off because a **weightloss camp could be whut I need** to loose the weight that I want and If I can do that I wouldnt want to gain it back so **I would keep the same habits I learned at Fat camp.**

➜ if money wasnt an issue and my parents let me i would love to go to weight loss camp, **you we be with others in the same situation as you.**

➜ It wuld be **great to see people that are like you**

➜ I am going this summer! I am SO excited! This is **exactly the jumpstart I needed!**

➜ I want to have fun during summer .....**swimming can help me lose weight** and isnt embarrising

➜ I **WOULD TRY MY HARDEST** ATLEAST!

➜ I would go to weight loss camp because it would be fun, and **you get a little vacation where you don't gain weight.**

➜ i think it weight loss camp is a great idea, although it would be kind of embarrasing **if i could go with a friend i would really enjoy it.**

➜ at least i'd hope to keep the weight off.Anyway **if the weight loss camps were cheaper i could afford to go to one.** oh well.

➜ if i could afford it..................... ;-(

Wouldn't go:

➜ **I didn't need a fat camp to lose 180 pounds** and be slim. I went from 11 years old and an immense 350 pounds,and am now 170 pounds and slim. I dieted and exercised; it's slow and hella hard but it worked and i know ill never be huge again

➜ No definetaly not! **We should be able to help ourselves!!!!! We dont go to a camp everytime we want to lose weight**

➔ cause i dont need to even if i am 58 pounds overweight. **ill just gain it back!!!!!!!** **duuuuuuh**

➔ They **won't give me the food I enjoy.**

➔ I believe that **different bodies require different weightloss plans** in order for them to be permanent. I don't think a weight loss camp would see to that.

➔ I wouldn't because I would feel bad **because I'm being treated like I'm a fat looser.**

➔ I would be too **embarassed** in front of my friends and i wouldnt want to be away from home

➔ I would **rather join a gym**. I just wouldn´t like to go to a weight loss camp.

➔ It would be so **embarassing**. What if I was the fattest there, or I couldn't do things that others could, that would mean I could even do what other fat people could do and would make me feel crap! ESPECIALLY if there were guys there!!!

➔ I would only go **if i knew someone else hu was goin** b cuz im a verry shy person

➔ its **stuipid**

➔ but thats an american thing! we don't have them in the UK! Would have to be far from home so you could have some discretion in what you're doing.

➔ it will **embarrase** me and **i will gain it back and alot more**

➔ because I would be too **ebarassed**

Weight Loss Buddies

Very early in the history of the site it was observed that the kids, on their own, sought weight loss buddies on the bulletin boards. They highly value the support of a web buddy in their struggle to lose weight, as they may not receive support from their family or friends. They email each other or chat live in the chatrooms or interact via 'instant messaging,' which is a one-on-one private chat. They share ups and downs, tips, and help to motivate each other. The following posts illustrate the search for a weight loss buddy:

From Kacey, Age 19 - 1/8/08
Ht. 5'6", Start: 300 lb, Current: 300 lb, Goal: 140 lb - I've tried dieting a lot before but it never ever works out. **I don't get any support from my family** and **my boyfriend**

doesn't really know how to help me out either. **I'm looking for maybe like a "diet" buddy** or someone who is my age or around my weight that can help me and encourage me.

From Kim, Age 15 - 07/12/09
Ht. 5'5", Start: 240 lb, Current: 245 lb, Goal: 150 lb - Ok, so I have tried to lose weight and I think I may make it this time, but **I just need support and advice so if you would like to be my weightloss buddy around my weight and goal** email me at bored_without_a_cause@hotmail.com... Thank you if you would help...

From Molly, Age 13 - 10/26/08
Ht. 5'1", Start: 150 lb, Current: 150 lb, Goal: 120 lb - hi my names molly.i am fat.i get called fat alot .my brother calls me fat my model sister calls me fat my mom calls me fat my friends call me fat.all i ever wanted was to be thin .my best friend is so pretty,every time im with her guys always come up too her and tell her shes hot.i hate my body .i have strech marks on my side.i love swimming when i was younger i used to swim every day ,i used to be on swim teams.but know i dont swim no more becocouse mt thies are so big.i sut started my diet today.hope it works. ps.i **realy need a friend to talk to….we can give each other advice** ..love molly

From Courtney, Age 19 - 12/27/07
Ht. 5'8", Start: 207 lb, Current: 180 lb, Goal: 135 lb - hi everyone. i met someone on this website a while ago and to we set goals and lost weight together. **we emailed eachother andit really helped me** focus on my goal. I lost almost twenty lbs, but still had alot more to lose. when she achieved her goal **she stopped emailing me**, i guess it was because she was done with her weight loss. **after that i coulnt lose the weight** as easily, so im back here again. I really want to find a person who is serious about losing their weight. please reply i you are interested, **its seems to be so much easier, when u have a friend doing it with you…**

This is SILVIA'S question:
Lucy, i live in **Australias** capital and i am obese and finding it almost impossible to do anything about it because my motivation is very low. **i know that if i had a companion in similar position any age it would be a lot easier.** (for the both of us) **wht can i do find a fat friend?**

From Ashley, Age 15 - 11/21/05
Ht. 5'4, Wt. Too scared to check. - Hey… I'm new here and I was looking for someone to be my **weight loss buddy! Preferably a girl, because in all honesty... it'd be weird otherwise.** If you're interested, you can email me..

Age 13, female, Ht: 5`9, Wt: 200 lb
I think haveing a weight loss buddy is great. I have one and i have lost 60 lbs. **We can**

talk to eachother abou anything. And if one of us wants to go off the diet we can talk and not do it.

From Mel, Age 15 - 11/18/03
Ht. 5'6", Wt. 14 stone 4 - Hi guys! im a 15 year old girl **from England,** im sick of bein so fat. i would like to find a diet buddy, of around the same age and weight as me. if u want 2 chat some time, or just need some motiveation...**i need help, i cant deal with this alone!**Lotsa luv melxxxx (Note: **14 stone 4 is 200 lb.)**

Age 10, female, Ht: 4 feet 6 inches Wt: 88.5 lbs
I think **it's great having someone to help you and support you,** and someone able **to tell you "Don't worry, you can do it!"** I think that's just what we all need.

We asked kids about their use of weight loss buddies in a poll
(http://www.blubberbuster.com/cgi/poll_new_39_percent.cgi):

What do you think about a weight loss buddy to help you to lose weight?

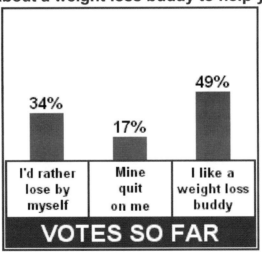

118 Kids Voted

Half of those who voted would like a weight loss buddy. About one sixth of the kids say their buddy abandoned them. This is because one or the other of the pair either reached his/her goal weight or simply gave up. A third of the kids say they would prefer to lose weight by themselves.

From Jeimi, Age 17 - 12/27/07
Ht. 5'2", Start: 240 lb, Current: 228 lb, Goal: 120 lb - hey everyone i've felt a little helpless latley i've messed up yesterday and today... idk **i feel like i'm never going to lose weight and it makes me really upset** ....this site is the only way for me to get this out o and **my weight loss buddys always stop emailing me for some reason** i feel like i'm never going to lose this weight just had to get all that out.

From Joanna, Age 15 - 07/22/06 -
Ht. 5'2, Wt. 184 - ... Idk anymore, I am depressed like major. and this week has sucked so much i just want to cry my eyes out. **I need help. A buddy thats true and will not stop emailing?** similar to me. or not it dont really matter. ...

As the posts in this chapter reflect, the life of an overweight child or teen can be very discouraging. Most dislike or hate their fat bodies. They struggle with the physical problems of large size and carrying extra weight, such as not being able to fit in desks or participate in sports. They have difficulty finding clothes, particularly popular styles. Being overweight is especially hard in the teen years, when acceptance by peers is of prime importance. Most are quite sensitive to disapproval and teasing. And they desperately search for a way to lose weight that does not require giving up the food they find irresistible.

A research study published in the Journal of the American Medical Association in 2003 echoes the unhappiness of overweight kids presented in this chapter. That study found that severely obese kids are as unhappy as kids diagnosed with cancer. [Schwimmer et al. 2003]. So, if overweight and obese kids are this unhappy because of their weight, why then don't they cease overeating and lose the weight?

What's actually going on here? Are kids overeating due to unmet needs? Is the health profession community failing to ask the right questions (see Chapter 6 - Health Professionals)? Why do parents find it so difficult to help their overweight children (see Chapter 5 - Parents)? How can kids attain and maintain a healthy weight?

In their quest for answers, many overweight kids have banded together on the web to help each other. Those who post on our site say that they rarely ask anyone for help - parents, siblings, friends, teachers, counselors, or even health professionals. They keep their weight problem a secret. Why is this? The next chapter presents what kids say about secrecy and shame.

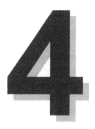

4 | Secrecy & Shame

Secrecy

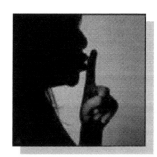

Secrecy plays an important role with overweight kids. Typically, they keep their weight issues and weight loss efforts a complete secret. Why is secrecy so necessary in the minds of overweight kids?

Everyone can see that a child or teen is overweight. But it's rarely talked about. Overweight kids don't talk about it, their parents don't talk about it, their friends don't talk about it, and even their doctors don't talk about it. Why? Is everyone too ashamed or embarrassed? Is it the old "elephant in the living room" situation, which refers to "a question, problem, solution, or controversial issue that is obvious, but which is ignored by a group of people, out of embarrassment or taboo?" That phrase is commonly used in addiction recovery terms to describe the reluctance of friends and family of an addicted person to discuss the person's problem, thus aiding the person's denial (http://en.wikipedia.org/wiki/Elephant_in_the_room).

Shame

Even though the Internet is anonymous, many overweight kids still feel tremendous shame about interacting with other kids, as the below posts relate:

From Kristin, Age 14 - 11/18/02 -
this is embarrassing but please dont laugh when you read this i am **14** and **i weigh close to 265** pounds **i am so ashamed** of my self so before you decide to make a rude reply i could really use som help with dieting thanks

From Naomi, Age 16 - 02/24/08
Ht. 5'9", Start: 303 lb, Current: 301 lb, Goal: 175 lb - **Okay(wow this is hard) speaking honestly, I have been on this site before but have used various names to cover up my shame from other people I may know.** My story is a little long so bare with

me, I have been overweight/obese my entire life. I was never really teased or anything just hurt, when i use the word hurt most people ask why, but its because I have had self-esteem issues since i was a child. When I grew up and headed to high school was when i was teased and began to have low-self-esteem issues/problems. ..

From Lola, Age 10 - 1/8/08 -
Ht. 4'7", Start: 9 stone 2, Current: 9 stone 2, Goal: 6 stone 00 (Note: 9 stone 2 is 128 lb.)- I am overweight and i have felt overweight since about 3 years old when my aunt said something bad about me and i realisied that I was fat. At school they call me fatty. one girl said an elephant would look like an ant compared to me. I don't cry in front of them but it hurts inside when they say bad things about me and call me names. **I am horrible and discusting**. i felt fat in my new clothes at chistmasand I don't like anyone to see me eating. One day I was wearing a dress that was too tight around my tummy and i heard my dad say to my mum is that all her? and he said he hadn't known how big i was getting and that my mum shuld make me loose weight. i REALY wish i could loose weight and be skinny.**I am too embarrased to tell anyone** but i know they all think i am fat and discusting.

From whatever, Age 17 - 12/11/07
Ht. 6'0", Start: 261 lb, Current: 261 lb, Goal: 179 lb - im 261 pounds I am seventeen years old. I hate my body. I'm 6 feet tall. I dieted I lost 35 pounds , then gained it back. **I'm ashamed. I a compulsive overeater.** I need help. **I'm suicidal.** I just want to be normal. I'm a prisoner. =/// I'm so happy. I have hope , but I'm falling apart. someone help me. =///

Overweight kids even say they feel invisible. People don't want to embarrass the overweight child or teen by looking at his/her body, so they look past them, as if they are not really there.

From Lacey, Age 16 - 06/21/06
Ht. 5'6, Wt. 150 - So there's this guy I've known for a long time ... **i feel invisible when im around him!** he only looks at me when im not looking.

Secrecy from friends

Overweight kids are embarrassed that their friends might discover their efforts to lose weight.

From Vinnie, Age 13 - 09/27/03
Ok i'm 13 years old **5'1** and weight almost **200 pounds** i want to lose at least 70 pounds but **i dont wanna be embarrased in front of my friends my eatting healthy and stuff**...

From Jennifer*, Age 14 - 11/26/05
Ht. 5"0, Wt. 159 - ....Alright today I just got a myspace and I want ppl to send me a comment, just **dont mention u met me on BB cuz then everyone in school will know that i am tryin to lose weight!** Just say u met me in a chat room! I know that might sound weird but plz dont Much luvin

This is MARIHA's question
hey im **12 and 4 9 and I weigh 136** i need to lose it before 8 th grade please help me and **I dont wont any one to know this** or this be shown on the web sigth thank you. i hope you can help me being on an diet i have already tryed

This is BRITTANY's question:
Hi im brittany im 13 5 5 and 220 lbs i have always struggled wit my weight? i just want to kno if u could help me wit thinkin of an exercisin program so that i can work out everyday **witout my frinds knowin cuz i would be really embarrassed if they found out**.if u could just help me wit that that would be great thanx a lot bye.

This is ALISON's question:
How do I loose weight without being embarrassed in front of my friends?

We asked kids in a poll if they keep our website a secret from their parents or friends. (http://www.blubberbuster.com/cgi/poll_new_48_percent.cgi)

> **Do you keep this site a secret from your parents or friends?**
>
> **YES: 97 votes (72%)**
>
> **NO: 37 votes (28%)**

135 kids voted

Nearly three fourths of 135 kids responding indicate that they keep our site a secret from parents or friends.

From Rebecca, Age 14 - 07/23/09
Ht. 5'6", Start: 320 lb, Current: 320 lb, Goal: 160 lb - Where do I start? Let's see... I have always been a heavy child for as long as I can remember. I hate it. People calling names, not being able to do a lot of the things other kids do (like amusement park rides, and certain sports) and having to be disgusted every time I look in the mirror... **I**

really hope it helps being able to talk to other overweight teens online helps, if it doesn't I don't know what else to do. I don't feel comforted talking to my mother or anyone else about my weight in person, I am afraid to talk face to face with others.

Why do these kids feel the need to keep their weight loss efforts a secret from their parents or friends? We asked kids about this in a poll:

If you keep this site or weight loss a secret, what is the reason you do so? (vote for one)

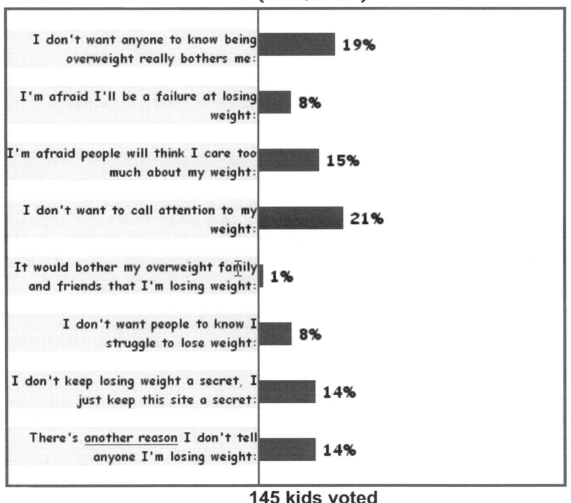

145 kids voted

The two main reasons why these kids keep their weight loss efforts a secret are: 1) so as not to call attention to their weight and 2) so that no one knows that being overweight really bothers them. If other kids know that being overweight bothers the overweight child or teen, he/she is then vulnerable to teasing. Plus, overweight kids feel shame, which they don't want anyone to know about.

In another poll we asked from whom specifically the kids keep their weight loss efforts a secret:

If you keep your weight loss attempts or this site a secret, from whom do you keep it a secret? (check all that apply):

Doctor:	52.8%
Friends	76.8%
Siblings:	70.4%
Parents:	80%

145 kids voted

The 145 kids responding keep their weight loss efforts secret mainly from their parents, probably because their parents are the most critical. However, it is distressing that more than half of these kids keep their weight loss efforts secret from their doctor. Kids may keep their weight loss efforts a secret from parents and health professionals because they fear failure in the eyes of those people and criticism.

From Taylor, Age 16 - 07/14/07
Ht. 5'5", Start: 275 lb, Current: 272 lb, Goal: 125 lb - do any of you ever feel like you don't want to set goals or say you're going to lose weight and get in shape, because everytime you have ever said that before you don't? ...**when it doesn't happen, i feel like a failure.**

Discussion about weight loss failures and alternative strategies offers another opportunity for healthcare providers to intervene, although many don't. Is it that the doctors don't ask, or that the kids don't tell? Do overweight kids believe doctors are critical of them?

From Courtney, Age 15 - 10/15/09
Ht. 5'5", Start: 224 lb, Today: 224 lb, Goal: 130 lb - Hey :) well ive always tryed to loose weight. But have never got far... **Ive noticed i do good untill i tell someone im trying to loose weight...then i stop, so i plan on just keeping this to myself well besides on here :P**

The kids keep their weight problem a secret from friends and family out of fear of being teased, as the poll's additional comments describe:

Age 11, female, 5"3', 160 lbs - **at school i tell people i dont care about my weight if they ask me.. but i really do.. am i dont wanna draw the fact to me, people will make fun of me more.** - I keep this site or my weight loss a secret from parents,sibs,friends,doctor

Age 13, female, 5'7, 169 lbs - People would make fun of me if they find out I'm over weight - I keep this site or my weight loss a secret from parents,,friends,

Age 13, female, 5/3, 140 lbs - i wouldnt want my friends to kno iim using this website because its to personal nd really there not all good friends . . even my best friend i dont tell her because shes a dancer nd she has a six pack nd shes SKINNY and ii dont want to be embarrased =[. . . nd if other people wud find out they wud laugh =[- I keep this site or my weight loss a secret from parents,,friends,doc

Age 16, female, 5'7, 180 lbs - My mom knos I come to the site but none of my freinds I feel dumb and i dont want my friends to think that im really self concious bout my weight so im tryin to be happy with who i am even if im not im tryin - I keep this site or my weight loss a secret from ,sibs,friends,

Age 12, female, 5'7, 170 lbs - i do it because my family says i am to young to be worried about my weight but in scool thay are always joking about it so i do it. - I keep this site or my weight loss a secret from parents,,friends,

Age 15, female, 5'7, 250 lbs - Im just tired of my mom getting into my weight business, so i come here for help. - I keep this site or my weight loss a secret from parents,sibs,

Age 13, female, 65, 182 lbs - i dont want anyone to think i am losing weight for how i look. i am content of the way i look. the only reason i want to lose weight is my heath. my parents also tend to annoy me and consistently push me to lose weight. i want to do it without their help and nag.ing - I keep this site or my weight loss a secret from parents,,,

The Burden of Keeping Weight Loss a Secret

Loneliness

Obesity has been described as a 'disease of loneliness.' The need for secrecy adds to the loneliness. The kids say that this website helps.

From Chiku, Age 15 - 02/10/09
Ht. 5'3", Start: 160 lb, Current: 160 lb, Goal: 110 lb - I'm going to lose weight, I m tired of being made fun of.I don't want to be called fat anymore or be picked last in P.E!! I'm gonna show the girls in my class that I can be skinny too! And I hope I can make it, and **I found this site and it seems like a lot of teens are in here and I don't feel so lonely anymore** ☺

From anastasya, Age 17 - 5/15/04
Ht. 5'5, Wt. 260 lbs - OMG!!! **my mom doesn't LET ME EXERCISE ENOUGH. she doesn't care about my weight** - she herself is extremely sedentary all her life and **buys junk food** too. **she says that looks are not important (maybe that's why my dad divorced)**and i should focus on school and academics.i hate her 4 this - talk to her every freakin day- she doesn't understand. i can't do much against her, but she makes me wanna die. **i'm very lonely and have no friends.i'm considering running away or going to foster home.** plzzz help.

Weight loss programs in school

Our site offers an online weight loss system, which schools may use to help their overweight students. School is the ideal place to positively impact on the overweight problem, as kids spend 180 days a year there, the school has a relationship with the kids, and tackling overweight is in fact an educational process. Sadly, a major barrier to announced weight loss programs in schools is that overweight students fear their weight struggles will be revealed.

We did a poll on this (http://www.blubberbuster.com/cgi/poll_new_66.cgi):

What do you think about an announced weight loss program in school?

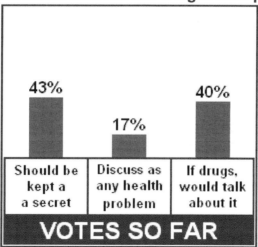

120 kids voted

Nearly half of 120 kids responding feel a school weight loss program should be kept a secret. Almost as many feel that overweight is as important as 'drug abuse', which is openly discussed. Slightly less than one fifth feel overweight should be discussed openly like any health problem. Most would like a weight loss program in their school (see results on following page).

> **Would you like a weight loss program in your school?**
>
> **YES:** 74 votes (62%)
>
> **NO:** 46 votes (38%)

Comments from kids about this poll:

Those who do want a school weight loss program:

Age 17, female, 5'8, 230 lbs - **We need to get health programs for schools so over weight kids can get back in shape.** - I want a weight loss program in my school.

Age 11, male, 5' 1", 150 lbs - I want to lose weight but it's harder than it looks. **I wish my school had a support system, it would help more people than just me.** - I want a weight loss program in my school.

Age 12, female, 4'9, 110 lbs - my school is all full of thin people we only have 4 overweight children out of 50 kids so **it would really single us out** - I want a weight loss program in my school.

Age 16, female, 5'7", 289 lbs - I'd be much too embaressing, maybe not has much in high school but in the younger grades, those kids would get tortured - not a good idea. **I like the idea of the school specially contacting overweight kids and keeping it a kind of secret within the school...you don't need to announce it.** - I want a weight loss program in my school.

Age 17, female, 5'7, 150 lbs - I believe that **schools should offer support to overweight kids so that if they are looking for help they know where to find it.** - I want a weight loss program in my school.

Age 11, female, 5'5", 160 lbs - **They should have a private program, but nothing that is embarrasing.** - I want a weight loss program in my school.

Age 13, female, 5'4", 196 lbs - **It may be embarassing, but it's helping to solve the problem.** - I want a weight loss program in my school.

Other topics are talked about openly in school, why not weight loss programs?

Age 15, female, 5'9", 131 lbs - **We talk in Health Classes about drug addictions, STD's, asthma, and every other health subject; why not obesity and ways to help?** - I want a weight loss program in my school.

Age 16, female, 5'8'', 168 lbs - **Most of the kids in my school have an acholol problem and my school is always talking about it.** But lately my school has been talking about a weight loss program. We have boot camps before formals to loss weight. We have to weight lift rooms you can use when ever you want. - I want a weight loss program in my school.

Age 17, female, 5'2, 62 kgs - **It's important to talk about it openly,** why mind others say? **What's important is our health. Being overweight is not a crime.** Everybody can be overweight. - I want a weight loss program in my school.

Kids have good ideas, why not ask them and involve them in coming up with ideas and plans:

Age 15, female, 5'6", 163 lbs - **I think that being overweight is just a health problem** and I think it'd be a great idea to have weight loss programs at school because kids are getting so overweight these days. **It'd be cool if they also had like after school excercise clubs because not everyone likes sports.** I'd like to excercise with people not just at home by myself doing a workout dvd or magazine workout all the time it gets old. **I'd really like to take a dance class or something!!!** - I want a weight loss program in my school.

Age 13, female, 5ft. 5 in, S: 184 N:167 G:145-150 lbs - I said I wanted a "weight loss" program, but **what I man by that is simply more activity, not a "special" whack diet club or anything like that.** People want to dance or something! We have sports teams, but I only like softball, so **I'd be great if we had our own little "other" activities club. Better yet, how about discount memberships to dance studios or a free yoga session at a gym?!** - I want a weight loss program in my school.

Below is an example of school health staff inappropriately handling the overweight issue and reinforcing embarrassment.

Age 14, female, 5'9, 196 lbs - I think **it should be an open thing. The only problem I have is singling out the larger kids. I've had a nurse approach me when I was** around other people at lunch and she openly said we should go and discuss a diet for me because I was "looking a bit heavier" and I was "already heavy on the scale" at **the beginning of the year.** - I want a weight loss program in my school.

Those who don't want a school weight loss program:

Age 13, female, 5'2, 121 lbs - **they will get maked fun of** - I do not want a weight loss program in my school.

Age 10, female, 4''11', 287 lbs - I am very fat. **It would be embarrasing** - I do not want a weight loss program in my school.

Age 13, female, 5'7'', 198 lbs - I REALLY want to loose some weight, but **I am afraid to do it in school becuase I think it would be embarrasing.** - I do not want a weight loss program in my school.

Age 13, female, 5'00, 290 lbs - **i would get bullied more** - I do not want a weight loss program in my school.

Below are additional examples of how kids fear staff could be or already are insensitive about their overweight:

Age 11, male, 4'10, 86 kgs - It should be kept a secret especially at my school. **The principal would say " And the students in the weight loss program are......."** - I do not want a weight loss program in my school.

Age 10, female, 5'4, 168.4 lbs - **that is just rude if schools anounce a weight loss program.** - I do not want a weight loss program in my school.

Age 12, female, 5ft, 173 lbs - **duh im so fat its like my fattness is already a huge topic even the teachers have told me if i wanted a "special desk " cuse i dont fit.** - I do not want a weight loss program in my school.

Age 12, female, 5'1, 146 lbs - **As if we dont already feel awkward in school! We dont need it announced!** - I do not want a weight loss program in my school.

Overweight kids seem to want a weight loss program in school, but schools need to be very sensitive to the embarrassment factor and the need for privacy.

Recruiting school kids for weight loss programs

We asked kids how school recruitment for a weight loss program should be handled (http://www.blubberbuster.com/cgi/poll_new_45.cgi), as shown on the following page:

What is the best way to recruit school kids for a weight loss program?

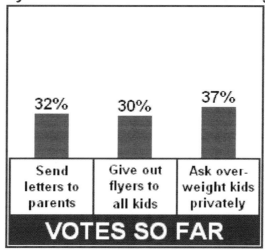

105 kids voted

Responses to the above poll were about equally divided among sending letters home to all parents versus passing out flyers to all kids versus recruiting overweight kids privately.

Comments from kids about this poll:

Age 16, female, 5'8, 178 lbs - **this is soooooooooooooooooooooooooooooooooooooooooooooooooooooooo insulting to fat kids**

Sending letters

Age 13, female, 5'4, 129 lbs - When I was overweight, **I would be emarased if my weight was talked with me. My parents would not care about a letter.**

Age 16, female, 5'7, 177 lbs - I think **if the parents now they are doing this at the school they will be more then happily to help out at home** and would be aware and its a great idea

Age 13, female, 5'7", 220 lbs - I think sending a letter to the child's home would be best because **it would be the least embaressing.**

Flyers to all

Age 15, female, 5'7'', 158 lbs - **Then everyone has an equal chance of doing it and no one feels singled out or pressured into it.**

Age 11, female, 4 ft. 9 in., 77 lbs - **If you did flyers, all the kids would pick on the overweight kid. If you asked them privately, they might be really embarassed.**

Ask privately

Age 11, female, 4'11, 105 lbs - they shouldnt announce it in front of everyone cuz then the skinny ppl will look at all the fat ppl n make fun of them so they should privately have a conversation w/ either the kid or parents

Age 13, female, 5'5'', 157 lbs - Asking ppl privatly would really help and it wouldnt embarrass anyone.

Age 15, female, 5 10, 200 lbs - dont anouce the people...keep it secret meetings...like not durning school when everyone knows who goes and who dosent cause most kids will get embarassed...i know i would

Age 18, female, 5'8 1/2'', 240 lbs - I believe that if the school has **nurses and PE teachers privately ask each child that is overweight if they want to participate, it will give them a more personal feeling that someone cares.** Not to mention if the childs parent asks them, it might make the child feel hurt. **Someone confronting you with being overweight can sometimes cause a very negative reaction. Also, it might be a good idea to both do this and pass out flyers. Give them a chance to do it on their own before having someone speak to them about it.**

Not ask privately

Age Mar, female, 5"6, 185 lbs - singleing them out will only make them feel worse about their problem, and resist to any form of help offered to them!

Age 13, female, 5"6, 130 lbs - It would be pretty mean to come up to certain individuals and say "your fat sign up"

Age 13, male, ?, ? kgs - i don't think that privately asking each overweight child or teen if they would like to participate is a good idea because they could get embrassed if that are the only one in there class who gets asked.

Thus, all three of the above recruitment methods have advantages and disadvantages.

Experience with a school weight loss program

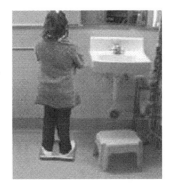

We learned very quickly that kids participating in a school weight loss program didn't want to be seen weighing in on scales or using our website. For our schools' programs we therefore developed wireless scales, located behind closed doors (bathroom at right), which automatically transmit the child's or teen's weight to their

website chart. Computer screens used by kids are turned so that no one else may see them.

We had the best success recruiting kids in a school in Alaska, where a very inspirational PE teacher publicly proclaimed the weight loss program to all the kids in his classes, as a way to become "fit." Suddenly, dozens of overweight kids and parents signed up for the program, whereas few had signed up until that point. The program no longer had to be kept a secret. Plus, it is more socially acceptable to be labeled "out of shape" than "fat."

Health classes

Again, tackling the overweight problem in kids should be an educational process, e.g. school health classes. What about including the topic of overweight in school health classes? Below are results of a poll on this (http://www.blubberbuster.com/cgi/poll_new_37.cgi):

Do you think overweight should be covered in school health classes?

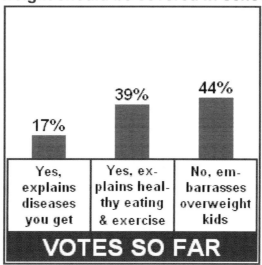

135 kids voted

Nearly half of the 135 kids responding feel that overweight shouldn't be included in school health classes, as it would embarrass and humiliate overweight kids.

A lot of kids commented about this poll, both positively and negatively:

Positive comments (overweight should be included in school health classes):

➔ **just like other issues of violence or sex or whatever, it's important** because overweight and obesity affects us all despite the fact that not all of us are overweight. **By learning more about this, you learn how to support people who are overweight instead of making fun of them.**

➔ i think it is a good idea to teach about weight problems in school because **it would help kids and let them know what being overweight can do.**

➔ **So overweight people will have to know how to deal with stress and stuff and for the non overweight people to know what it feels like to me called fat and names because you are fat and just are depressed all the time**

➔ It's not fair to ignore the weight issue because **some people, both fat people and not fat people, might really want to know about how to be healthy and stuff.**

➔ **A lot of kids never even grew up eating healthy so they don't know what right nutriton is.** I am struggling with this now. **If people have classes in their school teaching how to eat right and recognized obesity as an evergrowing issue, then a lot more kids would be able to fight it and not be ashamed of their hardships.**

➔ i feel that if i had been taught more about health and how to remain at a healthy weigth earlier on while i was in school i feel i would not have got to the weight i am now

➔ Yes it should because **not very many people or kids really know what the benifits are of not being over weight. A lot of over weight kids do not know what healthy eating and excirsing is. If it were more of a concern to the school like drug and acholal is than a lot less kids would be overweight.**

Even though the below kids think it would be embarrassing to cover overweight in health classes, they believe it's important for everyone to learn about being healthy.

➔ I chose yes because, even IF it does embarrass you (knowing from experience), it is still a very important issue that kids should know about.

➔ Yea, it may embaress overweight kids, but it also teaches them about why they are overweight and how they can become a healthy weight!

➔ I think that it will really help people out if it was taught on healthy eatin and excercise more people would want to be healthy and they me think it is fun and not as embarrased if othr peole do it to. well just my 2 cents.

➔ I think so, it also helps kids who don't know that they're overweight relize that they are.

➔ Even though it sometimes embarrases me when anybody talks about there weight...i believe that it should b tought in health classes so nobody else would b overweight too.

➔ Though it can be humiliating, it is necessary.

Negative comments (overweight should <u>not</u> be included in school health classes):

In the eyes of the overweight child or teen, the way health classes are currently taught only singles them out, fosters embarrassment, encourages teasing, and humiliates them.

➔ Fat kids get enough abuse without our health classes showing those durn films on obesity;i mean we're already fat why give the slim mean kids more ammunition to use against us....

➔ If a child is over-weight and the teacher takes the child aside or uses the child as an example, the child might get more humiliated than needed.

➔ I hate talking about being overweight because it just plain is embaressing. People stare at you and stuff. Ahhh! NO WAY!

➔ i hate talking about it during class because when we do start talking about be overweight and over eating, everyone turns around stares at me. i hate it

➔ its embarassing whenever i watch a health video about how obesity is sweeping the nation. I mean here i am fat, listening to people saying i'm fat. it also gives skinny mean kids things to laugh at us about

➔ everytime it cums up in health i feel like every1s lookin at me...

➔ we have to do that and every1 looks at me and they make jokes and its reall embarrising

➔ I used to be overweight and i remember how awful i felt when we talked about healthy food...the kids in my class would look at me like i was clearly one of the people who was eating all the "bad" foods. It was horrible and no one should have to go through that!

➔ i really think you shouldn't. students now days like to tease about anything

➔ I am overweight and people tease me about it all the time, if we had a class about it then people would be like "ya, this class is for you!".

➔ i would die if that happend!

➔ I'me 320 and age 14, so its hard to listen to that, although alot of kids in my school are obese(and when i say alot, i mean almost all). I'm probably the fattest and I HATE it

➔ I dont want other kids looking at me when the teacher is talking about it

➔ It shouldn't be a topic in school

➔ when im in my classes im usually one o the only "fat" kids and i feel like everyone is staring at me.

➔ i feel like i will be a target or teased in the classroom

➔ that is sooooo wrong, i mean, all of the skinny good looking kids will makefun of all the fat people and embarress them

➔ that would be wrong because letsay there was 3 overweight kids in the class who weighed 250pounds and every one else was like 90pounds how ebaressing would that be

➔ everytime a teacher brings overweight up... its so embarassing to me and my friend ana.. ana's fater but no one talks to her but me and acouple other ppl. but everyone talks to me.... and makes fun of me. not my friends, but if they hear it.. sometimes they laugh.

Perhaps kids could learn about overweight privately via school online computers, so that they wouldn't be sitting in the midst of others? Or, maybe it's the approach to teaching about overweight in schools that needs to change or be re-evaluated. Similar to the above PE teacher's method of labeling his program as a way to become "fit," perhaps health classes could disguise overweight topics as "ways to become healthy." Listening to what overweight kids say and including them in the planning of school curriculum and how courses are presented might make such programs more successful.

School weight screening

Weight screening kids in schools is a useful method to detect kids in need of help for overweight and has been proposed as one strategy to address the childhood obesity epidemic [Nihise et al. 2007]. Some school districts conduct weight screening annually on all students and send the results home to parents. In one study, "There was considerable parental support for school-based BMI screening and parent notification programs." [Kubik et al. 2006]. However, the state of Arkansas had to scale back its annual school weight screening in 2007 to every other year, due to parental complaints.

Several kids on our site have posted that they have major issues with school weight screening because of their embarrassment and need for secrecy.

From Beth, Age 15 - 04/05/04

I'm getting weighed in school this month (or possibly next month) and I'm terrified. Never once have I been weighed at school without some idiot in the background looking over my shoulder and laughing at my weight. I'm on a diet now and I'm losing a lot of weight but **I'm still going to dread this experience.** How can I get through this?

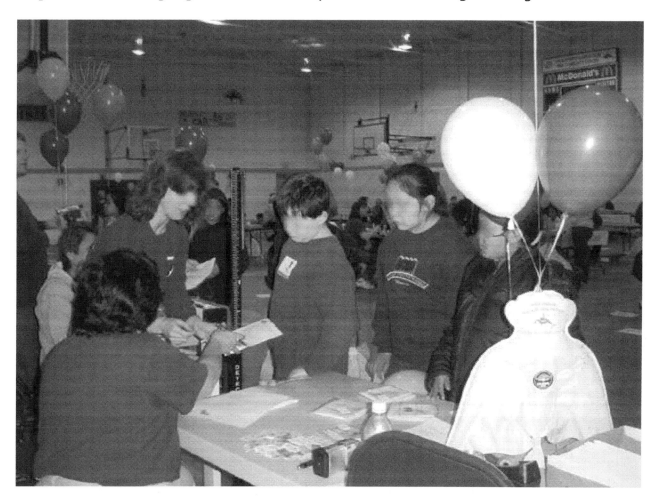

From meg, Age 14 - 03/05/06

Ht. 5'1, Wt. 160 - hey everyone i am due to get weiged in front of the whole school 2moz and i dont want to as i have gained loads of weight and **if you are over weight or have gained to much weight thenthey read out your name!** help me!

Reply from V, Age 14 - 03/21/05

I went through the same thing, it was this thing for health, and I already knew how much I weighed and everything, so it just bugged me. What I did, is **I just snuck into** the crowd and was like oh yeah I already did it, and just wrote down my weight in private...

We asked kids about this in a poll:
(http://www.blubberbuster.com/cgi/poll_new_29_percent.cgi)

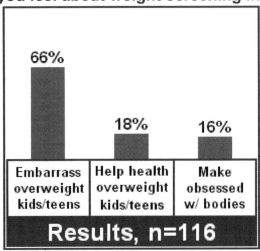

Most kids responding feel that open weighing of kids in school is too embarrassing.

Comments from kids about this poll:

Negative comments:

➔ **i know lots of people that refused to get on the scales at school,** the teacher just guest how much they weigh.

➔ **They do it at my school...its so horrible I don't sleep for like a week before it happens and I try to eat like practically nothing which doesn't work and I end up bingeing anyway and gaining more weight. Its horrible it causes so much stress...even the super skinny girls at my school stop eating lunch and stuff no one likes it!**

➔ **I think weighing kids at school is a bad idea. Even tho it will help overweight kids realize they are not healthy, it would embarrass most of us. I am really overweight and would hate to be weighed at school because I feel bad enough being fat. I don't need people at school (other students or even the nurse) teasing me about it or telling me that I need to lose weight. I know I do, but it would still be embarrassing. I think that most heavy kids would feel this way.**

➔ That is by far the stupidest idea I've ever heard of!! It's as if the gouvernment wants the overweight kids to be even more bullied and teased than they already are!!

➔ That is wrong. The only way that would be right is if it was confidential.

➔ They weighed our class at school and I was so embarrassed i'm not overweight but I am chubby and I feel so sorry for a boy in my grade who is dangerously overweight and everyone was teasing him I felt so humiliated!

➔ How embarrassing would that be!! how much you weigh is a personal thing, and nobody else should be allowed to know how much you weigh when you dont want them to!!! that is appalling!!!

➔ hey do that to me and i weighed 155 in 5th grade the kids made fun of me all year its so embarissing

➔ Last year they had me weighed at school. They told me that I was heavier than the heaviest of the 17 year olds by more than 50 pounds. They said it in front of everyone and i was so embarrased.

➔ its not the schools business

➔ ts embarrassing.... we had to do that in my school once. i made myself throw up so i could go home so i would get to do it in the nurses office where no one would see but the nurse and me. ughh, embarssed still!!

➔ they did that at my school as well as that pincher fat thingie and it made me feel bad because i was always one of the heaviest and the ones with the most fat

➔ Everyone in my class is kinda fat but Id still be humiliated

Positive comments:

➔ Well I think it is a good idea only if they can do it in privite so they dont humiliate students. I am overweight and I think that might help me to loose weight and want to eat healthy. I wouldntwant to do it though if everyone was watching. So maybe call one student in at a time to a little privite office during gym. That way students won't be embarassed...

➔ Hello? My school weighs us twice a year and we never die from it. We just diet like we're all going to be supermodels soon.

➔ WEIGHT IS A PROBLEM. Its not a fashion problem about "thin-is-better" . Its about your HEALTH - living long and keeping your body in top condition. Looking good has nothing to do with being skinny, because the best you is the healthy you. **If little kids are at risk of getting heart problems or diabetes, just because they have too much to eat, then this might put enough pressure on parents and the kids to get real. Screening might cause humilitation, kids might become a little body-obsessed, but if truth be told, who isn't body obsessed already anyway? We're bombarded left right and center with conflicting messages: "EAT, McDonald's, EAT" then "Stick-Thin is SOO in! Just look at our models and celebrities..." At the end of the day, I'd rather be humiliated a little if that's what it takes to keep me from dying young because of some serious health complication.**

➔ i kinda wish that schools would do this, i also wish that schools would have a class for weight loss that you could get a credit for

➔ i think it is a good idea because it will help the health of overweight children and teens, but also i think that indeed it will embaress some of the students. We get weighed at my school in pe though.

*There is a way to conduct school weight screening without humiliating overweight kids. As one teen suggests above, "...**maybe call one student in at a time to a little privite office during gym.**" Another great suggestion is, "...**that schools would have a class for weight loss that you could get a credit for.**"*

Getting help

To avoid isolation with their problems and get help, overweight kids need to talk to someone.

We did a poll on this issue, as shown on the following page. *(http://www.blubberbuster.com/cgi/poll_new_18.cgi):*

Have you ever talked to someone about your weight problem?

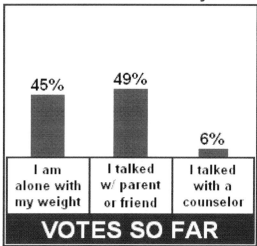

126 kids voted

Nearly half the kids responding say they've not talked with anyone about their weight, and hence they deal with their problem in isolation.

Comments from kids about this poll:

Alone with weight problem

➜ i have never been comfortable talking to anyone about my weight problem

➜ I'm too embarassed to tell anyone especially my parents.

➜ Yeah, Ive always been pretty secret about it.

➜ too fat to talk

➜ I always try to hide it

➜ i am embarressed to talk to anyone about my extreme fattness

➜ it sucks im the only fat one in my family :(

Talked to parent or friend

➜ It always feels better when you talk with a friend

➜ When I waas over weight my mom really helped me to feel special, and beautiful even if I was overweight and my friends helped too, they said I had a really pretty face :)

→ only with friends, we joke about it...

→ but they're no help

→ I have talked to my friend jon about my weight back in gr.7 when i was 230 pounds, and he understands because he is kinda chubby too.

→ I speak with my closest friend about weight problems.

→ Yes, But it's hard !!

→ i wouyld never dream of telling my parents, my friends r always there for me though

→ I talk to My MOM she trys to help but it never worked because my brother makes fun of me for being over weight.

→ ya I have talk about it to my mom and i was happy because she helped me the process also by making sure i exercise every day

Talked to counselor or doctor

→ I've talked with a doctor when it became ridiculous. That was when I was up to 200lbs and don't be embarrassed if he tells you to take off yer shirt or anything, because he's a doctor. He also suggested some good diet plans which have helped me lose 21lbs.

Even though it's embarrassing, parents and health professionals must ask overweight kids about their weight. Simple non-judgmental questions are, "How do you feel about your weight?" and "How does your weight affect your life?" That gets the discussion going without laying blame. The discussion might include asking the child what they would like to do about his/her weight or offering suggestions on what you can do as a "team."

Secrecy & shame as barriers

Secrecy and shame are significant barriers to attaining a healthy weight for overweight kids. First, overweight kids are ashamed and embarrassed to ask for help, for fear of criticism and ridicule. Second, their loneliness and isolation may contribute to lower self-esteem and depression, which often results in comfort eating (Chapter 9), stress eating (Chapter 10), and vicious cycles (Chapter 13).

In addition, parents may be embarrassed to discuss overweight with their kids. Parents don't want to insult their kids by bringing up the weight issue, as the below posts from parents relate:

From Patrica, Child's Age 14 - 6/22/04
..My daughter is always complaining about how fat she is. I know she is overweight but I'm not exactly sure how much. **i don't want to embarrasse her and just say get on the scale or say how much do you weight to her**. How can i get her to tell me without making her feel bad!!!

From Olivia, Child's Age 8 - 6/10/04
My 8-year-old stepdaughter is 4 feet tall and 125 pounds. **Her Dad (my husband) is completely embarrased to be seen in public with her.**

From Shari, Child's Age 7,11 - 01/20/02
I have two children who are both overweight. **I also, am overweight.** My son, age 11 tips the scales at 195 lbs and my daughter, age 7, 115 lbs. I am 34 and weigh 250 pounds....I want to do something about it, but, **without creating an atmosphere where "fat is bad" and have them get a complex about it**. This is such a thin line...

Parents may be uneasy about being overweight themselves and therefore not bring up the weight issue with their child.

From Jessica - 09/15/04
how can I help my daughter understand that being overweight is not good if **I am overweight and she thinks the world of me?**

Or a parent may not be overweight but is upset by the child's or teen's weight.

From Lindy, Child's Age 14 - 1/9/05 -
My daughter has always fit in well in her school, despite her size... Last night I brought up ... how I think it's un-healthy for a 14 year old who's **5'5"** to weigh **214** pounds. **She started crying because she thought I only wanted her to lose weight because I was embaressed of her. She didn't want to listen to me and I am to scared to bring it up again...**

The child or teen may then conclude that the parent doesn't love him/her and may thus feel isolated. Even if the parent doesn't bring up the weight issue, if the child senses that the parent is upset by the child's weight, the child may feel isolated. As a result, the child may seek comfort in food, in other words a 'vicious cycle' (see Chapter 13).

Sometimes kids say they want a "little push", as the below post describes:

From Rachel - 01/26/04

... For my entire life I have been a heavy child, I weighed 155 pounds when I was 12. ...Mostly from sneeking the food my mother told me I couldn't have. I would cry myself to sleep at nights, thinking my mom loved my brothers more because they could have desert after supper. ...I am now 129 pounds and 5' 6". .My advice is to stand behind your kids, celebrate every little step, and never give up on them. ...**Believe in your kid, they will lose when they are ready, just give them a little push**.

In the next chapter kids talk more about their parents...

5 | Parents

All parents want their kids to be healthy and have a healthy weight. Nevertheless, many, if not most, parents are unsure how to deal with overweight in their children. How does a parent motivate a child or teen to be a healthy weight? How does a parent even talk to an overweight child about his/her weight? Does nagging or embarrassing the child help? Many parents fail to support their child's or teen's weight loss efforts, either knowingly or unknowingly. Some parents even sabotage their kid's efforts.

What do overweight kids say about their parents?

Nagging is counterproductive.

Reply from Melissa, Age 15 - 01/07/09
Ht. 5'4", Start: 173 lb, Current: 173 lb, Goal: 130 lb
…**My mom said to me today "Melissa...if you just lost some weight, you'd be drop-dead-gorgeous." Comments like that don't help one's self-esteem.** So **talk to your parents** about it, tell them you want to lose weight, and that **comments like that make you feel insecure**...I just finished discussing with my mom on how things like that and comments like that are hurtful. And she apologized and said she'd start buying healthy food to help me, and the family. So get your family in on it...

From Trip, Child's Age I'm 16, bro - 1/16/05
Really, parents. **Yelling, threatrning, and punishing your kids over their weight and eating habits......is just gonna push kiddo away and piss them off, too eat even MORE.**A calm and rational approach.......concern over kiddo's health,and happiness......is always best. And eventually your young one will wake up to the realization that SOMETHING about all the weight must be done, and he/she will begin to take the matter seriously...

From Katie, Age im 17 - 4/7/04
To all you parents - … from personal experience I know the child has to be ready before they start losing weight - **my mum put me on a diet aged 7, and all I made of that at**

the time is that **SHE thought I was fat and ugly**, but this year that changed and I was ready and my parents support really helped.

From Molly , Child's Age I'm 14 - 10/21/06
If your child is overweight dont force them into losing weight. my mom never really said anything to make me lose weight; ...My mom has supported me a little, she buys me the food i want, but at the same time she makes it harder by still buying junk food for the rest of the family and herself. ... so its not impossible i used to be 5'1" 174.4 lbs. and now i'm 5'1" and 122.8lbs. ... **if you really want your kids to lose weight take them to the doctor and have them talk to your child, trust me that was my breaking point.**

Shaming or embarrassing a child in front of friends or family, in an attempt to motivate them to lose weight, hurts a child's self-esteem, is counterproductive, and may result in a vicious cycle of the child seeking comfort in food, more weight gain, more shaming by parents, and so on...

Can't talk to my parents

Tragically, numerous kids say that they are unable to talk with their parents about their weight.

This is RACHEL's question:
how do i tell my parnets that i want to lose weight when their way more overweight then me?? - rachel

From Ben, Age 13 - 6/19/08
Ht. 5'7", Start: 227 lb, Current: 225 lb, Goal: 155 lb - ....one think that I'm concerned about is my diet. We don't have the most nuitricinal\healthy stuff in my house, and **I can't really talk to my parents about me losing weight very easily. I don't know why, I just 'can't' do it....**

From Katie, Age 14 - 07/04/03
Hey everybody!! I was wonderin if anyone wanted to be my **weight loss buddy!!** i really need someone to talk to about it cuz i **don't really feel comfortable talkin 2 my family and stuff** so yeah that would be great! if you post a reply with ur e-mail address i'll send u an e-mail back:) thx a lot:)

From rach, Age 13 - 02/26/07
Ht. 5'3", Wt. 134 - **how do i tell my parents i want 2 lose weight?** there overweight and they'll say "u dont need 2 lose weight but i do and bla bla bla " i dont want 2 b mean or anything but **i dont want 2 end up like them!** lostya <3

This is CARL's question:

Hi. My name is Carl. I am **11 years old** and I weigh **200-210 pounds**. I need help. **I am too embarrassed to consult my mom or dad about this**... I am going to 6th grade. I really need help please. I wanna lose weight on my own. I really want to be 90-130 pounds by the physical fitness test in october. ... Bye

Depressed and embarrassed

carl

From ben, Age 12 - 10/06/07

Ht. 5'5", Start: 220 lb, Current: 220 lb, Goal: 137 lb - Hello. I am going to try to lose some weight -- with obsticals

1. I am currently injured in my foot, and I cant run or jog.

2. I don't have many places to exercise

3. I dont want help! Personally, that is. **I dont want my parents to know that im trying to lose weight**

but I have to. I want a weightloss buddy around my weight and age

Thanks, ben

This is KATHLEENA's story:

Hi i am almost **15 i am 5ft6in** and i weigh **178 pounds**!! help me **i dont want to talk to my parents they don't understand** i don't know what to do I caonstantly feel fat there is a lot of fat on my stomach and thighs please help!

From Ben, Age 13 - 01/23/09

Ht. 5'8", Start: 234 lb, Current: 213 lb, Goal: 150 lb - ... So, me and my family have been going through some very hard times...(we're dirt poor)

And, I really want to lose weight..

But **I don't know how to talk to my parents about it.**

They're both obese and unhealthy...especially my mom.

Really, I know how to lose weight...

But I can't get motivated...

How can I tell my parents that I want to lose weight?

From sara, Age 12 - 12/22/08

Ht. 5'3", Start: 178 lb, Current: 198 lb, Goal: 130 lb - so if you noticed i gained 20 pounds... in like 4 months.. i got more strech marks... right in the front of my stomach and on my thighs.. i feel really fat.. **i added some material to some of my pants cause im too embarased to ask my mom for more**... help me.. **im so depressed and i just keep eating**

Kids even hide our website from parents, as the chat on the following page relates.

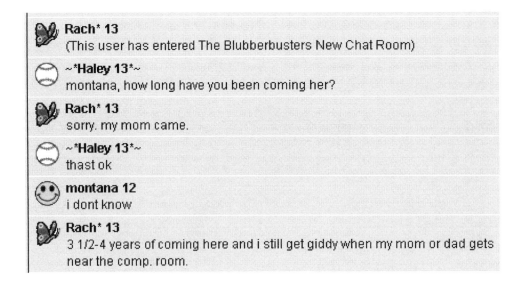

Rach* 13
(This user has entered The Blubberbusters New Chat Room)

~*Haley 13*~
montana, how long have you been coming her?

Rach* 13
sorry. my mom came.

~*Haley 13*~
thast ok

montana 12
i dont know

Rach* 13
3 1/2-4 years of coming here and i still get giddy when my mom or dad gets near the comp. room.

From ??????, Age 11 - 05/14/05
Has anyone looked at the poll for this month??? **I just now realized that I was not the only one to get on without my parents knowing**.LOL. As a question, does anyone else have to **go this this website very early in the morning, or while your parents are out?**

Why do kids hide their weight loss efforts from their parents? They may fear being ridiculed about their weight, particularly if they fail at losing weight. Or they may fear that wanting to lose weight may threaten their parents, if the parents themselves are overweight.

Lack of support or sabotage

Parents may not support their child's efforts, and they may even sabotage them, as the following posts relate.

From Lekira, Age 12 3/4 - 11/29/05
Ht. 5'5'', Wt. 180 - hi **how do I tell my mom i want to see a dietician or see a weight loss doctor?** (she weighs as much as me, by the way, so shes a bit overweight herself) shes always like "if you want to lose weight get off the darn computer and go on a bike ride!" i want more support than that. I want to lose 40-45 lbs. she wont even let me get a scale! she keeps saying "i wont let you get a scale, i am afraid you get obsessed with it!" and **when I say i want to go on a diet, she says "I don't want you to go on a diet because i am afraid you'll lose weight (ummm...duh....)** and diets are really stupid" **SHE WILL NOT LISTEN TO ME!! SHE WONT EVEN LET ME BUY BOOKS ON DIETING!!!!** Please someone tell me how to reason with this woman!!!

Age 15, female
Ht: 168 cm, 74.5 kg - If your **parents are obese**, you eat what they cook so you dont really think anything is wrong **untill you get into your teenage years and relize your not**

healthy and that you are eating and doing the wrong things and are bigger than everyone else.

This is HAILEY's question:
ill be **12 in 2 weeks** and i weigh lets say a little bit over **170**. i hav 2 little bros and **my mom gets them all these snacks that r bad 4 u and i eat them and i cant stop** can i hav som tips on how to stop!!!! please!?!?!?!?

This is a girl's question:
im fifteen and im **5'1** and i way **152lb** and i hate it **i feel like i have no support at home because my mom is smaller then i am** and i dont know how to loose weight 20 pounds would be great but i dont know how to do it..

From Michelle, Age 14 - 09/03/08
Ht. 5'6", Start: 254 lb, Current: 268 lb, Goal: 154 lb - ... I've tried about a million diets and treatments and I just can't do, I've had no help, **my parents are always too busy to support or help me in anyway and although I say I'm on a diet they still continue to cook foods that are bombarded with grease and fat** can anyone give me any tips?

From JJ, Age 14 - 2/27/05
Wt: 225 lb - **My mum constantly buys crap food.** I have said to her, look, mum we're really dangeroulsy obese stop buying this crap. and she's like "ok I'll find a diet and then we'll follow it alright?? Good" Then she forgets. I keep naging and freaking nagging to her about tai chi or kick boxing or yoga classes, and I find places and all she has to do is say but she's always going on about "it's too far away" or **"we can't afford it"** (but somehow **we can afford all this other crap like better tv's and more and more junk food)** Do any of you guys know what I should do? Thanks! P.S This site rocks...

From Karmel-Ann, Age 13 - 4/18/01 -
If you think your life sucks, I bet you all I have that mine is a lot, lot worse. I have been fat since I can remember, and **currently weigh 324 lbs.** I have a set of scales in my room but most of the time I'm too ashamed to even stand on them. I don't even have a pretty face. **Whenever my mom drags me off to the shops I usually end up in tears surrounded by gorgous slim girls.** The other day I was in a store and I saw a blue summer dress I really liked. I got the biggest size and tried it on, but when I tried to get it off the zip got stuck. The asisstant had to come and try and get it off, but she had to come and get her friend to help her because it was stuck fast. I ended up running out of the shop in tears. Its even worse at school. They've managed to think up every mean name accosiated woth being fat that there is. **My mom is overweight too and says I'm being stupid when I try to diet, and fills the house with junk food which I can't resist.** You guys mean so much to me and any suggestions you come up with will really help. Thankyou!!

From Katie, Age 13 - 1/6/06
Ht. 5'6", Wt. too much - I wanna make a new diet, but **my mom won't help me with any of it! I wanna go to the gym to work out, and she doesn't care!** Ah, I hate being overweight. Wish me luck in the future..

From Jenny, Age 16 - 3/12/08
Ht. 5'2", Start: 190 lb, Current: 223 lb, Goal: 150 lb - I've been so much into eating the last half year that I've gained 33 lbs! **I'm so disgusting fat.** i just need to eat and eat... **my family is fat, too. my mother is buying all that stuff,** and i can take it from the cupboard. there's always enough there. **when i complain that i'm getting too fat she just says "you're right how you are".** then i don't feel that fat anymore and i just eat some chocolate. what can i do?

From rachelle, Age 16 - 7/26/06
Ht. 5'6, Wt. 235 - ... my parents by healthy food, but **they will not stocking up on the ice cream, potato chips, etc.** because **"they want to eat too."** but **having those foods in the house make it IMPOSSIBLE for me to eat healthy.** i have had countless talks with them asking them not to. so does anyone have any suggestions on how to not eat them?

From rach, Child's Age im 14 - 4/6/08
i am 5'4. and about 145 lbs. **both of my parents are overweight.(almost obese)** and we have chips and stuff in the house that my dad likes to eat.. all of. ..my mom usually cooks like fattier foods that i dont need.. i do have to get food somewhere. ya know? they're not very active. my mom is busy a lot and my dad has an office job..... my question is this. **why can't they start living healthier.. for me?** dont get me wrong i know they love me and everything, but it just makes it harder for me trying to live a healthier life style. **i really don't want to end up like they did,** i know that sounds bad..but yea. neither of my parents were overweight before o yea my mom eats not to bad, but too much. and whe n i try to cook she usually doesn't let me because she likes cooking. plleasee help mee

From Katraena, Age 9, female - 6/17/06
Ht: 4'11" Wt: 130lbs - ... I was eatting about 6 hot pockets a day or 4 corn dogs a day becuase **my mom was never home that much to cook...**

Enabling

Parents may directly enable the child's overeating habit. A parent revealed this in the parents chat room.

Sarah
sometimes when me and my daughter sit down with just piles of junk food and 4 hours later i look around and the amout of food and calories we have eaten amazes me.

Sarah
its like a drug for her and i, but she really is quite normal beside it all.

Children comment on how parents and grandparents enable them.

From Rina, Age 16, female - 8/10/06 -
Hey Everyone, I just thought i'd share with you some of my experience about being overweight. I was overweight from the time I was 3 or 4 til 14. **My mom used to enable me by making fattening foods such as cookies, chinese and any kind of dessert.** Overtime it stuck to me, literally, **I ended up weighing 313 pounds when I was 14...**

From Amanda, Age 15 - 2/2/06
Ht. 5'4'', Wt. too depressing :'(-... i live with my mom, brother and grandparents.. and my grandparents love junk food, not to mention theyre the ones going shopping.. so basically i have to choose to pic the sad carrot over the box of donuts or bag of chips.. plus the soda.. i love soda, and i drink like so much.. but thats all **my parents buy.. and they wont give up their junk food habits for me.. so basically i wonder if i should just give up and eat myself into the grave.. its like putting a drug addict in a drug house and telling them to stop the drug abuse!**

From JJ, Age 13 - 11/15/04
Wt: 225 lb - My mum is such a b*tch!!!! **I asked her "can you please stop buying junk food,** I really think it would make us healthier and we might lose a little weight" you know what she said?? "No, I need it" **I said she sounded like a drug addict and she agreed!!!!** (she is majorly obese[as am I])I told her "please stop buying the junk food, I have no will power and you always offer it too me. We aren't healthy and I think this would be a good idea" **she goes "if you want to lose weight we should find a plan and stick to it, I'll find one, until then I'll eat my chocolate bars"** that was two months ago!!!What can I do to stop myself from eating the candy and junkfood she CONSTANTLY buys??

From Shekina, Age 17 - 10/5/05
Ht. 5'3", Wt. Start:218 Now:207.5 - **I have a hard time staying away from fast food and resturants because my mom gets us food from out to eat all the time. I am homeschooled,** so it makes it easier for her to go out and get something ratherthan just fixing something from around the house. And we always go out to eat on friday nights and Sunday lunch. I probably get to go out to eat 4-5 times a week. And my mom NEVER wants to go anywhere like subway, or any place where I can get fesh/healthy food. So **how do I tell my parents not to go out so much,** and all that stuff??? I know that's one of the reasons I gained 20 pounds last year.

From Olivia, Age 14 - 2/23/08 -
Ht. 5'2", Start: 360 lb, Current: 360 lb, Goal: 200 lb - ...My mom and dad are both really obese. Their too obese to work and so all they do is eat and watch the TV. I'm home schooled and **my parents let me eat whatever I want**. We only have junk food in our house I eat A LOT of it. But now I know how much I actually weigh I realise that **I dont want to end up like them** and so I wanna try lose some of the weight. ...and I love to eat. **How can i lose weight when all my parents will buy is junk food!?** I love eating so how do i stop eating so much?

From Hali, Age 15 - 02/01/09
Ht. 5'4", Start: 181 lb, Current: 174 lb, Goal: 166 lb - Okay, I have seriously done terriblely. I need a good kick in the butt. But **my father likes to stock the house with alot of unhealthy things and of course I eat them**. Oh well, I guess i have to start over....again, this is seriously getting me down.

A reply defends enabling parents.

> **Reply from Melissa, Age 15 - 02/01/09**
> ... people **don't blame your parents** for your weight problem. **They may buy the food, but that doesn't mean you have to eat it.**

But are kids able to control their eating if exposed to tempting foods?

Relationship with parents

We've conducted several polls asking kids about their relationship with their parents. (http://www.blubberbuster.com/cgi/poll_new_74.cgi)

Have you asked either of your parents for help with your weight?

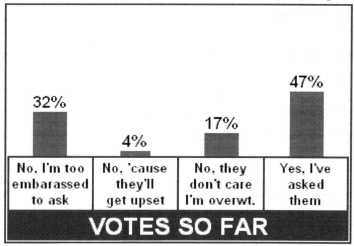

93 kids voted

Is either of your parents overweight?

YES: 59 votes (63%)

NO: 34 votes (37%)

Slightly less than half of 93 kids responding have asked for help with their weight from a parent. About a third say they're too embarrassed to ask and about a fifth indicate that their parents don't care. A small percentage feels that their parents would become upset, so they haven't asked. Most have at least one overweight parent.

These results compare to the poll presented on pp. 53, where nearly three fourths of kids responding indicate they keep our website a secret from parents or friends. In another poll, less than a fifth of the kids keep only our website a secret; most keep both weight loss and our website a secret (http://www.blubberbuster.com/cgi/poll_new_49.cgi). Thus, the vast majority of these overweight kids appear to have difficulty asking for help from their parents.

Comments from kids about poll #74 above:

Age 15, female, 5'5, 263 lbs - **they dont real feel that im serious or really dedicated.** - One or both of my parents is overweight.

Parents Support Weight Loss Efforts:

Age 13, female, 5'5", 140 lbs - Neither of my parents are overweight. They are both athletes. My mom is a dancer and she used to run **a dance school** and I was the best one in the class. **Since it shut down, i never picked it back up again. Thats when i gained the** weight. **They support me and wish that I could start dancing again.** - Neither of my parents is overweight.

Age 9, female, 4'4'', 73 lbs - My mom always helps me with stuff like this like **encouraging me to eat better and cut down on the food.** - Neither of my parents is overweight.

Age 45&42, male, 6 1&5 4, alot lbs - they tried to put me on a diet but **it didnt work** - One or both of my parents is overweight.

Age 17, female, 5'4, 171 lbs - My mom signed me up for **weight watchers!** - One or both of my parents is overweight.

Age 13, female, 5.6, 210 lbs - **they care alot but i can never lose the wight.** - One or both of my parents is overweight.

Age 18, female, 5'8, 197 lbs - I told my mom I wanted to try losing weight, and **she supported me and asked me what kinds of foods she should buy at the grocery store. Whenever i lose a single pound she's always proud of me.** - Neither of my parents is overweight.

Age 14, female, 5'7, 215 lbs - **MY MOM HELPED ME AND SHE LOST WEIGHT TOO** - One or both of my parents is overweight.

Age 16, female, 5'7", 278 lbs - **They have tried to help me but nothing has been very long-lasting or helpful because they are also overweight and are often unable to overcome their own weight/eating problems to help me with mine.** - One or both of my parents is overweight.

Age 14, female, 5"2, 130 lbs - They have bought healthier foods, **but havn't really gotten into it.** - One or both of my parents is overweight.

Age 14, female, 5'2, 150 lbs - i asked my mom, **she said that she would do anything to help me, except buy me diet pills. and my dad laughed at me.** - Neither of my parents is overweight.

Age 19, female, 5'6", 155 lbs - **they want to lose weight too.** - One or both of my parents is overweight.

Age 13, female, 5 3'', 130 lbs - i asked my mom and **ive tried to loose weight but she was the one doing it she lost about 80 lbs.** - Neither of my parents is overweight.

Could it be that when parents do support their child's efforts to lose weight (and often wish to lose weight themselves), they nevertheless often lack the knowledge of how to go about it or lack motivation themselves. Who should be helping these parents?

Parents Don't Support Weight Loss Efforts:

Age 14, female, 5ft.4in., 135 lbs - thye said only i could change that. **they wont help me!!!** - One or both of my parents is overweight.

Age 9, male, 5'1, 205 lbs - **I live with my dad, he is really fat. He thinks i am OK** - One or both of my parents is overweight.

Age 14, female, 5'3", 135 lbs - **They say I don't have a weight problem and I don't need to diet.** - One or both of my parents is overweight.

Age 14, female, 5'2, 169 lbs - **but their really don't want to help me** - One or both of my parents is overweight.

Age 12, female, 5' 5", 172 lbs - **My mom makes fun of my weight** - One or both of my parents is overweight.

Age 13, female, 5'5", 301 lbs - **I've asked them to buy healthier foods and cook better.** - One or both of my parents is overweight.

Age 13, female, 5'5", 278 lbs - **They respect me for being overweight.** - One or both of my parents is overweight.

Don't Ask Parents for Support in Weight Loss Efforts:

Age 16, female, 5'3", 249.6 lbs - **i just get too frustrated when they try to help. i like doing everything on my own, unfortunatly.** - One or both of my parents is overweight.

Some parents actually seem to block or sabotage their child's efforts to lose weight. Why would parents do this? Perhaps these parents struggle with their weight themselves and have no motivation to tackle their own issues, let alone their child's. Or perhaps they are threatened by the possibility that they may have to give up having certain foods in the house, 'junk food' for example, which they use to cope?

Hence, parents may support, ignore, or even obstruct their kids' weight loss efforts. We asked kids further about this. (http://www.blubberbuster.com/cgi/poll_new_13_percent.cgi)

How do your parents treat you in regard to your weight?

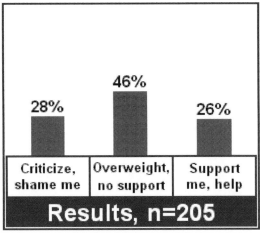

205 kids voted

Of 205 kids responding, only about a fourth indicate that they receive support from their parents in regard to their weight problem, a fourth of their parents are critical or shaming, and nearly half of their parents offer no support and are overweight themselves.

Comments from kids responding to this poll:

Positive:

➜ My parent are really supportive and **do what ever I ask of them when it comes to loseing weight.**

➜ **my mom is the best and she helps me!**

➜ **my mom is more supportive now that i'm actually trying instead of just saying i want to lose weight!**

Somewhat Positive:

➜ **my mom supports me but my dad doesnt because he is heavier than i am**

➜ **they do not support me but they do not teese me,** somethimes i ask my mother if i'm fat and she says, work out, and do lots of exersise,and do diet, but she never answers my question

➜ **My grandparents and my Dad are the ones who tease me but my Mom doesn't**

➜ I wish my folks would be more healthy, i try to get them to exercise with me, but they don't. I think its because they're overweight too.

Negative:

➜ Always poking my belly and stare when I eat.

➜ They call me mean names like fat and fat b!tch but my mom is also overweight

➜ My mom always tells me that i am fat and i need to loose weight. If i eat somehting not on my diet she goes well now u blew your diet and you will never loose weight

➜ My dad just can't stop buying junkfood! Well he was raised that way, so that is what he bring home to us. We never really sit down as a family to eat, and most of the time we are eating fast food, or trying to finmd something to eat around the house. I finally put my foot down tho, and I found soemgood thing to eat arounf=d the house, and I'm making my mom go grocery shopping and I keep telling her that if she doesn't go shopping I will cuz I have the money to do it and I WILL do it! **My mom and dad don't like me to have to pay for things like that, like clothes and food, stuff I need, so when I say I'm going to do it myself that ususally gets them to do something. Anyway, almost all my family is overweight…**

➜ my dad and my brother are mean to me and sometimes my mom and dad call me a Fat Little Bitch i don't like it.

➜ My dad calls be "Marshmellow" and I know he's just joking around, but sometimes it hurts.

➜ They criticize me.

➜ my grandparents and father make fun of me they tell me everyday your too fat

➜ All they do is blap about how overweight I am, like I've never heard it anymore and if they havent notice....IT ISNT HELPING MUCH !!! What they need to do it physically help me and start something instead of telling me how much I weigh as if I didnt know.

➜ My mom always teases me so much about my stomache

Negative comments from parents, with little or no encouragement, is a tough obstacle for kids struggling to attain a healthy weight. Kids need support from parents, and they need help forming a plan.

If kids sense that their parents do not support them, they may not tell their parents about their weight loss efforts, particularly if the parents themselves are overweight. (http://www.blubberbuster.com/cgi/poll_new_35.cgi)

If your parents are overweight, how do they act if you try to lose weight?

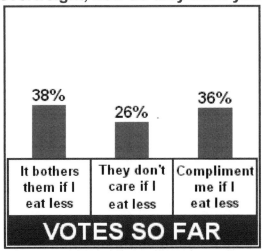

125 kids voted

Slightly more than a third of 125 kids responding say that it bothers their parents if the child eats less. Slightly more than a third of the kids indicate that their parents compliment them if they eat less. And about a fourth of the kids indicate that their parents don't care if they eat less.

Comments from kids about this poll:

Compliment Child About Eating Less

➔ my parents are overwieght also and they are so proud of my that i try to loose weight!

➔ my mom and i are both in the middle of our weight loss. we are on different routines but we still keep each other's motivations up!

➔ they tell me that I'm doing a good job, adn that i'd be looking great soon"!

Negative to Child About Eating Less

➔ I think parents just get jelous if their child starts to lose weight because they think their kids will look better than them.

➔ My mom seems to think I starve myself which I don't. In fact, the reason that I'm overweight is because I overeat. It makes me angry when she accuses me of not eating.

Neutral/Don't Care if Child Eats Less

➔ my mum dont care.. she trys to help me even tho she lives all the way in virgina.. and i live in another state.... my dad, i dont tell him cause hes a jerk about that stuff.

➔ my mom is alot skinnyer then me, and i hate it, me and my mom are close, but when she looks at me, she allways has sorta a pitty look, and sadness feeling in her eyes, i want to lose weight for mostly her, i weigh 253, and she weighs 175.

Overweight parents may be threatened by kids who try to lose weight. Or they may try to help the child avoid the same lifelong problem, which the parents have struggled with. If the parent is overweight, the parent and the child might work together to lose weight.

Comments from parents greatly affect the emotional state of the child. Positive comments, such as "they are so proud of my that i try to loose weight! " *make a major difference in the child's or teen's weight loss efforts and self-esteem.*

Parents as role models

Kids very much want their parents to be role models of a healthy lifestyle, as confirmed by the results of a poll. (http://www.blubberbuster.com/cgi/poll_new_63_percent.cgi)

What do you think would reverse the growing overweight problem in children and teens?

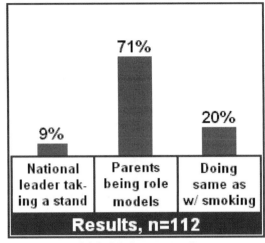

112 kids voted

Overwhelmingly the 112 kids responding feel that parents being role models would have the greatest impact on reversing the growing overweight problem in kids, versus a national leader speaking out on the childhood overweight problem, or attacking the overweight problem in the same way as the smoking problem was addressed. Most worry about overweight shortening their lives (results below):

Do you worry about overweight shortening your life?

YES: 72 votes (64%)

NO: 40 votes (36%)

Comments from kids about this poll:

Age 16, female, 5'7", 289 lbs - The majority of overweight kids have overweight parents as well. I believe overeating is a learned behavior. If we see our parents doing it when we are young, we are likely to follow in their footsteps.

Age 12, female, 5' 1'', 108 lbs - I feel that parents often think that their kids are not overweight and do not see the problem that is probably growing.

Age 12, female, 5'1, 132 lbs - I think being overweight can be partly be your fault and your parents. Parents:they are sometimes responsible for packing your lunches,buying the food in your house. Also,their habits can rub off on you. Yourself: It's your choice to eat right or not.

Age 17, female, 5'3, 130 lbs - **Parents have everything to do with the overweight/obesity problem in America. They are enabling their kids to eat junk food non-stop. Even if they don't force it on their kids, they should at least set a good example for the kids. If parents are overweight, what message is that sending to their kids?** I'm not saying everyone soould be stick thin, but at least at a weight that's not life-threatening. My mom went completely organic, vegetarian, and everything else, and I followed since that was really the only thing in the house. Yeah, occasionally I do splurge and go buy something like a candy bar or some chicken or something. But once a month is better than all day everyday, right?

Age 17, female, 5'4, ??? lbs - **If kids and their families would just join a family activity where they all could get active kids would be eager to join and do more and healthy eating habits should be tought from the beginning if you let you kids start out eating horribly then thats all they know and it becomes harder to put the proper eating habits into their heads.**

Age 16, female, 5'4, 130 lbs - **parents have alot to do with children being overweight. My mom... making fattening foods such as cookies, chinese and any kind of dessert.. I ended up weighing 313 when I was 14...**

Age 13, female, 5ft. 4", 169.8 lbs - **Authority figures have already tried lecturing kids. FOr the most part, it doesn`t work. People who care about you should try to be good role models!**

Age 19, male, 6'2, 294 lbs - **look on the t.v show called " Hunny we killing our kids"**

Although many parents suffer from the same weight issues as their kids, the kids say that a parental role model is inspirational. How can parents be positive role models?

Actively talking about healthy eating as a family, researching and learning about healthy foods, planning menus together, shopping together, cooking together, eating family meals together at home, and doing activities together are ways for parents to be role models for their kids. In order to help their kids, parents must look at the reasons they overeat themselves. Fast food and junk food are very tempting, and parents as well as kids can get hooked on comfort eating and stress eating (see Chapters 9 & 10). Learning how to cope with life, without seeking comfort in food, is a skill which kids learn from their parents.

Foster care?

What about parental responsibility and even foster care for severely overweight kids? There was a recent case of a 200 pound eight year old in the UK, which has been much debated by childhood overweight and child abuse professionals. There have been similar cases in the

U.S. We asked kids what they thought about this.
(http://www.blubberbuster.com/cgi/poll_new_71.cgi)

Should extremely overweight kids be taken away from their parents?

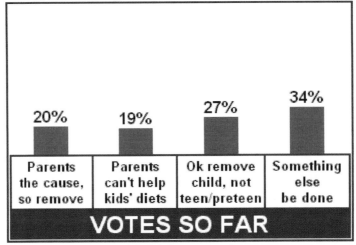

83 kids voted

Were your parents part of the cause of your becoming overweight?

YES: 37 votes (45%)

NO: 45 votes (55%)

Even though many of the kids feel that their parents are at least partially responsible for their becoming overweight, few feel that severely overweight kids should be taken away from parents and placed in foster care.

Many kids commented passionately about this poll:

Age 16, female, 5'8, 178 lbs - take the kid away for a while until it looses weiht and gets healthy, **but if the parents makes them feel bad by calling them fat and huting their feelings then the kid is gonna get depress and eat more, so in that case you should take the kid aay and help raie its high esteem and have a very happy life,** with some other parents that love im and that eat healthy, and the kid is gonna be happy, and not be depressed and be eating all of the time, so parents sometimes(not all the time) have to do a lot with the kids weight, but some parents just give their children whatever they want... - My parents were not part of the cause of my becoming overweight.

Age 11, female, 5ft.4in., 135 lbs - **Wow! That is really terrible. The parents are totally responsible because they control the portions, not him.** - My parents were part of the cause of my becoming overweight.

Age 9, male, 5' 1, 200 lbs - **maybe help them in their house, cook good food with the parents. I want to live with my dad-he is fat too** - My parents were part of the cause of my becoming overweight.

Age 10, female, 5ft 6.5in, 137 lbs - **parents are the ones who buy the food. the kids just eat it because all there is is unhealty foods in the refrigorator. they cant just not eat.** - My parents were part of the cause of my becoming overweight.

Age 16, female, 5`10, 200 lbs - I think that they shouldnt necesserly be taken away from their homes, **but if thats impacting the health of a young person, then extreme measures should be taken.** The parents dont realize that they are taking valuable years off their childs life. - My parents were not part of the cause of my becoming overweight.

Age 13, female, 5'6, 200 lbs - i think that connor should stay in his house **there should be something done like makine him exersise and eat better** also in most cities there should be gyms built just for kids - My parents were part of the cause of my becoming overweight.

Age 16, female, 5', 153 lbs - THe parents are responsible for how their children grow up. allowing them to stay inside or letting opportunities come up like sports and clubs. **They are responsible but care for the child in nother home could make things worse and will not help at all.** the whole family should be doing things to promote good helth not just the kid. - My parents were part of the cause of my becoming overweight.

Age 13, female, 5'3, 150 lbs - i think instead of taking him from his parents permentaly, they should send him to a camp to help overweight kids, and then give the parnets another chance. - My parents were not part of the cause of my becoming overweight.

Age 11, female, 5 2, 140 lbs - thats not fair at all! **the parents should start out by going on walks, not eating some junk foods** and hopefully get healthier - My parents were part of the cause of my becoming overweight.

Age 13, female, 5'2", 145 lbs - **The kid AND the parents were both responsible.** It's bad that he's that overweight that young but taking him away is very extreme. **The kid and parents should have gotten outside help for the kid's weight problem and the parent's parenting skills.** - My parents were part of the cause of my becoming overweight.

Age 15, female, 5"9, 280 lbs - I do believe its the parents fault,but I don't believe foster care is the answer, **they should assign him a dietian and work out plan. They should make it mandatory** for the parents to take him to the meeting and should help him along the way and change his eating habits. - My parents were part of the cause of my becoming overweight.

Age 16, male, 5'11", 235 lbs - **i think that they should try to help the parents and child in their controled living areas.** - My parents were not part of the cause of my becoming overweight.

Age 14, female, 5'4'', 141 lbs - i think that **it all depends on the age of the kid. if they are a preteen or a teen, then the parents don't have very much say over what they eat or don't eat.** but, like in this story, the parents choose what the kid eats for every meal except for snack which the parents let them either eat or not. So **i think that the boy in the story should either go to diet classes and learn how to eat healthy or if they aren't willing to do that the boy should be taken into foster care.** - My parents were not part of the cause of my becoming overweight.

Age 14, female, 5ft. 5 1/2 in., S: 184 N:162 G:145-150 lbs - Putting overweight kids into foster care is the LAST RESORT!!! Although **I think that some people who neglect their kids let them spin out of control and that's when things become ridiculous and dangerous.** An 8-year-old kid should not weigh almost 200lbs! **Parents are supposed to at least try to set a healthy example.** - My parents were not part of the cause of my becoming overweight.

Age 18, male, 6'5, 320 lbs - **It's not fair to remove the child, but some kind of intervention should be implemented.** - My parents were part of the cause of my becoming overweight.

Age 15, male, 6'0, 282 lbs - I think that it's really unfair. I mean, what's so wrong with the kid being fat? **Most people in the united states are overweight. Is the government just gonna force them into diets or weight-loss camps?** I say that they let the kid eat what he wants. - My parents were not part of the cause of my becoming overweight.

Age 17, female, 5'2, 125 lbs - **it is only fair if they can prove that the parents are the cause that the child eats so much...**say if they keep pushing the food at the child or threning them if they don't eat everything.. - My parents were not part of the cause of my becoming overweight.

Age 13, female, 13, 134 lbs - the kid should getr a dietitian and a trainer. not a foster home! this isnt an issue of abuse! **there are a lot of other children in worst situations in** need of foster care. this kid needs 2 go 2 a camp or something! - My parents were part of the cause of my becoming overweight.

If parents were giving cocaine to their child, we'd certainly have a problem with that. But few people seem to find fault with giving a child excessive food to the point of obesity, which can be nearly as damaging to the child's health. Parents may significantly contribute to a child's weight problem, but similar to what kids say above, foster care for such is highly controversial.

How do we teach parents to be positive role models for kids? Giving tips to parents on how to approach the issue of overweight in their children is often a missed opportunity for health professionals.

Two households

Living in two households many times contributes to the overeating of the child or teen. Parental divorce itself is a common cause of comfort eating (see Chapter 9).

Parents have posted the following regarding their children and two households:

From Mark, Child's Age 14 - 11/6/04 -
I am **divorced** and I live in California. My daughter and ex-wife live in New York. **My ex-wife feeds her like no tommarow and ignores the fact that she is totally unhealthy.** From June till August she was staying with me. When I first picked her up in June, I could not believe my eyes! She had gained so much weight since I last saw her (which was a little less than a year ago). Her stomch was buldging over her jeans and her arms had stretch marks on them. Of course, I didn't say anything, but it hurt me so much to see her so unhealthy. When I needed to send her to a local day camp and they needed her medical form I called my ex-wife to send it up. She was only **5'5" and weighed 243 pounds.** Those numbers jumped out at me, I would never guessed she weighed over 200 pounds, more than me! She gained 39 pounds in one year. Later that week when my (new) wife took her to get jeans at gap, she had trouble finding some, because the biggest size they had (16) did not fit her and they eventually had to go to a Lane Bryant. **Is there any way I can help this issue thousands miles away?** I've discussed this with my ex-wife, but she weighs proably over 400 pounds so 240 doesn't seem like much. **She also got really offended when I told her that Jenny looked un-healthy.** Thanks in advanced! –Mark

> Reply from *Ray*Ray*, Age 13 - 11/11/04
> Gap goes up to size 20. Try Old Navy for jeans and stuff too. As for the healthy eating, **just try to talk to your ex-wife, unfortunatly there's not much you can do since you're so far away.** *Ray*Ray*

From Teresa, Child's Age 16 - 5/16/04 -

My **16 year old step son is extremely over weight**. I would say **at least 75lbs**. I brought up his food choices today and asked him how he felt about how he looked. He says **he does not care**. I really think that that is a farce. He has no self-confidence, walks slouched over looking at the ground. Does not face people when he is in front of them.**He lives with me and his father. Every time he goes to his mother's for a week or more he put on more weight.** He has gone through two pant sizes this school year.**At home we have healthy food and buy diet drinks** but he has a problem with his portion sizes and on his own he chooses sugared colas. **At his mom's he basicly eats all he wants and sits in front of the tv all the time.**His mother also has a weight problem. They make fat jokes about their problem. I commented that I did not think it was all that funny to do that and he replied that they do so because they "accept their bodies"When I talked to him today I tried to talk to him **about health problems, he won't listen** because right now he doesn't have diabeties, or heart disease or the like.What do we do????

Reply from Dan's mom, Child's Age 13 - 5/20/04

My son never had a weight problem until the divorce. **Going from house to house makes it tougher, and I know they don't eat well at his dad's. I've tried to get the other parents to cooperate, but they just get insulted, so I gave that up.** ..My son was open to losing, because he gets picked on. I was quite surprised how little he knew about nutrition and healthy choices. (How did I think he would get it? Osmosis?)... **You can't do it for him, but don't believe for a second he is happy with his weight. Try not to dwell on it with him. Talking about it too much just makes him feel worse about it. He may even eat more just to get back at you. Teenagers are like that.** For now, just get the junk out of your house, and wait for an opening when it appears he might be willing to listen. If he tried it for just a week, the loss would keep him motivated.

From Tara, Child's Age 4 - 2/5/03

My son is **4 and 1/2 years old, he's 3'11" and weighs about 76 pounds**. It hurts so much when he comes home from prescool/day care and tells me that the kids make fun of him because of his weight. He lives with his dad, and each time I see him he gets bigger. He goes through clothes like people go through tissues... At this rate, he'll be wearing men's clothes in no time. He loves food and his **father is forever giving him fried chicken and pizza** and he doesn't make our son drink water. It's always juice, punch or whole milk, even though I've told him to give him water or at least skim milk and cut out the junk-food. But **his father lets him eat whatever he wants**. If my son sees someone eating something, he wants it...even if he just finished a meal...

What can a parent do to prevent overeating when their child is in the second household?

Reply from Katie, Age 13 - 2/17/03

...**do some research on what can happen to your child because he is overweight, Show them to your ex-husband, and ask him if he really wants to hurt his child.** Your son doesn't know any better, he thinks "hmmm yummy food.... i want some". Your need to **have a serious talk with your exhusband .... make him understand that he needs to be a rolemodel in his sons eatting habits.** Remember young children are just like the saying 'Monkey see, Monkey do'.

Parents as barriers to weight loss

Even without actively enabling a child's weight problem, parents may be barriers to a child's or teen's weight loss because: 1) the parents themselves are overweight and are unsure or unwilling to deal with their own weight issues, or 2) the parents are not overweight but are upset by the child's or teen's weight, which may result in one or both parents being nagging and less loving. This may cause the child or teen to seek comfort in food, in other words a "vicious cycle" (see Chapter 13).

Parents of overweight kids need to: 1) look at their own weight issues and what effect this is having on their child's health and self-esteem, and 2) look at how they are reacting to overweight in their child and whether their disapproval is contributing to the problem. Again, what an opportunity this is for health professionals to dialogue with parents!

Parents may not know how to talk to their kids about weight. But parents may do everything possible and still end up with a frustratingly overweight child, as the mother below relates:

From juliet, Child's Age 12 - 11/18/03

today my daughter weighed herself and she has put on another 8 pounds in a month something i didnt think was possible while she is eating healthy well at home anyway and i make her lunch for school.**i am fed up with everyone blaiming parents when i really do try my best. i have another appointment with the doctor on thursday but can anyone tell me what a doctor can offer apart from a dietician who the doctor even admitted cant tell me anything i dont already know** my daughter needs help but i dont know what else to do. she told me yesterday that she feels so heavy and ill all the time its breaks my heart.someone please give me advice

In the next chapter, kids talk about their health professionals.

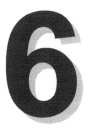

Health Professionals

Why talk about health professionals? Health professionals have the unique opportunity to discuss with children, adolescents, and parents the importance of a healthy weight, with open communication about feelings, such as stress, depression, and boredom, and associated overeating. There is the importance of guiding and supporting kids in their struggle to lose weight, and the fact that if we health professionals don't speak up, children may obtain incorrect information from inappropriate sources. Physicians may feel uncomfortable discussing overweight issues for various reasons, such as embarrassment or not having the knowledge to deal with the problem. They may pass such discussions off to dietitians, nutritionists, personal trainers, etc., although such additional professionals also may not have the needed knowledge.

What do overweight kids say about their health professionals?

What do overweight kids say about their doctors?

Many overweight kids say that they are embarrassed to talk to their doctors.

From Scared, Age 15 - 7/8/08
Ht. 5'2", Start: ? lb, Current: 195 lb, Goal: ? lb - guys I'm really scared for the past two years I face been gaining a ton of weight and trying to get it off mymomis very mean about it and I have a physical tomorrow and of course she has to be there I dont want to weigh myself and **I am embarresed to go to the doctor** HELP??

> Reply from Beth, Age 15 - 03/31/04
> **No, no, no. He does not need a doctor. He can get on just fine without spending a fortune on a doctor who's only going to tell him to get out more and start eating right. Any of us can tell him that...**

This is DANNIELLE's question:
hi i am fat and i dont like it, **i dont want to go to the doctors** and i need to know how to lose 1 pound a day, please email me why ,

From annonnomous, Age 13 - 03/30/08
Ht. 5'1", Start: 190 lb, Current: 191 lb, Goal: 130 lb - Hey guys... **Do you ever feel embarassed when you talk to your doctor?** (Four replies are below)

> Reply from Jeimi, Age 17 - 03/31/08
> yea sometimes i feel like all their going to say is lose weight and when i go and i've gained weight **i feel so ashamed** but watever that's wat wahy they're there to help us so i guess there's no reason

> Reply from Erica, Age 15 - 03/30/08
> yes...**it will go away** when you not as self contious about yourself.

> Reply from becky, Age 13 - 03/30/08
> i don't like it when my doctor show me that chart...and says normal ppl are here...and you are here. and i am way above the line

> Reply from Jessica, Age 13 - 03/30/08
> **I do...**

It seems that many overweight kids fear disapproval or criticism from their doctors.

Do kids ask their healthcare providers for weight loss help?

We did a poll on this (http://www.blubberbuster.com/cgi/poll_new_2_percent.cgi):

Have you asked for help on your weight from a doctor or dietitian?

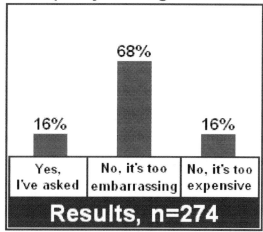

271 kids voted

A large number of kids responded to this important poll. Even though kids say they want help with their weight, it appears that most are too embarrassed to ask a healthcare provider for help. Are healthcare providers likewise embarrassed to bring up the subject with overweight kids or their parents, because: 1) the provider fears insulting the patient/parent, 2) the provider is unsure how to treat overweight, or 3) the provider him/herself is overweight? If so, this type of open dialogue is a missed opportunity for healthcare providers.

Below is a post on this subject:

From Callie, Age 14 - 01/02/09
Ht. 5'4", Start: 263 lb, Current: 263 lb, Goal: 120 lb - ... I admit, I need help. **I dont feel comfortable to talk to my family about my problem, not even my own doctor**. In the begining of the new school year, I played Volleyball for my hs team, and i was losing alot of weight. but it all seemed to come back. i was totally,depressed. I thought i sticked ou of my team like a big pimple! all the girls so skinny..except for a couple,and i was one of them! :[...

A child or teen may want to lose weight, but who is there to turn to if they can't talk to their family or their healthcare provider?

The below post offers information on what parents of overweight kids feel about their healthcare providers.

From juliet, Child's Age 12 - 11/18/03
today my daughter weighed herself and she has put on another 8 pounds in a month .. i **have another appointment with the doctor on thursday but can anyone tell me what a doctor can offer apart from a dietician who the doctor even admitted cant tell me anything i dont already know** my daughter needs help but i dont know what else to do. she

told me yesterday that she feels so heavy and ill all the time its breaks my heart.someone please give me advice

What else do overweight kids say about their doctors?

Positive Comments From Physicians Definitely Help

From renee, Age 13, female - 1/31/02

hi guys, i have **lost 18 pounds** in 3 months, i still have a long way to go. i weighed **207 now i am 189**.... what makes me so angry is that **when my mom first took me to her doctor, he said " oh, she's just a big tall girl" and acted like it was no big deal. later my mom found a pediatrician and she basically said the same thing.** but i had to go back for a booster shoot and saw a different pediatrician and she agreed that i weighed way too much. at first i was angry that my mom keep bringing up my weight to every doc i saw, but now i'm glad she didn't give up. **this doc is great** she sees me once a month to weigh me and **she is like my biggest cheerleader.** last time **i lost 9 ponds in one month and she hugged me!!!! she always asks about how i feel about the weight loss and she really cares,** sometimes i feel like if i gainred any weight i would disappoint her. but she only wants me to lose 4 pounds a month. because if you lose it too fast it is easier to gain it back. and any more than that is not healthy. i've already lost 6 pounds since i saw her and i can't wait to weighed in now. so if you follow what my doc says, no soda, no junk fod, eat fruit when you crave sweets, walk (which i dont do) and portion control, one plate of food at meals, take what you can fit on that plate and no more! but i think the biggest thing is support from people who care about you!

From Shannon, Age 12 - 12/27/06

Ht. 5'1", Wt. 146 - today I went to the **doctor's for a physical.** ... She told I was 5th percintile in height, and 96th percintile in weight. She then asked me an unexpected question. **"Do you care about your weight?" I just looked at her with my mouth open. "Of course I do. It's just..well nothing EVER works.** I lose weight, then it comes right back. After awhile...you just get hopeless." Then she told that she knew it could be struggling, but think of the payoff. Then we started talking about how I should lose weight and all that stuff. ..she told me I should cut the sandwich I have at lunch in half and save the other hald for the next day. Also, she said to drink plenty of water. (which I already do) Well, then I just kind of snapped. This is what I said, "IT'S NOT FAIR! .. My doctor calmed me down .. then **she surprised me by saying, even if I didn't lose a lot of weight, but maintained it, I could still look good...**

Negative Comments From Physicians Don't Help

From katie, Age 13 - 08/13/08
Ht. 5'2", Start: 402 lb, Current: 402 lb, Goal: 130 lb - i have a big problem my peditrician said if i gain more i can die my mom started sobbing when she said this so did i ... **at the doctors they took me to a different part as the scale in the kids area didn't go high even that was emmbarrising.**

From Katie, Age 12 - 05/26/03
Help! i am the fattest pig ever ! **i weigh 247** and **i am only 12** almost 13 **my doctor picks on me! he said that i could lose some weight and then he says at least you'll stay warm in that winter with all that flubber!** oh was i mad so i starved imyself down to a 213 and then i always got dizzy ! help me so bad i am fatter than the eqautor help me i am a blob of usless ness

Reply from Ray Ray, Age 12 - 05/29/03
Hey Katie. I weigh about the same as you **I'm 5'6 230 pounds.** I know what you mean when you say your doctor makes comments...mine does too. **my doctor will outright tell me that I am fat.**

From Michelle, Age 13 - 10/16/07 -
Ht. 5'8", Start: 227 lb, Current: 219 lb, Goal: 140 lb - tia i am mad with myself... i want to play soccer but im to fat i get out of breath running in my house ahhhh!!!!!!!!!!!!!!!!!!!!!!!!!!!!!!!!!!!!
most of the other girls are like 16 or older who weigh 200 something not me 13 and **im sick of being judged** for being this size **even my doctor(the skintyest man on the earth)judges me** im sick of every thng about being fat

From Lily, Age 11 - 09/26/09
Ht. 4'11", Start: 130 lb, Today: 130 lb, Goal: 88 lb - ...Kids make fun of me. I want to weigh 88 pounds. ...Anyway **the doctor embarresses me by saying I'm fat**...I'm to fat and lazy to exercise. what should I do! love Lily P.s. in your next weight update please tell me what to do!I'm hopeless!

Reply from Amanda, Age 19 - 6/24/08
yeah **doctors can be a pain in the a**. i dont know whether theyre hard on us to motivate us to lose weight, or because theyre giant arseholes.** either way, i like to think its for our own good. but he should be really pleased with what youve done...

As the preceding posts relate, healthcare providers need to be sensitive to how they approach the weight topic with kids and what they say.

Are we healthcare providers good role models?

From Rae, Age 13 - 4/19/05

Hey everyone! I am **13 years old I"m 4' 9" and I weigh 143 pounds!** My BMI is 30.9. ... **My doctor told me I need to loose 12 pounds** but I've gained one pound. So now I need to loose 13 pounds. I really want to loose 43 pounds, and I have to do this by august 15th. **My doctor didnt give me weight lose tips he just told me to loose it. When he was talking to me I felt really uncomfortable because he was probably 70 pounds overweight himself.** He looked like he was living on dougnuts, and sugar. ..

What help do healthcare providers offer to overweight kids?

From lucy, Age 14 - 07/20/05

Ht. 4 11, Wt. 142 - Hey guys **im 32 pounds overweight according to my doctor.** I've been overweight since I could remember. **my doctor didnt tell me what to do on how to loose weight.**

From AJ, Age 15 - 12/8/00

Ht: 5'6 Wt: 260-275 lb. ...I have tried to diet and excersize but i cant do it alone. When I do it with some 1 eles it motervates me to do it. But all my friends are skinner than me, and I don't feel comefretable. I have a lot of stress. A bout a half a year ago I was dissed by my mom. I tried to kill my self. Now I am liveing with my grandparents. When I lived with my mom she called me things like "Fat @$$ and other names. For a hole week I wouldn't eat. **I have it in my mind that the reason my mom and dad(I never met my dad) don't want me is because I am fat.** I wear size DDD in bra. That hurts. And size 24 in pants. I keep getting bigger and bigger. I think 1 day I am going to explode...(not really) I look at my self in the mera, and I see a beautiful smile, glowing eyes, and then a nasty, peice of fat, that covers my body. **I have been to the Dr. and all she did was send me to the nutrinest. That didn't work.** I have tried to get help. I cant run bc it hurts my brest and my legs, back, and my feet, just hurt so bad. I can hardly breath now... but when I am doing things like that It is also hard to breath. I don't know wut to do. I am so mad at me, bc all i do is give up. I have no good immage about me. I am afraid that my b/f is gonna break up with me bc im so fat. pelase help me.

From Jess, Age 14 - 05/01/05

I think I am overweight. I look at calculators & ask **my doctor...they usually say I am at risk!** I am in the **140** range. I am about **5'3**.

Reply from Julie, Age 17 - 06/06/06

The **average doctor gets only 2-3 hours of nutrition education in their whole training. Im not sure how much you can rely on them for nutirtion advice...**

But overweight kids do understand the value of their healthcare provider.

From Isabella, Age 13 - 10/23/06
Ht. 5 ft. 5in., Wt. 166.6lb. - To Shannon (and everyone else): Okay, I'm going to be honest with you! **First of all, you should talk to your doctor to see how much you should weigh!** On this site it said I should be in the 130s but my doc knows my parents and knows I'm meant to be larger and healthy, not thin and healthy!

From tammi, Age 15 - 08/03/03
to all of you guys who are saying i am going to make my self throw up..dont do it i used to do it and it really messes you up..**just talk to your doctor ok**...be safe about it...really just talk to someone dont become sick like that its reallly no fun...and it really messes you up..just think about it first..**see your doctor guys!!**

Do doctors detect and advise overweight kids?

We conducted several polls about this and other issues with their doctors:
(http://www.blubberbuster.com/cgi/poll_new_46_percent.cgi)

If you're overweight and saw your doctor, did he/she mention that you're overweight?

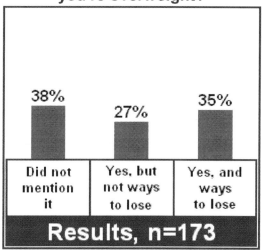

173 Kids Voted

Although this poll is not scientific, in view of the large number of kids responding, it does appear that more than a third of their doctors did not mention that the child was overweight and only about a third of their doctors provided any information on weight loss.

Here are comments from kids responding to this poll:

Age 13, female, 4'11, 165 lb. - my docter is not that smart and is over weight him self

Age 13, female, 5'2, 195 lb. - My doctor always says that I'm at risk for obesity and that's all that she talks to me about!!!

Age 12, female, 5 foot, 308 lb. - when i came in he stared at me disgusted for a second but did not say anything

Age 12, male, 4\9, 200 lb. - He never told that i was overweight but i knew he was lying to me so i cried and cried.

Age 13, female, 5'8.5, 200 lb. - he said that I should take a double dosage of the anti biotics as i was a 'big girl'

Age 16, female, 5'5, 185 lb. - he told me a have gotten way to "fat" for a teenage girl and need to lose a lot if i want to ever have a relationship...

Age 11, female, 5'4, 200 lb. - i metioned it but she showed no intrest

Age 13, male, 5'4" , 142 lb. - I AM ANNOYED HOW DOCTORS WILL STRAIGHT AWAY COMMENT ON YOUR WEIGHT PROBLEM BUT WILL NOT HELP YOU WITH IT...

Age 12, female, 5ft 2 in, 155 lb. - he just said to eat healthier

Age 13, male, 5'4, 449 lb. - my doctor blames every illness i get on me being fat

Age 16, female, 5"7, 198 lb. - my doctor doesn't help me at all and i have low self estem

Age 13, female, 5'4, 165 lb. - my doctor didnt answer but i asked him and he suggested that i go on a diet

Age 16, female, 5"3, 237 lb. - My main problem is portions and sugar. I would love to loose this weight but I don't know how. All my doctor says is to exercise...

Age 13, female, 5'6, 159 lb. - I think he should have suggested ways to lose wieght.

Age 12, male, 5'0, 155 lb. - my doctor just said im ''overweight for my age'' and whent on to the rest of the stuff

Age 14, male, 5'5", 154 lb. - **My doctor only said something once when I was 4... now I'm 14**

Age 13, female, 5'4, 163 lb. - **only if i ask him**

Age 12, female, 5'0, 140.5 lb. - **My doctor said like I wasent even there she said she is very FAT**

Age 13, female, 5'4", 147 lb. - **I think that doctors are cruel and should gain weight to c how it feels**

Age 14, male, 64, 165 lb. - **My doctor has helped me lose alot of weight. I'm glad he was always there to help me with this cruddy mess!!**

Age 13, female, 5ft. 5", 168 lb. - **My doctor mentioned it once or twice, not in a mean way, and I wasn't hurt becuase I knew it was true. However, I didn't take him seriosly until I decided it was time to loose weight for myself! Then I went back he was completely impressed, I finally got the courage to ask for some advice so we had a nice conversation and I feel great. :0) I know others aren't as lucky becuase my doctor is a really nice, funny guy...**

More should be learned in regard to how doctors feel about talking to overweight kids. Do doctors actually get little nutrition training in medical school, as kids seem to believe? What are the current programs in medical schools regarding this? A survey in 2006 of U.S. Medical Schools found: "The amount of nutrition education in medical schools remains inadequate." [Adams et al. 2006]. How can doctors in practice obtain adequate training in this area?

Anger from kids about doctors

Some of the above postings by overweight kids express anger about their doctor being overweight and giving advice on overweight health risks and how to lose weight. Consequently, we did a poll on this to find out more about how kids feel. (http://www.blubberbuster.com/cgi/poll_new_82.cgi)

How do you feel about overweight doctors, nurses, or dietitians advising kids about a healthy weight?

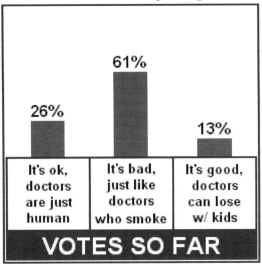

62 kids voted

Of the 62 kids responding, most disapprove of overweight healthcare providers giving advice on overweight health risks and weight loss, similar to healthcare providers, who smoke, giving advice on smoking health risks and how to quit. About a fourth of the kids feel that doctors are only human and may have weight problems like anyone else. About an eighth feel that doctors could lose weight along with the kids and thus serve as weight loss role models.

Is your doctor, nurse, or dietitian overweight?

   YES: 19 votes (31%)

   NO: 43 votes (69%)

Commendably, most of the kids' healthcare providers are not overweight.

Comments from kids on this poll are below. Some comments are pretty angry.

Age 17, female, 5'5'', 107 lb. - **I think it's stupid for someone to give advice and not even follow their own advice.** - Neither my doctor, nurse, nor dietitian is overweight.

Age 12, female, 5'2, 120 lb. - **It's disgusting and its the same for everyone... Doctors should know that if they tell us to lose weigh and they need to also, they should first.** - My doctor, nurse, or dietitian is overweight.

Age 11, female, 50 in, 148 lb. - **they're hippocrit's.** - My doctor, nurse, or dietitian is overweight.

Age 15, female, 5"6, 219 lb. - **I agree with it being hypocritical, however, health professionals have to do their job, and so should be respected in their position. Just like anyone else, they have to make their own choices** - Neither my doctor, nurse, nor dietitian is overweight.

Age 15, male, 5', 170 lb. - **I think if they are, they should talk about how "we" can do these things together and both of will try to lose weight.** - Neither my doctor, nurse, nor dietitian is overweight.

Age 12, female, 5'2, 163 lb. - **they call us fat look at them** - Neither my doctor, nurse, nor dietitian is overweight.

Age 17, female, 5'3, 172 lb. - **how can a fat doctor tell me to loose weight if his also a big fat as, get lost** - Neither my doctor, nurse, nor dietitian is overweight.

Age 10, male, 4'11, 190 lb. - **My dad is a fat doctor, he is 400 pound, but he works with old people** - My doctor, nurse, or dietitian is overweight.

Age 12, female, 5', 94 lb. - **it's like they're saying do as i say not s i do. that's just idiotic to me.** - Neither my doctor, nurse, nor dietitian is overweight.

Age 11, male, 5/11 three fourths, 78 lb. - **It shouldnt matter what they think. If they want to be overweight, thats their choose. All that matters is if you want to be overweight.** - Neither my doctor, nurse, nor dietitian is overweight.

Age 13, female, 5,8, 153 lb. - **Personally I don't think it matters how the health professional looks. If the patient is really serious about losing his or her weight, then he or she will listen to exactly what the doctor says and not judge by what they see.** - My doctor, nurse, or dietitian is overweight.

Age 11, female, 5'0, 140 lb. - **most doctors i see are overweight** - My doctor, nurse, or dietitian is overweight.

Age 10, female, 5'2'', 139.2 lb. - **I would feel a little bad about the doctors, nurses, etc. because they might give advice they use but does not work and it could discourage the kids because they think it works but it does not.** - Neither my doctor, nurse, nor dietitian is overweight.

Should overweight health professionals exclude themselves from treating overweight kids? That seems extreme, but they should be sensitive to the fact that many overweight kids have a problem with overweight health professionals. On the brighter side, though, the poll results below suggest that overweight kids overwhelmingly prefer health professionals who have previously been overweight and have lost weight.

Who should treat overweight kids?

Perhaps the results of the below poll were predictable, but we were looking for any surprises. (http://www.blubberbuster.com/cgi/poll_new_65.cgi)

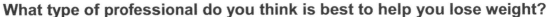

What type of professional do you think is best to help you lose weight?

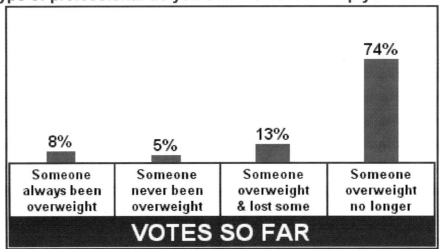

126 kids voted

Nearly three fourths of the kids voting prefer a health professional, who has been overweight but is no longer, to help them lose weight.

Comments from kids about this poll:

Age 16, female, 5'7", 289 lb. - **They know what it's like to be there, and they know what the journey is like, and they know what they had to do to change things. They would understand the situation from more than just a nutritional level...they'd understand it on an emotional level as well.**

Age 11, male, 5' 1", 150 lb. - **I think some that used to be but still is and losing is the best, because they've done some losing, but can support you because they know what its like.**

Age 13, female, 5'2'', 131 lb. - **People who are fit and have always been fit are better. They can have really good tips(I know from experience)**

Age 13, female, 5'3, 220 lb. - I am on a weight loss program and which the peroson who is helping me was overweight, and has lost the weight.

Age 11, female, 5'3", 118 lb. - they were sucessful so they could help you be

Age 9, female, 4,9, 76 lb. - They know what we've been through.

Age 11, female, 5'5", 160 lb. - This way shealready knows how to do what you are trying to do and has gone thru the same things.

Age 11, male, 5'2, 118 lb. - My youth minister at church is overweight but he has lost a lot. He is a very good role model because he is overweight but he is losing weight not gaining or staying where he is at not caring. He is very brave to be telling other people about his problem!

Age 14, female, 5'8", 145 lb. - Someone who has never been overweight can not really help you as much because they don't know what it's really like.

Age 15, female, 5'1, 216? lb. - I wouldn't want someone that has always be perfect helping me.

Age 12, female, 5ft 6.5in, 200 lb. - i would feel better with sum1 who has been through what i am going through now

Age 14, female, 5'6", Too much :(lb. - They could definately help someone if they've been overweight and got to a healthy weight. I think they would be a great person to ask for advice. One of my teachers told us about his weight loss. A couple years ago he was like 60 pounds heavier but he lost it through diet and excercise. We were talking about goal setting. My goal is to lose 10 pounds. I am going to ask my teacher for advice next class I have with him.

The results of the above poll are as expected, but it does show that kids identify best with someone who has been through what they are going through, has succeeded, and can pass on advice about how to do it. Therefore, it is productive and reasonable for parents to ask children's weight loss professionals if they have ever been overweight.

How are we going to treat all of the overweight kids?

The 2008 NICHQ National Congress on Childhood Obesity issued the following challenge: "Treating obesity requires frequent contact and skilled counseling; there are too few specialists available to meet the demand. How can effective treatment be done in community or primary care settings?" One possible solution is technology and the Internet. We asked

kids what they thought about this idea.
(http://www.blubberbuster.com/cgi/poll_new_31_percent.cgi)

Can you lose weight without face to face visits with a health professional?

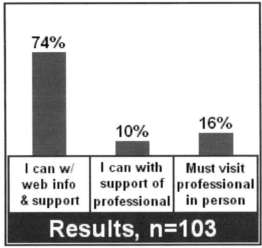

103 kids voted

Nearly three fourths of 103 kids responding feel that they can lose weight without a health professional. Less than a fifth of the kids feel that they must visit a professional in person. This overwhelming result may originate somewhat from most kids being embarrassed to talk to a healthcare provider about their weight. The last comment below expresses the embarrassment factor.

Comments from kids about this poll:

I can lose without professional help:

➔ I lost like 30 lb. and I did it all by myself. I didn't visit a doctor or anything! I went with what I already knew and found information in magazines and on the net so it worked.

➔ I can do it with help of friends online and support thats why i like blubberbusters so much cuz it really helps me out a lot and i think everyone should like blubberbusters also

➔ You dont need professional help to lose weight. Just put ur mind to it, and you can do it!

➔ I have never used a health professional to help me lose weight~~and i've done it~~~~it's not impossible

➔ I know i can do it by myself!!!!!!!

➜ i have never visited a dietion etc, and i lost 10lb..

➜ I lost 40 lb. over the summer without anyone to help me.

➜ I have lost maore then 5 pounds and I do not even have a doctor like that!

➜ I could probably lose weight by myself if i really set my mind to it.

➜ I think anyone who is really overweight should see a health proffesional, but otherwise, you can do it by yourself

A professional is not really the answer:

➜ You don't need information to lsoe weight, just motivation. Everyone knows to lose weight you have to consume less calories then you burn.

➜ You don't need to see help just to lose weight!

➜ Beleive Me its hard anyway you challemge it!

➜ no...... too embarressed!

There were no comments that a health professional is essential for weight loss.

Health professional critics

Health professional critics have objected to children and teens on our site self-assessing themselves as overweight and sharing tips with each other on diets, exercise, and weight loss. Our bulletin boards and chatrooms are monitored by registered dietitians and nurses, who promptly remove any unhealthy posts. Furthermore, the weight calculator on our site uses the growth chart data files of the U.S. Centers for Disease Control and the CDC's definitions for overweight and obesity in children (http://www.cdc.gov/obesity/childhood/defining.html). This information is available to kids on the CDC's site as well as on our site. Many overweight kids on our site say that they're too embarrassed to ask for help from a health professional, or that their doctor doesn't provide them with weight loss advice. Furthermore, health professionals' criticism of Internet self-care by kids is in contrast to the fact that there are too few specialists available to take care of the estimated 25 million overweight kids in the U.S. [NICHQ 2008]. Is 'no care' thus better than Internet self-care?

What's the take away message for health professionals?

Many, if not most, doctors, nurses, dietitians, PE teachers, and other health professionals are not aware that overweight kids are embarrassed to ask for help with their weight. Health professionals themselves may be hesitant to bring up the weight issue for various reasons. At the American Academy of Pediatrics national conference in 2007, several pediatricians confided to me that they don't bring up weight issues with overweight kids because they fear the parents (and kids) would be insulted and leave the practice. This may be more commonplace than we think. As noted previously, health professionals also may feel uncomfortable due to lack of knowledge or embarrassment about their own weight problems. Thus, there are many reasons why health professionals may be missing opportunities to intervene.

Parents should bring up the weight issue with their overweight kids even if their healthcare provider doesn't.

At some point overweight kids may decide that they want to try to lose weight, with or without the help of a professional or their parents. The next chapter presents what kids say finally motivates them to try to lose weight.

7 | Motivation

This is KATIE's story:

I realy want to loose wheight but i have no motervation. Like this morning i thought i will get up go for a run and come home and have a realy healthy day but this morning i said i'm to tired or i'll go for a walk instead but i just end up in frount of the t.v.**Please help me to be more motervated?**

Despite feelings of hopelessness, lack of support, and secrecy, overweight kids tend to reach a point where they are motivated to try to lose weight, either on their own or with the help of others. This chapter discusses what it is that motivates them and keeps them going.

Reply from Winona, Age 17 - 2/29/04 -
I think youve realise **the number 1 reason people fail diets- motivation.**

What motivates kids to try to lose weight?

From Quincy, Age 11 - 03/19/09
Ht. 5'3", Start: 190 lb, Current: 220 lb, Goal: 175 lb - i am about to be in the 6th grade and i don't feel comfortable about my body. **i want to loose weight because I dont want a short life of health problems. I also want to loose weight because iwant to feel better about my self and i don't want to get picked an because of my weight.**

From Ellie, Age 12 - 7/7/08 -
Ht. 5'3", Start: 165 lb, Current: 163 lb, Goal: 120 lb - I would like some help in a diet plan that has a lot of protein because I am a vegetarian. **I'm tired of being fat and at junior high this year we have to egt undressed in front of other girls, and I would like to do it comforabtly.** If I can get to 120 or 123, I will be just at the healthy weight. **Plus, this guy that I like,** Sal, likes me a little, and **I think if I lost some weight, he would like me even more.**

From Jennifer, Age 14 - 06/13/09 -
Ht. 5'2", Start: 195 lb, Current: 185 lb, Goal: 160 lb - okay, so how bad is this. **My reason to lose weight is to show my EX bf, that just broke up with me**, how awesome im gonna look when school starts again :D!

This is NIKITA's question:
hello,i am **13** years old and weigh **12st 4lbs [172 lb]**... **i have a pony and she is a small horse and it is very hard to ride her at the moment because of my weight andi get very upset about it because when i do ride her i know it hurts her**,.. please would you be able to give me some advice at excersises and things that i should eat please..

Here's a great tip on motivation:

From sabina, Age 16 - 11/07/06 -
Ht. 5'6, Wt. 157 - **THIS OR THAT**: Taco bell or size 00? Second best chubby girlfriend or the girl your man's friends wish they had? The girl self conscious in her tankini or the one showing off her bikini? The one worried about her thighs rubbing together or the one who cant keep her boyfriends hands off them? Chubby sitting on the couch or thin enough to sit on his lap?
I read that everytime i feel like giving up. It is a real pick me upper

What specifically motivates them?

1) To attract the opposite sex...

From Karry M., Age 15, female - 6/7/02
It really stinks being overweight for many different reasons but one big thing is not having a boyfriend, but someday i will. Right now i wear about an 16 to 18 in jeans and i plan to get to a 10 or 12.

From Claire, Age 19 - 09/15/08 -
Ht. 5'4", Start: 210 lb, Current: 177 lb, Goal: 150 lb - I'm losing the weight for the right reason. I always have been but **lately I've been thinking about guys.** I've been having **dreams about guys** (one that I've been crushing on since I was 14 and one that I've been crushing on since Feb) they were nice dreams...some of them, we're I was with either one of them and get this--**in the dreams, I was skinny.** It just makes me wish that I was skinny so that they could notice me because I know that's what it is. Of course i don't want a guy who just wants me because of my body (those types are jerks) I want someone who wants me for my heart but still **in order to FEEL beautiful around a guy, I want to to be thin and healthy. I want to feel comfortable** and not have a guy struggle

to put his arms around me. I want to have a guy be able to take me in his arms and lift me off my feet. I want to be lighter than a guy and not heavier..you know what I mean? ...

From Rachel, Age 14 - 5/19/08
Ht. 5'6", Start: 320 lb, Current: 299 lb, Goal: 150 lb - So, I started off good. But well lately, I have let myself just fkc up all over... But **this past weekend was a real eye-opener. I went to an amusement park and I just fit to be buckled on the rollercoasters.** I will go to Six Flags for my eighth grade trip in about a month, and I would like to loose atleast 10 pounds by then. **I do not want to grow up to be some old fat lady living alone in a tiny apartment with 50 cats.** I also have my eight grade graduation dance, and I would like to feel a little more confident. I know what to do the only problem is just sticking to it and not always messing up.

From Flower Fawn, Age 15 - 7/1/08
Ht. 5'5", Start: 184 lb, Current: 178 lb, Goal: 150 lb - Hey guys. Well **I became really motivated today because I was thinking about how I was too embarrassed to go to mixers at nearby schools this year becuase of my appearance.** Well...I want that to change. I want to be able to go to a mixer and feel confident and meet people, not hide in the corner and be the see-through fat girl. I'm SO SICK AND TIRED of that.I'm not sure if I really look bad or it's just how I perceive myself, but **I just want to be able to relax and have fun without having to worry about my appearance.** I really want to be 165 by December so that I can go to holiday mixers and my school's Christmas dance looking better than I did this year. ...

 Mikayla 15
I have motivation other than health that is making it really easy for me to keep going

 Mikayla 15
In 2 months I turn 16 and when i am 16 i get to date

2) For school...

From Ben, Age 12 - 5/5/08 -
Ht. 5'5", Start: 209 lb, Current: 227 lb, Goal: 155 lb - Hey. I've been on this site for awhile now.. But I never really got motivated to doing it. Honestly, I REALLY want to lose alot of weight before 7th grade... **Because you have to get undressed infront of everyone.** I also want to lose weight **to be healthy.. I worry myself.** I just can't find a way to get motivated. :/ ~Ben

From Zach, Age 15 - 01/31/08
Ht. 5'5", Start: 260 lb, Current: 260 lb, Goal: 240 lb - ... now im in highschool and **wut really made me wunt to lose weight was the fact that i barely fit in my desk anymore. And i feel like people are looking at me.** So please give me some good exercise routines and tip on losing weight. I need, Cuz im tired of bing fat.

From Lisa , Age 16 - 6/28/08
Ht. 5'7", Start: 184 lb, Current: 184 lb, Goal: 150 lb - OKAY so i just found this websitee and i think its absolutaly amazing! reading everyone's posts is so encouraging and helpful and i love how everyone opens up=P i think ill be writing here often but just to get started ill say that its summer time now and **i really need to lose some weight especially for school in september .. its my last year in highschool and i really want to look good for it!** alrighty i guess that means i start todayy. Wish me luck!

From tia, Age 16 - 6/5/08
Ht. 5'6", Start: 225 lb, Current: 190 lb, Goal: 160 lb - hey guys! my school just got out! and i sort of restarted my diet i HAVE to lose weight **im gonna be a senior and i CAN"T go to prom being fat!!** tips anyone?!

From sarah, Age 16, female - 4/12/02
...Just keep thinking about your future and wheather you want to be fat and lazy and depressed or healthy and beautiful. i am telling you when you are a healhy weight you do not have to be so self concious that your top is too tight or your belly is hanging out. I hope this story has inspired you so just excersize and keep healthy!!

3) For health reasons...

From Katherine, Age 14, female - 8/3/01
I am overweight-I am 14 and I weigh 240 puonds! I feel so shy around people at school or in a new place because I am overweight. Just recently I started a diet. I feel GREAT! Even though you may look the same **you feel different, like the earth was released from your shoulders!** I lost 10 punds in 5 weeks! I am so happy, I feel like I can do almost anything and everything. To me, I have more confidence to talk to people I want to meet. Now I have more friends than ever.

From Annie, Age 23, female - 5/24/05
Hello, I am a 23 year old female and I have always been overweight. My mother was abused as a child and made a promise to God that her children would not have to go through what she did. SO, **food was LOVE**... Mom would make this HUGH meals, and we, my brother and sister would eat away, and ask for seconds. We all grew large. I however grew above everyone else. I am now 23 and 368 lbs. It hurts just to write that down. I am looked through by everyone. No one see's me. **It is such a horrible feeling to be denied things**

because I am overweight. **It kills me everyday**... I am now 368 and I feel helpless. I wish I was thinking about a diet at 12 like some of you, I might not have the problems I do now. **All I can tell you is keep it up, stay healthy, because I can't tell yo how much I wish I could go back to being 12 and lose the weight then. I never had a boyfriend; this made me have low self esteem** and I got with the first person who saw me. 5 years, 2 children and a abusive relationship later, here I am, 368lbs. That's my story, and I never hope to hear one like it... All I can tell you is keep it up, stay healthy, because I can't tell yo how much I wish I could go back to being 12 and lose the weight then....

From storm, Age 16 - 3/5/07
Ht. 6'2", Wt. 373 - Today I went to go get my **yearly physical for track**. I'm a thrower so we don't do much but pump some iron every once in a while and work on our legs. Well **I went into the doctors office** and did all the usual bs, but I noticed my weight had jumped a lot!!!! I've never been so embararased in my life! well he procided to take **my blood pressure and it was high to. 164/90!!!!** I'm obese! He told me he would not clear me for track and I about died right there! track is my way of being with every one and doing some athletics. Now he wants me to go see a health care person to have test done on me. I've never been so scared in my life and I came home and bawled my eyes out *right now* and the only thing that keeps running thru my head is "**I dont' want to die young**"...

This is ZOE's story:
hi my name is zor i am 11 years old and extreamley over weight im am 213 pounds i need your help **so i can be healthey agian**

manda 14
my grandma was big and she died from kidney failure and heart failure and i dont wanna die like that!

4) Body appearance...

From Justin, Age 15 - 12/9/07
Ht. 5'7", Start: 305 lb, Current: 305 lb, Goal: 175 lb - i need some thoughts on this- ive gained about 20 lbs since the beginning of this school year and people are starting to notice- people have been poking me in my belly and this part is really embarrasing but **they make fun of me because i have man boobs that jiggle when i walk- thats the worst** and i wish people would stop

From Lauren, Age 16 - 6/19/06
Ht. 5'8, Wt. 181.5 - well this is to do with being overweight bt also not! im like 14lbs overweight and since ive become overweight ive had an **embarassing problem**,which i have never told anyone before now. I have dark areas of skin on ma groin, neck and armpits! i

just thought it was because i was fat and not washing properly but now ive jus found out **its a medical condition called acanthosis nigricans - its associated with being overweight. So if you lose weight you loose the dark skin!** i am so happy to find this out! if any one else has this problems just do a search on it to find the information out! i hope ive helped!

5) For a special event...

From Katie, Age 16 - 3/22/08
Ht. 5'9", Start: 160 lb, Current: 175 lb, Goal: 150 lb - Hey guys,... **Prom is coming up and i'm wearing a dress** I wore to another prom last year...but **I've gained weight! so its not gonna look too hot**...i have the exerise down, but **i need help with the food thing..because i love to eat..:(** **Help!** ps: as you can see..i've gained 15 pounds..

From Sam, Age 17 - 10/16/08 -
Ht. 5'5", Start: 235 lb, Current: 199 lb, Goal: 130 lb - I really hate being overweight. this sucks. i want to lose around 20 pounds by december. is that possible? i **want to be a semi-lighter and slimmer person by the time i see my cousin.** its been like 2 years at least since ive seen her. i want to have memories of that time. what can i do to get this weight off. im sure im like everyone else and want a quick fix that will last forever...

From molly, Age 17 - 11/18/08
Ht. 5'7", Start: 210 lb, Current: 210 lb, Goal: 162 lb - so according to doctors I am obese ! Gosh I hate that word. So I need to make some sort of a change and with thanksgiving next week I'm sure this is gonna go over well. So **my goal or big reveal is to look absolutely breathtaking for prom** witch is in April . I need to lose 44 pounds in all to be at a healthy weight. Does anyone have any motavation tips?

From Arturo, Age 13 - 11/22/08
Ht. 5'7", Start: 180 lb, Current: 180 lb, Goal: 110 lb - I need some HUGE tips.. This year I will be promoting from a junior high to a high school and **yearly they have a trip to the water park while at the water park i would like to take my shirt off and be proud of myselff**.. i mean i dont want killer abs i want a flat stomach.. nnot a huge gut sticking out..please write back with GREAT tips..

From Kim, Age 17 - 04/02/08
Ht. 5'7", Start: 191 lb, Current: 175 lb, Goal: 145 lb - So me and my bf broke up early today because hes in Iraq and its kinda hard being 17 and dating someone whose 3000 miles away from you. We found that out the hard way it...So we want to get back together when he gets home in Feb. of 09. So **when I go and pick him up from the**

airport **I want to surprise him weighing 145 lbs.** I'm 172 right now. ...Starting tomorrow I'm cutting sweets out of my diet including pop and energy drinks (which im addicted to)...

We did a poll asking kids what motivates them to lose weight.
(http://www.blubberbuster.com/cgi/poll_new_3.cgi)

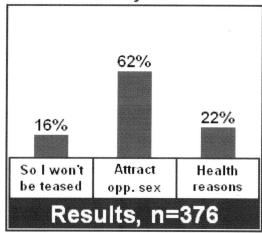

What is the main reason you want to lose weight?

376 kids voted

This is an important poll. Of the three choices, the 376 kids responding overwhelmingly voted for, "So I can attract the opposite sex." "Health reasons" was a distant 2nd, followed by, "So I won't be teased."

What does this suggest? Does it mean that they don't understand the health risks or don't care about later life, just live for the prom, etc? Is this a missed opportunity to teach about the risks/benefits of a future healthy life? What about all the later year events - to be healthy for college, grad school, marriage, etc.? Nevertheless, attracting the opposite sex is what mainly motivates kids to lose weight, and we should keep this in mind in designing weight loss and prevention programs for kids.

What Keeps Kids Motivated?

In a word, 'success' keeps kids motivated. Once kids have been able to lose even a few pounds, this adds greatly to their motivation to keep going, as demonstrated in the post below:

Roxie, Age 21, 10/16/08
Ht. 5'8.0", Goal 165.0 lb, Start 207.0 lb, Last 202.0 lb, Today 199.4 lb - I Feel great ! this is the first time in 2.5 years that i have been under 200 ! **This is pure motivation to me i want to keep going !** i wanna get to 165 ! i doing great so far !

Here's what successful kids say about their motivation to keep going:

✮ **Reply from Amanda, Age 19 - 8/2/08**

i know how you feel. **i lost 55 pounds so far** and i have another 20 to go, and **i feel discouraged all the time so i give up.** the thing is though, **we need to rethink why we're doing this, and become motivated** to push on. even though it comes off slowly, in the end it adds up, and **after a year if you're only 15-20 pounds lighter, its still 15-20 pounds that won't be coming back.**

✮ **From Alexis, Age 15, female - 9/5/01**

Hello to all. I weigh **210** and... 1 to 2 weeks ago, I weighed **220**... I made a promise to loose my weight, and keep this diet. **The reason is because I want to look and feel better about myself, and not be ashamed of my body any longer. I cover my stomach, wearing a jacket or sweater, and I'm tired of feeling sorry for myself...** My mom went through the same thing her freshman year, and she succeeded tremendously. She was about the same size I was, and lost over 70 pounds...The big thing is, I have such a pretty face, and I want a pretty body...

✮ **From Marina, Age 13 - 4/27/01**

.. I'm **currently 5ft 6in and 118lbs.** I used to be like everyone else in here....i **weighed 207lbs.** But **one day something came over me....i knew that this was unhealthy for myself.** I didn't want to lose weight to look better....but to be healthy. But there are only 3 things you need to lose weight, three important things: sensible foods, Exercise & Will power. with these three things you'll have the most ideal weight. at first you'll feel that it takes too long and be discouraged....well i'll be honest, yeah it does take long....but if u work at it now....by the summer time you'll be feeling a lot better than u do today. I used to be so negative about my weight but then one day i realized that if i just sit around & complain, i won't be accomplishing anything, so right then and there...i got up off the couch and took my dog for a long walk....then it developed into a jog....then a run. so each day twice a day i was not only taking care of my pet, but i was also helping myself.If you start thinking the way I did.....you'll be losing weight in no time.....but also u must eat sensible foods!!

✮ **Reply from fara, Age 13 - 8/2/08**

whenever you feel discouraged think about **how great you'll look when you lose some weight, how everyone is going to think your totally hot,** and **how anybody who ever made fun of you is going to regret it.** thats what i do and it really helps

And as one overweight girl put it:

"i wanna lose weight cuz it will give me more self of steam."

So, once kids are motivated to try to lose weight, what happens next? Kids talk about their struggles to lose weight in the following chapter.

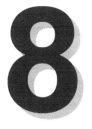

The Struggle

What happens when kids try to lose weight?

From Kt, Age 15 - 8/15/06
Ht. 5'4", Wt. 143 - **how long do you think it will take me to lose 20 pounds if i normaley mess up a lot**

> ➤ *The degree to which overweight kids struggle to lose weight is striking.*

The Struggle of Trying to Lose Weight - Step by Step

1. They don't know where to start

From Panic at the disco luver, Age 14 - 5/3/08
Ht. 5'5", Start: 187 lb, Current: 180 lb, Goal: 130 lb - This is a bad thing;; ... i took pics with my friends on my camera and **i look huge. I mean huge too.** i have been trying to loose weiht for a long time now ... and **i don't kno were to start beacuse im so overwealmed**

From Anna, Age 14 -3/20/08
Ht. 5'2", Start: 191 lb, Last:172, Today: 173.2 lb, Goal: 165 lb - **I don't understand why I can't lose weight**

From Claire, Age 19 - 7/17/08
Ht. 5'4", Start: 210 lb, Current: 176 lb, Goal: 140 lb - ok again..the only thing that can sum up **how I feel is this Beatles song:** HELP! I NEED SOMEBODY! HELP!!!!!! NOT JUST ANYBODY! HELP! YOU KNOW I NEED SOMEONE! HELPPPPPPPPPPPPPPPP!!!!

2. They feel helpless and overwhelmed

Kids may have no one they feel comfortable talking to about their weight or their desire to lose weight, so they start dieting or exercising without much information or help from anyone.

From Gabrielle, Age 14 - 3/22/08
Ht. 5'7", Start: 155 lb, Current: 180 lb, Goal: 155 lb - **It's not that i dont know how to lose wieght** exercise and watch wat u eat. **But it's so hard to do and i feel so helpless when i start like im wasting my time nothings going to work.** Next year im going to high school and **i actually want to get a boyfriend for the first time in my life.** Also i play volleyball and wear spandex and **dont want to have thunder thighs.**

From nikkita, Age 10 - 11/25/08
Ht. 4'11", Start: 179 lb, Current: 175 lb, Goal: 120 lb - i ate to much today **i hate myself cry cry cry cry cry crycrycrycrycrycry**

From Jeimi, Age 17 - 2/15/08
Ht. 5'2", Start: 240 lb, Current: 224 lb, Goal: 180 lb - HELP **i really don't know what to do anymore i feel like a failer** can u guys PLEASE give me some TIPS i really could use all the help i can get..

From Sara, Age 17 - 5/3/08 -
Ht. 5'9", Start: 330 lb, Current: 286 lb, Goal: 150 lb - **I hate being the fattest girl** on this site.. **I want to be slim and its so hard.** I cry just being this heavy......Help me please...

Age 15, female, 5'4, 174 lbs - I'm trying so hard but **losing weight is the hardest thing that anyone would ever have to go through**

From Kabey, Age 16 - 2/10/08 -
Ht. 5'5", Start: 155 lb, Current: 155 lb, Goal: 115 lb - Okay, I am past being exasperated. I am past being mad. I'm am past being COMPLETELY discouraged. I don't know what to do. **I'm downright hopeless.** I'm supposed to be traveling this summer to Italy, Greece, and Barcelona, and no hot guy's going to even look at me twice when I go! I need HELP. ... **And cravings?** Forget them. **I give in to them EVERY time.** I'm starting to feel like I'll be this size forever.

3. They lack motivation

Or kids are motivated for only a short time or for a particular short term reason, such as a school prom, or event.

From Mikayla, Age 16 - 4/4/07
Ht. 5'6", Start: 197 lb, Current: 175 lb, Goal: 130 lb - **I am so sick of being overweight.** I've been overweight since I was a little kid. **I have so much to lose weight for** (prom, senior year, family weddings, confirmation, etc), **but I still seem to lack motivation.**

 *Ray*Ray* 14 in 8!!!
Lucy - Do you have any tips on motivation? I know how to lose weight, I just can't seem to stay focused. And people say, if you really wanted it you could do it...but it just doesn't seem to be the case. I want it so, so bad...but I can't stay on track.

4. They lack control

Many overweight kids feel that their eating is out of control.

They may not understand that their lack of self control is a common problem and that controlling eating is a learned behavior, one that takes practice and repeated efforts. They become depressed over their failure to stick with a diet or weight loss program. So, they may give up.

From Ishie, Age 15 - 6/22/05 - Ht. 5'1, Wt. 147.5 - **Does anyone ever feel reckless around food?** Like, i'll describe the feeling. I do very well in dieting until midday when i see food i really want. i take a bite. another bite. i stop, and when everyone leaves the room, i **cant stop**_looking at the food. i can like hear my heart beating, not any faster or louder, i just notice it more. **i feel like i have the shivers**, i stuff my face with the food, it only makes it worse. i keep stuffing, gorging all i can in my mouth, when i realize i just ruined my diet. i eat more, and i give up exercising for the day, because i know i've already ruined my diet. i feel like bursting out crying and i dont feel in the mood to do anything about it. the thought of getting together with friends just makes me feel fatter, grosser, guiltier. I hermit from friends and family for the rest of the day, eating more, crying more, feeling like im going to burst, but i cant stop, i wont stop, something inside me wont let me stop, i lock myself in my room, i fall asleep, and then i get in trouble for everything that i obviously ate, not only with my mom, but with myself and my weight. i think im psychotic. if i'm not, reply, if i am, reply, but really if i am i can deal with it myself. really, just... HELP!

This is KATHY's question:

it's really hard for me to stop eating so much and **even when i'm not eating, i'm thinking about it**. how come it's so hard to lose wieght, when the food is sitting right in front of you???

From julie, Age 15 - 8/20/07 -
Ht. 5'4", Start: 200 lb, Current: 200 lb, Goal: 150 lb - hey guys :) this is my first time here. why is it so hard to lose weight? **i've tried so hard to say no to food.. but i just cant for some reason..**

From kitty, Age 16 - 01/29/09 - IP#: 24.125.150.xxx
Ht. 5'4", Start: 215 lb, Current: 209 lb, Goal: 140 lb - **god i can't stop eating. after i eat i keep feeling hungry.** this is so retarded and **i can't handle it** :(

From Danielle, Age 17 - 2/21/08
Ht. 5'6", Start: 190 lb, Current: 190 lb, Goal: 165 lb - I'm having the heardest time becomming motivated, it's nuts. Lately, **as soon as I get motivated for a bit, I blow it by going home and eating so unhealthily.** I know I need to make better choices, but **i'ts like i don't have control**. Even when i tell myself no i will still go into the frige, then i feel gross and full. Guys, how do i get control back...

From Jane, Age 16 - 09/13/08
Ht. 5'7", Start: 196 lb, Current: 196 lb, Goal: 125 lb - I'm almost in the 200's. I'm so fat, I think I'm going to cry. I've lost all motivation, I just can't find any. I go out with my friends and avoid having pictures taken with them, because I look so fat all the time. My clothes only just fit. **The trouble is, with me it seems to be all or nothing. I can eat nothing at all, but if I start eating, I won't stop. I need serious help.**

From Amanda, Age 19 - 09/20/08
Ht. 5'8", Start: 225 lb, Current: 166 lb, Goal: 150 lb - GOD. okay so i keep trying and then messing up. all i want is to weight 164 to be considered a normal weight, then to get down to 160. those are attainable goals, but **i can't control myself!!** ... but good luck everyone and wish me luck! **i need some self control** lol byee :)

From Julie, Age 16 - 1/5/08
Ht. 5'6", Start: 185 lb, Current: 185 lb, Goal: 160 lb - im doing horrible. **i need control but i feel like i cant do this. i need motivation**, but i guess i also really smarten up. lol. i got a free ice cream cake from my work yesterday and i had a slice of that tonight :(and i had a burger around 11:30 this morning, but it was just the burger and the cheese, and then i had crackers around 2 or 2:30, and for supper i had pizza :(hopefully tomorrow will be a lot better. NO MORE CAKE!

From Morgan, Age 13 - 10/22/08 -
Ht. 4'10", Start: 107 lb, Current: 123 lb, Goal: 100 lb - **I have no self-controll.** Please i need to do something to stop myself. **Its horrible. Its like everytime i c food i EAT IT. That is not right.** There must be an easier way.

From michelle*, Age 17 - 1/17/08
Ht. 5'3", Start: 170 lb, Current: 180 lb, Goal: 132 lb - **I CANT DO IT!!!** Im sooooo hungry You know what Im doing im on google looking up ALL of my favorite foods and just looking at them in AGONY Im STARVING I NEED FAT I WANT FAT! but Ive been doing so good on this diet this is my third day and I realllyyy want to stick to it I keep telling myself that its not gonna be worth the five minutes of HEAVEN but **Im just sooo tired and hungry** cause of this diet I need something to keep my mind off of it I need help anyone please give me some advice!

From Brittany, Age 15 - 3/21/08
Ht. 5'5", Start: 263 lb, Current: 302 lb, Goal: 120 lb - Hi im Brittany ive been on here for awhile and i started out weighing 263 which was already horrible for a 15 year old. **I dont like being overweight and i wish i could stop eating but i love food and cant stop myself i dont kno wat to do.** i weighed myself today and im now 302 lbs!!! its crazy ive gained so much weight but i eat nonstop... **plz someone help me figure out how to stop eating i cant keep gaining weight like this im miserable**...thank you!!

From Jenny, Age 16 - 3/12/08
Ht. 5'2", Start: 190 lb, Current: 223 lb, Goal: 150 lb - I've been so much into eating the last half year that I've gained 33 lbs! **I'm so disgusting fat.** All my jeans are too tight now. **But i can't stop eating.** I eat a full bag of potatoe chips and feel very full and stuffed afterwards. But I cna't stop it. **I'm always thinking "tomorow i'll stop eating so much crap", but then I do it again.**

Bingeing and bulimia and loss of control

Bingeing and bulimia seem to especially exhibit this loss of control. Bingeing is eating large amounts of food very quickly. Bulimia is using extreme methods (purging) to rid the body of consumed calories, such as self-induced vomiting, laxatives, starvation, or intense exercise.

From Claire, Age 19 - 7/19/08
Ht. 5'4", Start: 210 lb, Current: 176 lb, Goal: 140 lb - Ok so **my binging has gone out of control. Like completely out of control! I feel like I can't control myself.** My brain just switches off and I eat everything I see and thats why **I hate it when people leave the house and leave me alone and I go to the fridge and just eat everything like a pig.** I feel like if I don't stop this I'll be back to where I was and that's the last

thing I want! I can't get back to something that horrid! everytime I tell myself to not do it, I binge. It's like I don't listen to myself. **It just happens like a reflex and I can't stop it**. ... I have to get my binge under control because that's whats made me gain the 18 lbs over the past year. Wish me luck, please guys. And good luck to you all

From Claire, Age 19 - 05/15/09 -
Ht. 5'4", Start: 210 lb, Current: 174 lb, Goal: 140 lb - just had a crazy **binge** on Ritz crackers. **Feel like complete and utter crap!!** :(

From Anon, Age 15 - 3/19/08
Ht. 5'8", Start: 232 lb, Current: 195 lb, Goal: 150 lb - **I have been bulimic for about a month**, or a little longer, and I need help stopping! **I can't control myself! I eat too much and feel so guilty afterwards!** I need help to stop eating so much!

From Lucee, Age 16 - 3/14/08 -
Ht. 5'8", Start: 147 lb, Current: 183 lb, Goal: 140 lb - OMG i cannot believe it. I have GAINED ... 37lbs since August. That is freakin crazy and **its all down to bulimia. I am so out of control it is unbelievable and it feels like i am never going to regain control of my life, my weight or my eating.** The binges are becoming so frequent im consuming way too many cals to purge or exercise off so as a result i am gaining weight like crazy. In my attempts to lose weight i have become overweight. I feel so ugly, fat and depressed..even my aunt said to me the other day that i was looking rather fat (does wonders for the self esteem dont it?!?) **Its so annoying because i know that if it werent for the binges id be losing weight like crazy because i exercise for an hour everyday without fail and i have a lot of knowledge about healthy eaing, calories etc. so i know how to eat to lose weight and i do eat like that 80% of the time but because the other 20% is just bingeing i cannot lose weight**..just gain it. Anyways i am vowing as of now to make a rigid effort to stop bingeing, ...**when i was losing before i was posting on here regularly so i think it helps to keep me focused**

From Pam, Age 16 - 10/25/08
Ht. 5'5", Start: 170 lb, Current: 150 lb, Goal: 130 lb - oh my god.. i ate an entire batch of rice crispie treats today.... plus all my other meals. gah...
i feel so terrible!

5. Weight loss plateaus

Many kids have initial success and then are unable to lose additional weight. When kids plateau or level off in their weight loss, they do not understand the physical and psychological reasons that cause plateaus, so they may become discouraged and often quit their weight loss plan. They need to know ahead of time that plateaus will occur.

From Amanda, Age 19 - 01/09/09
Ht. 5'8", Start: 225 lb, Current: 170 lb, Goal: 145 lb - i'm at a loss for words... i **cant GET OFF THIS PLATEAU!** ive been this weight since JUNE. i got down to 167 but i was BARELY eating this summer, then when i ate normal i blew up like a blow fish. ive lost 55 pounds already like as if i cant lose at least another 10. what am i doing wrong i count calories i eat healthy most of the time, and when i dont i include it in my calories. i exercise more than i used to and NOTHING. why do i even bother anymore like am i meant to be this weight or what. ugh sorry for the rant but im so tired of seeing the scale go up or stay the same.

From chelsea, Age 17 - 06/07/09
Ht. 5'6", Start: 208 lb, Current: 178 lb, Goal: 135 lb - **i have hit a COMPLETE plateau**i have neither lost nor gained in over 2 months and i am still trying very hard

What causes these plateaus? Is this a weight "set point" that they can't get beyond? Does their metabolism slow down when they lose weight? Kids lose weight when the number of calories burned up by exercise is greater than those from food eaten. As a result, even though these kids say that they are unable to lose further, they would lose if they were able to eat less and exercise more. There's the rub - they are unable to further resist what is driving them to eat, which is typically emotional (see the following chapters).

Also, as kids become lighter, they burn up fewer calories with exercise, because they are moving less weight around. Furthermore, when kids first lose weight, everyone compliments them and they feel encouraged. Thus, they tend to seek less comfort from food (see Chapter 9 - Comfort Eating). But then the compliments become less frequent, so the kids may once again return to food for comfort. Plateaus result from basically the same reasons that relapses do (see below).

6. Relapse

If kids are able to lose weight, unfortunately most seem to gain the weight back, and more. Why does this happen? Typically, relapses occur because the kids have not learned to deal with the reasons that drive them to overeat to begin with. These reasons include depression, stress, and boredom. These are discussed in the following chapters.

When kids relapse or go off their healthy eating plan, they feel like failures. They need reassurance that this frequently happens and re-enforcement that getting back on track is the best way to head down the road to successful weight loss.

From Tasha, Age 15, female - 4/28/02
On New Year's I vowed to loose 70lbs by the summer. I was 220 lbs, and I excersized for at least 40 mins everyday, followed a strict diet, and lost 10 lbs in a month. I was so excited! I kept going and lost another 5lbs until disaster struck . . . I became heavily depressed for various reasons. **I began eating out of depression and I gained ALL my weight back, if not more.** Recently I decided it wasn't worth it. I went back to my plan and I lost 10 lbs in 2 weeks, and I'm on my way again. I'm happier now, too. You just have to remember that nothing's worth making yourself feel even worse. Don't get careless and have fun while you're doing it, otherwise you won't see results.

From michelle, Age 14 - 10/09/08
Ht. 5'8", Start: 228 lb, Current: 200 lb, Goal: 150 lb - ok **so lost 10 pounds and i've gained it right back im so depressed right now agh** im going to be fat for the rest of my life

From kellina, Age 15 - 4/11/07
Ht. 5'6", Start: 157 lb, Current: 157 lb, Goal: 130 lb - hi ive been to this site before and it really helps but **i have put weight back on and im really down on myself** i can never keep a good eating habit so if anyone has any sugestions plz reply im in desperate need of some weight loss Kellina

From alissa, Age 15 - 12/4/07
Ht. 5'0", Start: 187 lb, Current: 187 lb, Goal: 150 lb - okay ... so u can imagine how i look like a butterball turkey. lol...umm yeah well ... last summer i started going to the gym everyday with my parents. i managed to lose 10 lbs but i didint really change my eating habits. but then school came and **i gain all the weight back and more.** i felt so disgusting and cant believe i let myself go like that...

From April, Age 14 - 4/14/06
Ht. 5.4, Wt. 150 - I always do really good on my healthly eating, then i have something that messes up my whole day, then i start pigging out when i get home thinking that i am going to start to eat good the next day and i do then when i mess up it happens all over again and **i gain the weight back.** How do i stop?

From meghan, Age 13 - 5/5/08
Ht. 5'10", Start: 185 lb, Current: 178 lb, Goal: 159 lb - Grrr it seams like when i ever i say im going to start **i do good then do bad.**

From Jeimi, Age 17 - 2/22/08
Ht. 5'2", Start: 240 lb, Current: 225 lb, Goal: 200 lb - this week has bine horrible it's like **everytime i start well i mess up** i really don't know what to do anymore and **i feel like giving up it's hopeless** idk

From Sierra, Age 14 - 4/26/08
Ht. 5'2", Start: 140 lb, Current: 139 lb, Goal: 110 lb - I feel bad. **I broke my diet yesterday through tempation and laziness....I feel really awful.** and i dont know when I'm gonna lose any weight. I'll just have to keep trying despite temptations.

From Jennifer, Age 18 - 4/25/08
Ht. 5'7", Start: 331 lb, Current: 331 lb, Goal: 300 lb - ...if I tackle my goals in smaller portions I don't become so discouraged and give up. This week was such a mess, **I did good the first 3 days and after that it went downhill**, I just have to build on my will power because **I give in so easily to fatty foods.**

Despite the setbacks of relapses, many kids offer support to others that struggle with it, as in the post below.

Reply from Amanda, Age 19 - 10/09/08
don't get depressed girl, i gained like 6 or 7 pounds in the last 2 weeks because i just got completely sidetracked. but now im trying again and trust me, **its easiest to lose the weight you just gained if you do it right away**. you can definately do it!! i had the same mind frame as you last year, and ive lost about 60 pounds since then. so just keep on trying. who cares how long it takes. you'll be a thin person in the future. good luck :)

Cravings

Kids on the boards say they struggle to resist cravings for food, actually certain types of food. What are cravings? Cravings are what kids feel when they want pleasurable, comforting foods, such as junk food or fast food. Webster's dictionary defines a craving as: "An intense, urgent, or abnormal desire or longing." Webster's definition implies that cravings are not a normal desire. Cravings tend to be antsy, uneasy feelings, and kids may do almost anything to relieve them.

From Kabe, Age 16 - 11/28/07
Ht. 5'4", Start: 155 lb, Current: 155 lb, Goal: 120 lb - **OMG I'm getting so frusturated! It's like no matter what I do, I can't ignoe tha cravings.** I'm at the point where its like whatever. I keep hsving to start over

From sandy, Age 17 - 10/19/06
Ht. 5'6, Wt. 161 - i am new! i know what to do, i guess why i am here is for moral support. you know? sometimes i **just get really bad cravings and it's really hard to fight them.**

From Marshall, Age 12 - 12/01/03
Hi I just wanted to ask if anyone had tips on what to do to control cravings. I just started dieting and now I want chips and sweets more than ever! **My cravings are out of control! I control my cravings now by just not opening the pantry or** fridge. But I feel like I am torturing myself!

Cravings are different from hunger. A craving is an emotion - a desire. Hunger is a physical sensation - the growling, empty feeling in the stomach. Many overweight kids have never felt physical hunger, only emotional hunger.

Reply from Crystal, Age 16 - 12/08/00
Hey, im size 18 ... I want to be happy, and where i am, im not... I eat because im bored and depresssed, not because im hungry... **i dont think ive ever felt hunger in my life actually!**

Food relieves hunger for a much longer period than it does cravings. Cravings may return soon after the pleasurable food is eaten, so that kids continue to eat even when they are full, as the post below illustrates:

From Christine, Age 16 - 10/10/08
Ht. 5'6", Start: 210 lb, Current: 198 lb, Goal: 145 lb - ...I gained back 60 pounds last year and my weight keeps bouncing between 195-210, and my waist keeps going from 39 to about 44 inches -- **ouch!** ... **My problem is that I get TONS of cravings for everything.** I started keeping a food journal, and my calorie range is usually 3000-4000 calories a day, but **I can't stop eating when I'm full and pigging out between meals!** Anyone have any tips for cravings?

Kids don't like cravings.

From Stacy, Age 17 - 09/19/07
Ht. 5'4", Start: 179 lb, Current: 174 lb, Goal: 137 lb - I am having an **extreme craving** for one of the bite size chocolate bars down in my fridge....**UGH!!!!!! i hate urges!**

From Leena, Age 13 - 10/17/05
Ht. 5'6, Wt. 170-ish -....I really want to lose weight but it's really hard with what is in my house. I have no will power! Like, **if there is a candy bar in the** fridge, **I'll see it and be like "no, I don't need it....", then 10 minutes later I come back and eat it! It gets so annoying and I really don't know what to do**

What's causing all these cravings in kids? Cravings are typically seen with alcohol, tobacco, and drugs. How does this relate to food?

The struggle to stop overeating, knowing the dreadful effects of weight gain

Overweight kids say they struggle to resist cravings for food, typically high pleasure 'junk food,' in spite of being fully aware of the terrible effect that being overweight has on their lives and the pain of further weight gain. They feel disgusted after giving in to cravings.

From Anna, Age 16 - 4/25/07
Ht. 5'4", Start: 345 lb, Current: 321 lb, Goal: 290 lb - Okay , so I have been doing kinda bad lately.... **I have been having unbearable cravings, for anything. I just want to eat. so I do, and I feel gross afterwards,** And I've been feeling depressed.

From Jennifer, Age 18 - 3/27/08 -
Ht. 5'7", Start: 320 lb, Current: 320 lb, Goal: 280 lb - Hey guys! I'm not new to this site but I have returned to make a last and final attempt at losing this weight but first i'm not setting big goals anymore because I realize that I fail at that...**I am a sucker for candy, ice cream, pop and cookies, it is going to be soooo hard** but I'm determined to enjoy my sophmore year of college, **i'm tired of being the "fat girl out".**

From aimee, Age 13 - 1/2/08 -
Ht. 5'6", Start: 14 stone 7, Current: 14 stone 7 (203 lb.), Goal: 11 stone - hi, ireally need help. i've tried losing weight so many times i feel it'e impossible... **i think my main promblem is snacking, i snack in between almost every meal and i know i need to stop it's the temptation,** how do i stop the temtation exspecily in the winter, i need real help with this. PLEASE HELP ME!!!!!!

From Rachael, Age 16 - 4/22/08 -
Ht. 5'7", Start: 221 lb, Current: 213 lb, Goal: 180 lb - I have been wanting to lose weight for a while... Now I'm to the point where **it's making me angry.** I want it off more than anything... **My biggest problem is portioning**...it's how much of it I take and what I take. I'm eating too much of the wrong kinds of food... The biggest reason **I want to lose the weight is so I can excel in sports.**

This is KAELYN's story:
I get very depressed when I think about my weight and the doctor said that I am overwight for my age. I am a **15 yr old girl and weigh 190 pounds.** I want to weigh at

least 120 pounds but whenever I go on a diet, **I end up eating the wrong things.** I need help. **I get made fun of when I go to school because of my weight.**

From Nailpolish , Age 14 - 3/22/08
Ht. 5'5", Start: 187 lb, Current: 176 lb, Goal: 130 lb - oh **i don't know if i can do this any more.** I have gained a pound plus i have been excising like crazy. But **im always hungry now , and still can't stop eating during the day and night.** I think it will be better when i go back to school on monday cuz i was on spring break. I guess is i lose the pounds then its all worth it. ...I just hope that i can get all of it off by high school, becuse ever sceice 4th grade it was all like, you know kids were just mean. And now in middle school they don't call you fat, they just do it in different ways, so i want that to change in high school. You know also **im 14 and i have never had a bf. I think its cuz im fat, YEAH stright up im fat.** BLAH =[[[im just makeing my self sad. ugggh

These kids don't understand why they are unable to lose weight, even though they hate being fat.

From Jessica, Age 13 - 2/1/08 -
Ht. 5'0", Start: 153 lb, Current: 158 lb, Goal: 120 lb - Hi guys. I gained 5 pounds in 1 month... I'm about to start crying. **WHY CAN'T I LOOSE WEIGHT?** :` -

Anna, Age 14, 3/20/08 - Ht. 5'2.0", Goal 165.0 lb, Start 191.0 lb, Last 172.0 lb,Today 173.2 lb - **I don't understand why I can't lose weight**

From Jeimi, Age 17 - 12/27/07
Ht. 5'2", Start: 240 lb, Current: 228 lb, Goal: 120 lb - ...i've felt a little helpless latley i've messed up yesterday and today i just kept going and workedout really hard but idk **i feel like i'm never going to lose weight and it makes me really upset** i feel like i'm going to be this way 4ever and i don't want to it hurts when i mess up because this is something i've wanted since i can remember **i feel ugly and not worthy sometimes** i really want to loss weight to feel better about myself and messing up all the time doesn't help me confidence... just had to get all that out.

From Jeimi, Age 17 - 12/18/07 -
Ht. 5'2", Start: 240 lb, Current: 230 lb, Goal: 180 lb - hey everyone i did really good yesterday untill about 8 or 9 acolck came i sware idk what happen to me **it's like i couldn't stop eating** i mean i ate 2 plates of coco pebils i felt really bad but the worst part is that i feel like eating everything right now **i don't understand why i get this feeling i'm trying to fight it** i brushed my teeth and i just keep telling myself it will all be worth it at the end but it's so hard well i just had to let this out because **if i don't i think i would eat my whole frige.**

From Lola, Age 13 - 12/11/07 -
Ht. 5'0", Start: 156 lb, Current: 167 lb, Goal: 132 lb - Hi i am Lola and i am new here. As you can see i am very overweight over 40 pounds.and i really want to loose weight. **i just cant seem to stop overeating every time i eat i find myself eating huge portions and plates of them. i also got a huge sweet tooth and love junk food. i just cant seem to stop.**also i **have no phisical exersize whatsoever its too hard.**my daily diet is usually a penut butter and jelly sandwitch subble decker,and two eggs for breakfast, two pan self pan pizza and a bag of chips for lunch and then greasy greassy mexican food(home made from my mom)i also eat snacks between meals then my midnight snack is a tripel decker penut buter sandwhich and chocolate milk and two muffins and a big cookie. i know i know no wonder i am this fat! also i always have a choclate bar and some gum uring school too.please help me befor i get even more fat!!!

From Jeimi, Age 17 - 12/8/07
Ht. 5'2", Start: 240 lb, Current: 225 lb, Goal: 180 lb - omg i feel horbbile **i just can't stop eating as much as i try** i just went back to my old habbits i hate myself for it but i'm still going to keep trying i made a promise to myself that this is going to be a life style thanks for listening guys **i know i can always come here and write it really helps** ttyl

From *Sarah*, Age 15 - 11/27/07 -
Ht. 5'5", Start: 146 lb, Current: 150 lb, Goal: 130 lb - why can't i commit?! **if food is there i just eat it** and i get caught up in the moment thinking of how good it tastes. then **the next day i go to school and hate myself cause i'm fat.** please i need some kind of inspiration! i have tons of homework today but i'm gonna try to jump rope for 20 minutes later.

From Jeimi, Age 16 - 11/8/07 -
Ht. 5'2", Start: 240 lb, Current: 230 lb, Goal: 180 lb - **i really don't understand why i can't stick to my diets i'm so mad at myself and it's frustrating i really don't know what to do with myself. i just can't stop eating i hate it so much** but i'm going to keep trying because i really want to lose weight.

From Sophie, Age 17 - 11/17/07 -
Ht. 5'0", Start: 163 lb, Current: 163 lb, Goal: 106 lb - **I am about at the end of my rope. I am so tired of failing,** guys. I need inspiration and motivation. **I want to be skinny so I can feel better about myself and be healthier,** but how can I do that if **I'm always messing up?! I don't even know what to do any more.** Advice?

Above are many postings saying "I can't stop" or "I can't control myself." What the heck's happening here? What's the cause of all this? Is it the type of food these kids are exposed *to? Is it that there's just too much food available? Is it that the kids just don't **know** how to eat healthy?*

Barriers to kids' weight loss efforts

Junk food

Kids say that 'junk food' is especially hard to resist.

From Sam, Age 14 - 6/16/08
Ht. 5'0", Start: 150 lb, Current: 140 lb, Goal: 115 lb - okay well i guess ill start off with saying that i've been up and down the scale since i was 13.i lost 10 pds last yr,and i stopped and now,im trying to get back on track.well,i've been walking 2 miles everyday on the treadmill,but **i cant stop eating junk food.and it's totally killing me.**if anybody had tips or if u just wanna talk,post back and ill give you my email adress.or just post back and leave tips.ALL will be appreciated. thanks.

From Chloe, Age 16 - 1/9/08
Ht. 5'9.0", Goal 160.0 lb, Start 240.0 lb, Last 240.0 lb Today 240.0 lb - **Ive been eating lots and lots of junk food, i cant seem to stop eating it.** But ive teamed up with a friend and we are going to push eachother to lose weight.

From Anna , Age 14 - 11/8/07 -
Ht. 5'2", Start: 203 lb, Current: 169 lb, Goal: 125 lb - Did anyone watch the cma's last night. **I'm doing good on my diet until I see junk food then I'm horrible at it.** How is everyone else doing

From sabina, Age 16 - 10/28/06
Ht. 5'6, Wt. 157 - i was so bad today. i had been really good for almost two weeks then my mom bought pizza, and bought ice cream. you see the thing with dominos is one slice tastes good, but it never fills me up, so i keep eating and then the damn icecream was what nearly killed me. i have the worst **addiction** to strawberry icecream. my mother thinks the fact i'm on a diet is funny, and i should really just exercise. **Good i hate that junk food tastes good!!!**

From Lisa, Age 15 - 11/8/07 -
Ht. 5'6", Start: 175 lb, Current: 162 lb, Goal: 130 lb - WELL, I HAVE NOT BEEN DOING GOOD AT ALL....I HAVE TOTALLY GOTTEN OFF TRACK... I HAVEN'T LOST ANY WEIGHT AT ALL. **I JUST DON'T KNOW HOW TO TELL MYSELF NO TO JUNK FOOD.** I ALSO WANT TO GO RUNNING IN THE MORNING, I JUST CAN'T SEEM TO BE ABLE TO DO THAT EITHER! I NEED MOTIVATION

Holidays

Holidays are particularly hard on kids who are trying to lose weight or maintain it.

From Jill, Age 15 - 1/1/08
Ht. 5'0", Start: 155 lb, Current: 157 lb, Goal: 135 lb - Around the **holidays** I seem to gain a lot of weight. **There are just too many temptations. Sweets, pop, anything junk food. I seem to get drawn to it like a fly to a light.** I need to lose weight. It's really **hurting my self esteem** and **it's hard to concentrate in school**. I keep telling myself that I will start... but it never happens.

From Julie, Age 14 - 11/10/07
Ht. 5'6", Start: 166 lb, Current: 150 lb, Goal: 130 lb - ugh i feel so bad **i was doing so good and then i just ate a bunch of halloween candy. ugh.** im such a fat ugly pig! **i hate halloween!!!!!!!!!!!** And yesterday the guy i like went on this big rant in class on how he hates fat people and that we should tie twinkies to the end of tredmiles to makes us lose weight so i feel even worse now!!!!! ugh!

From sk8ergirl, Age 16 - 3/24/08 -
Ht. 5'2", Start: 221 lb, Current: 189 lb, Goal: 160 lb - I gained 3 pounds in three days! I am freaking out! My appetite got bigger! **I am eating way too much junk** and its all **thanks to easter! I HATE HOLIDAYS NOW!!!** I am back where I started last week! I NEED more motivation right now!!

From Jeimi, Age 16 - 11/21/07 -
Ht. 5'2", Start: 240 lb, Current: 230 lb, Goal: 180 lb - omg i'm so mad at myself i **ate like a pig.There was a thanksgiving share at my school 2day** and at first i didn't eat any food at all but when it came to the dissert i pigged donuts cookies cake i went wild **it's like couldn't control it** ... well thanks u guys always listen sort of lol

From Mandy, Age 16 - 11/23/07 -
Ht. 5'7", Start: 206 lb, Current: 160 lb, Goal: 135 lb - .... **im glad we dont have thanksgiving in australia i dont think i would b able to handle** it rigth now :/

From Jeimi, Age 17 - 1/1/08
Ht. 5'2", Start: 240 lb, Current: 225 lb, Goal: 180 lb - hey ya well yesterday was really bad from pizza to cake to cookies **it was just very bad but it was new years eve** so i can;t let it get to me ...my aunt made me feel bad this morning because she said if i were you i would get an operation i really do believe in myself and i think this is my year to make a change... happy 2008 everyone

From Jane, Age 12 - 11/08/07 - IP#: 24.2.157.xxx
Ht. 4'9", Start: 140 lb, Current: 136 lb, Goal: 110 lb - **I am worried about thanksgiving.** My grandparents always want us to eat more and more.

From Suzan, Child's Age 14 - 7/8/04 -
My teenage **daughter** is over weight and **she comes to me for help but I just don't know how to help her** and what to tell her to do. She did loose about 8 pounds for a little bit but then **she gained it back because of easter** and everything and she said that since then she hasn't been able to loose anymore.

Healthy eating information

Does teaching kids about healthy eating and exercise help in their struggle to lose weight? Currently, the primary professional approach for dealing with overweight and obesity in kids is healthy eating education and exercise programs. As discussed in Chapter 1, in 2007, the U.S. Expert Committee on the Assessment, Prevention and Treatment of Child and Adolescent Overweight and Obesity issued new recommendations, which included: 1) "Five or more servings of fruits and vegetables per day," 2) "No sugar-sweetened beverages," and 3) "Eat a healthy breakfast."

The below poll was also presented in Chapter 1 and is included here again to emphasize the point. (http://www.blubberbuster.com/cgi/poll_new_85.cgi)

Do you think information on healthy eating helps you to lose weight?

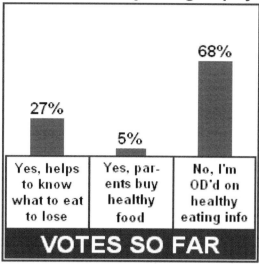

88 kids voted

More than two thirds of the 88 kids responding indicate that they're "overdosed" with information on healthy eating. They instead need information on how to resist cravings.

And most have learned healthy eating information in school.

Have you learned healthy eating info in school?

YES: 55 votes (62%)

NO: 33 votes (38%)

Consequently, healthy eating information does not appear to significantly help these kids in their struggle to lose weight and maintain it.

Further posts of the struggles of overweight kids may be found at:

http://www.weigh2rock.com/struggles

The puzzle

Why do overweight kids struggle so much to lose weight and to maintain it, even though they hate being fat? Why is losing weight so difficult? What's really going on here?

The posts in the next chapter shed light on this perplexing puzzle.

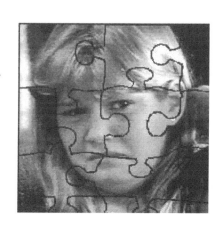

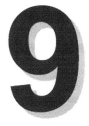

9 | Comfort Eating

Why do overweight kids struggle?

The previous chapter exposed the striking struggles of overweight kids trying to lose weight. Why do these kids struggle so much to lose weight?

Many of the kids say that they seek comfort from pleasurable food when depressed, sad, rejected, disappointed, angry, lonely, or anxious.

Age 14, female, 5'7", 280 lbs - **I eat to make myself feel better...its coping.**

Age 13, female, 5'7", 223 lb.: **Everyone I know practically soothes emotions with food!**

The problem is that the kids may become hooked, i.e. psychologically dependent, on this 'comfort eating' behavior and may be unable to stop, even though they become unintentionally overweight or obese because of it.

From ChElssEa, Age 13 - 04/03/05
I hate when I comfort eat but i do it alot and i just cant stop it that and i eat when im bored I DONT KNOW HOW TO STOP ITS KILLING ME

Comfort food

Age 12, female, 5' 1'', 108 lbs - **Junk food=comfort food. food listens to our problems. its like a therapist.**

What is "comfort food?" Comfort food is any food that soothes unpleasant emotions, typically foods that taste really good, sweet and creamy, like many so-called 'junk foods.' According to the Modern Marvels "American Eats" TV series, ice cream is one of the top comfort foods. When I was 8 years old I recall playing in my first little league baseball game, which was a night game. I was pretty nervous, and my parents were watching. It was the bottom of the ninth, two outs, the score was tied, and I was covering center field. Suddenly, there was a high pop fly ball. I looked up and tried to spot the ball, but I was blinded by the glaring field lights. The ball landed just behind me. Still blinded, I struggled to find the ball in the dark and finally managed to heave it to the infield. But by then the other team had scored, and we lost. I was devastated. After the game, I slowly walked up to my parents, head down. I will never forget what my mom said: "It's okay, we'll go get ice cream – that'll make you feel better."

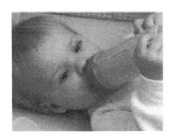

Parents frequently use a bottle to soothe an irritable infant. They may continue to use food to comfort the child, so that the child learns to use food to cope with bad feelings.

Or kids may learn on their own to use food for comfort, at any age, as the below post describes:

From Anastasya Izhik, Age 18 - 6/13/06
Ht. 5'5, Wt. 260 lbs - **i'm afflicted with emotional eating!!!**ever since 12 years old, **every time im stressed out or feeling down, uncool, i start eating** (binging on sugary/fatty stuff), even if i'm not hungry. right now i'm pressured to study for 2 exams, 1 test and write an isp essay. i cant deal with myself - deep into the binge of cheese, peanut butter and cookies. i despise myself, and feel like dying, way more miserable than before. every day i try to give myself another chance, a new beginning, and **fail miserably at the slightest thoughts of uncoolness.** i'm terrible, i know i'm a frigging pig and cant be respected. please gimme some tips against emotional eating or binge - eating disorder. i'm such a jellyfish, i have no will power or self control whatsoever. i'm probably going to eat myself to death.

Age 11, female, 5", 140 lbs - i eat all day even whens thier nothing else to eat. i'll make an food out of no food at all **m not even hungry just bored and depresed**

Numbing unpleasant feelings

From Stacy, Age 17 - 04/08/08 - IP#: 141.158.143.xxx
Ht. 5'4", Start: 184 lb, Current: 178 lb, Goal: 140 lb - … Im soo aggrivated with myself. I want/need to lose weight and yet **ill just keep eating those choc bars to numb whatever feelings i have at that moment.** Maybe its the weather. Maybe its stress from school and work. I dk. Im just upset. TOMORROW IS A NEW DAY! I SWEAR! I'M GETTING BACK ON TRACK!!!

Many kids say that they 'use' food to avoid feeling bad emotions.

This is KAY 's story:
I am **14** (turning 15 in june). **I weigh 330 pounds**. I was never the skinnest kid or anything when I was younger but I wasn't nessarrilly heavy either. Then about 5 or 6 years ago **my mom found out she had cancer. I got really scared and depressed. I started to use food as a krutch for my feelings.** I would give anything to go back and not do what I did but unfortunatly I can't...I can't do anything without worrying what people think about me. I hate shoping because mostly the cloths don't fit. I love to swim and Im good at it but I don't go to the pool because I can't find a bathing suit that fits. More than what people think or have to say about me I want to be heathy. I don't want to be the girl any more that has to take a break from running because my chest hurts and Im out of breath. I don't want to be the girl who just barely fits in the desks at school. I don't want to be the girl that can only go on certian rides at an amusement park because the seat belt won't fit. Im tired of being the fat girl. Im tired of being obess. Could you please help me?

From Megan, Age 18 - 3/23/08 -
Ht. 5'4", Start: 180 lb, Current: 175 lb, Goal: 140 lb - I am so tired of always being the fattest person. i always want to dress cute and things but nothing ever fits. I am tired of avoiding things because i'm not sure i can do it. **I am an emotional eater so i eat to avoid what im feeling**. sometimes food carries me through the day. my senior ball and graduation are coming up soon and i really want to be able to get a pretty dress as well as a date!!! I just can't force myself to lose the weight. any suggestions or thoughts?

From Whitney, Age 15 - 9/4/06 -
Ht. 5'4, Wt. 236 - I'm at the end of my ropes I just wanna die!!!! I hate my life life I'm just a dying cow and the world would be way better without me! My mom always tells me i'm fat and all my dad cares about is my perfect 5'6 115pound varsity soccer player sister........... **I take out all my emotions out on food**. I need help or i'll be dead soon!!!!!!!!!!!!!!!!!

From Kat, Age 15 - 6/22/06 -
Ht. 5,8, Wt. 183 - Well,i keep trying to loose weight but it keeps finding me..lol. I try over and over again but i just cant stick to a diet!..i **get bored.or sad and then BANG there i am gettin food again even when i am well over full ugh**

From tamara, Age 12 - 7/12/08
Ht. 5'6", Start: 166.6 lb, Current: 166 lb, Goal: 136.5 lb - I've been called fat all my life. **I have to suck in my stomac every time I see a boy**. I want to be small because I look at all my friends and it hurts me when people rather look at them then the big people. You normally cant get a boy friend when their freinds say behind your back "Look at the new kid she so fat Haha"! A small boy came up to me and said I was fat. You look at TV and see all the Thin, happy people that show off their bodies by bikini's and tight shrits. All the small kids dont know what It's like to lose weight. **I eat because my**

sadness and anger. My sadness was because back in VA kids would call me Ugly and fat right in frount of me and that makes me sooooo angery and sad more than thin kids think... I looked on the internet to see and everything ignored me, but I found this website and seeing all these kids and all the weight they lost and I actully cried because their problemly went through the same missery as I'm suffering and I thought I was the only one, but I'm not and NOW, THIS YEAR I'M GOING TO PROVE ALL THE KIDS THAT CALLED ME NAMES WERE STUPID AND WRONG were all the same inside, but soo diferent on the Outside.

This is SARAH's story:
Hi my name is sarah. I am 12 years old and in have been overwieght all my life i am realy over wieght i wiegh about **197 pounds** now i have alot of musel on my legs but people still tease me all the time it sucks going to the malll and the shirt you want being to small. i cant wear bikinis when all my other friends are wearing them... what ca i do to lose wieght i always tell myself i am going to lose the wieght but then **i get sad and i eat i alkways eat when i am boared or sad which is all the time** i live in california and my mom lives in virgina which sucks.

From krista , Age 12 - 3/14/06 -
Ht. 5"7, Wt. 273 - ppl i realy need help **evertime i think about my dead grandma i go to food for comfort** adn i dont wanna ruin everything i did ppl plz i really need help i think i am gonna just like starve myself

From Ashley, Age 17 - 2/11/06 -
Ht. 5'5, Wt. 190 - ... I have been overwieght for the majority of my life. I have tried to kepp high spirits but it gets hard when people say things that hurt your feelings. I love food there is no doubt about that but **i also eat when i am stressed or my feelings are hurt, kinda like comfort i guess...**

This is ANGEL's question: **I eat when i am tired, stressed out, angry, sad, and esp. board**, i dont know how to stop that. I dont like sports, cant find any jobs, friends are always busy, i do talk on the phone, watch tv, and stuff but it doesnt stop me from going int he cuboards. .. I dont know what to do i have so many problems and so many blank answers. I hope you can help me threw this even though you are busy!thanks for your time~

From Jason, Age 13 - 1/30/08 -
Ht. 5'2", Start: 203 lb, Current: 200 lb, Goal: 165 lb - I am very obese...The other kids in the locker room make fun of me. **This makes me very angry which makes me overeat alot.**

From michel'   ther, Age 13 - 1/3/00
Ht. 5'8", Star r: 227 lb, Current: 207 lb, Goal: 130 lb - ok i discovered something i
not only eat when im depressed but when im bored too how do i stop help.............taco luv

This is ALYSSA's story:
I cant stop   ating what do i do? **i eat when im bored and when im sad, im an emotional
eater.** i reall want to have a nice body! help me!

From Isabella, Age 14 - 11/12/07 -
Ht. 5'6", Start: 184 lb, Current: 180 lb, Goal: 145 lb - Hi! I know it's been months
since I've been on for those of you who might remember me. Life's been crazy, and my
weight has suffered as a result. Over the summer **I was going though a rough time with
a family so food became my crutch**... I'm really not happy with my body. I feel horrible
about myself... **I hate feeling being out of control around food.** It makse me feel like I
don't have power over anything.

From Bryce, Age 12 - 11/9/07 -
Ht. 5'5", Start: 157 lb, Current: 157 lb, Goal: 130 lb - Hey guys, I just found this
sight and my java connection aint workin so I can't use the chatroom :P I feel really
overweight. I wasn't always **it's just I got really depressed when my mom and dad died
and tried to eat away pain.** ..any tips or someone to help me please email me. I REALLY
want help, I'm desperate.

From Marisa, Age 10 - 10/12/07 -
Ht. 4'7", Start: 133 lb, Current: 133 lb, Goal: 100 lb - **I feel depressed! I think I
am en emotional eater. I eat whenever I feel sad.** There have been about 10 people in
my family that have died lately. My grandpa died last year and I miss him so much. I also
get made fun of at school becuase I am overweight. People call me names and say mean
things. I try not to let it bother me, but it does! I want friends who accept me for who I
am.

From Abby, Age 16 - 9/18/07 -
Ht. 5'5", Start: 170 lb, Current: 164 lb, Goal: 140 lb - **I know how to lose weight.
You eat less and exercise more.** I have gained and loss weight a million times. But right
now my biggest struggle is finding the motivation to lose weight. **I have been really sad
lately and have been overeating because of it.** I need some words of encouragement to
get me right on track. Anything or any advice will be greatly appreciated.

From Ashley, Age 13 - 5/28/07 -
Ht. 5'7", Start: 198 lb, Current: 195 lb, Goal: 170 lb - It's hard 4 me 2 lose weight
because when i go 2 the fridge and see something real good i have 2 eat it...**I do eat when**

i'm bored or depressed i have 2 do something 2 occupy me so i don't think about food... I want to be skinny so i can be able 2 weare bikins and stuff.Plus more guys would like me!

From mary, Age 15 - 2/13/07 -
Ht. 5'3", Wt. 158 - My family is driving me crazy!! **I am an emotional overeater, so when someone makes me mad, or if im sad, then i eat.** My mom made me soo made today that i ate like 10 hersheys kisses and 3 oreos. Im so **stressed out** right now. Ive already gained like 8 pounds the past 10 dayz cuz my dad has been back from a militry deployment so my mom bought a bunch of junk food. So, yeah im fat and **im stressed and im mad** at my mom, and **i want to eat**. Hope everyone else is doing dandy!

Age 12, female, 5ft, 150 lbs - **its hard for us fat kids to give up food!! its so good and comforting.**but i know i have to stop. - I'm worried about overweight shortening my life.

Cravings

The brain's need for comfort or stress relief can come out as 'cravings' for pleasurable foods. The pleasure or action of eating will satisfy this craving, although only briefly.

From megan, Age 14 - 6/5/05 -
Ht. 5'5", Wt. 168 - **I'm trying my hardest to fight the food cravings..** I keep picking it up and putting it back down again.. **It's when I get sad or stressed that I eat** :(wish me luck

Denial?

Some kids appear to be in denial that they eat for comfort. The below teen says, "i even gain weight when i dont eat." But she does believe that her overweight is due to depression.

From Jessica, Age 15 - 09/19/08
Ht. 5'4", Start: 195 lb, Current: 195 lb, Goal: 140 lb -...just last year i started gaining and gaining. & i dont understand because **i dont sit and stuff my face with bad food. i even gain weight when i dont eat;** and it just all makes no sence to me. ...i dont know what wrong with me. im rly athletic, so i dont know how i weigh this much. **i guess its from depression bc my mom has just got cancer, so i have been gaining like crazy.** people help, i dont want to be like this anymore!

Many overweight kids recognize that they eat for comfort - to cope with depression, fear, anger, disappointment, rejection. But, do they know what to do to avoid using food for comfort, so that they can lose weight, and does the health professional community offer suggestions for how to avoid comfort eating?

Food is my friend

Some kids say that food is their friend, even their best friend.

From Itzel, Age 13 - 5/13/07 -
Ht. 5'0", Start: 165 lb, Current: 190 lb, Goal: 118 lb - Have any of your Gym teachers made fun of you because your the slowest one in running? it happened to me today! we were running and my teacher said come on we want to loose weight or dowe want to be overweight like her? every one started to laugh i got so embaressed. then she said i'm just joking but should loose some weight. how rude am i right **i got home and started fealling depressed and eating a whole bucket of ice cream with two bottels of soda and cookies.**do you guys think that i will ever loose weight i dont think so i am just too lazy,fat,tired,and bord to make a big commitment like that.**i love food so much that i can never let it go i think it is like my best friend!**i constently think about it like what is for breakfast lunch and dinner and inetween meals i eat snacks all the time

From jane, Age 17, female - 7/5/06
I haven't always been overweight...Everything changed when I was 8 years old and moved clear across America. Without any friends, and both my parents always at work **I fell into a depression and used sugary foods, soda, and the television to comfort myself. Little Debbie Snacks, and Coke became my best friend since I had no real ones**... I had swelled up to a grand total of **240 lbs** when I entered my freshman year of high school... I am **5'5"**

Giving up comfort food often represents a major loss – essentially grief – similar to losing a best friend or favorite pet.

From Julia, Age 12 - 11/17/06 -
Ht. 5'5", Wt. 178 - I am so worried about **Thanksgiving. I mean, it'll be a MAJOR loss if I don't eat all those luscious foods**.... juicy turkey... creamy mashed potatoes... whipped creamed pumpkin pie.... oh ya! PLEASE HELP I'M GONNA GAIN LIKE 20 POUNDS!!! It's happened before. =(

Emotional eating idea may be offensive

Some kids are offended by the emotional eating idea as a reason for overweight.

From Ben, Age 13 - 01/23/09
Ht. 5'8", Start: 234 lb, Current: 212 lb, Goal: 150 lb - Well, **I never thought I was an emotional eater...I know that I'm a bored eater, but emotional, ugh...** I just...can't resist the foods my parents buy...I feel...mad when I know I have a stomach full of junk...and I'll get small portions of alot of things...Like, 2 cookies of this, a few table spoons of this, and a few chips, and then a few minutes later, I'll do the same thing...

From Mikayla, Age 15 - 05/22/06
Ht. 5'4, Wt. Too much - **I hate how the "school" on this website basically refers to overweight people as primarily "emotional eaters."** Even Lucy on the chat room does this. **Have they ever considered that stress and no free time to work off calories may have been part of it??** How about **genetics?** It annoys me how all the tips are for emotional eaters, when not all of us are. Does anyone else agree?

The below reply by a teen to the above post shows keen insight....

Reply from Shan, Age 19 - 05/22/06
stress is an emotion! And genetics is part of it but you need the lifestyle to become overweight. **If you don't eat emotionally, then why else do you overeat?** You don't need much food to stop being hungry. Also, this is what's wrong with the population so this is what the site focuses on... Sorry I don't wanna be rough these are jjust my opinions.

We therefore did a poll on this.
(http://www.blubberbuster.com/cgi/poll_new_61_percent.cgi)

What do you think about emotional eating as the cause of overweight in children and teens?

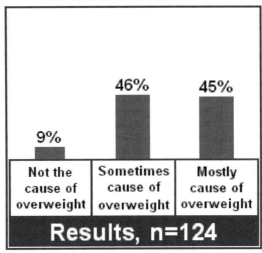

124 Kids voted

Nearly all of the 124 kids voting feel that emotional eating is sometimes, or mostly, the cause of overweight in children and teens. We further asked if talking about emotional eating offends them and if they themselves eat for emotional reasons.

Does talking about emotional eating offend you?

   YES: 12 votes (10%)

    NO: 112 votes (90%)

Do you think that you eat for emotional reasons?

   YES: 76 votes (61%)

    NO: 48 votes (39%)

The results of the above poll reveal an opportunity for health professionals to help overweight kids deal with emotional reasons for overeating. Most kids responding say they eat for emotional reasons, and those kids responding, at least, don't mind talking about it. Teaching kids to express their emotions and deal with them head on, instead of numbing them with the pleasure of food is a topic of discussion where health professionals could make a difference.

Addiction?

So, what's going on here? What's happening when kids seek comfort in pleasurable food and are unable to stop, even though they hate that they have become fat? What do kids say about this? Many kids actually say they are "addicted" to pleasurable food.

From Amanda, Age 15 - 2/2/06 -
Ht. 5'4'', Wt. too depressing :'(- ... i need to lose like 150lbs... before i always wanted to lose weight so people would like be but now i want to do it for myself, so ill like myself.. **i have a food addiction, im a binge compulsive eater** and this is my 1st time posting here.. it seems helpful and i hope it will help me but its going to be so hard..

From Laura, Age 17 - 8/29/07 -
Ht. 5'2", Start: 231 lb, Current: 231 lb, Goal: 150 lb - Hey everyone, I have finally realized that I need to take some serious action about my weight problem. I have tried so many times before to lose the weight and nothing has worked... **I love to eat, even when**

I'm not hungry I eat... once I start eating I just want more and more! **Food is a total addiction to me**, how do I stop it???

From Nailpolish, Age 14 - 03/04/08
Ht. 5'5", Start: 187 lb, Current: 185 lb, Goal: 130 lb - ..if i want to make a life style change like this then i have to take baby steps and im not going to give up everything at once. So i geuss i have to take that into consideration. Like right now i just want to go and raid the fridge. **I am addicted to food**. And honstly i think im going to get something to **eat after this just out of boredum its hard not too**. Its very late so maybe i just need to go to bed and see how i do tomarrow. Was it hard like this for everyone at first?

From Alicia, Age 14 - 9/10/06
Ht. 5'3, Wt. Idk - ughhh ive finally discovered my problem: **IM ADDICTED TO EATING**. For example, I'll have lunch..then eat a cookie..then a few minutes i'll go back and get another cookie..etc..i cant stop !! HELP?!?!

From Heather, Age 13 - 10/9/06 -
Ht. 5'0, Wt. 185 - I'm having a horrible time. Haven't lost weight in a few months. Starting to gain a few pounds. Now my clothes aren't fitting as nicely. I don't want to revert back to my old ways so I am going to force myself to start going on walks again with my dog and then do 30 minutes on the treadmill or eliptical with some weights and stuff. My eating was getting out of control too. **I haven't had junkfood in a few months, but i had some at a party and i've forgotten how addicting it can be.**

From Lexi, Age 14 - 8/26/07
Ht. 5'1", Start: 140 lb, Current: 180 lb, Goal: 100 lb - i try to lose weight but i just impossible **im addicted to food** i cant stick to a diet **wen people pick on me i eat loads** which is ever day ... **i'd got loads of stretch marks and i hate it. i look huge and i hate it**

From Claire, Age 18 - 5/29/07 -
Ht. 5'4", Start: 210 lb, Current: 162 lb, Goal: 130 lb - It's getting hot so it's beginning to get even harder to avoid ice cream. I put a little ice-cream (about 2 scoops) in a small bowl and then after that I began craving more and I tried to stop myself but I just found myself going bcak to the freezer and puting in 2 more scoops this time bigger. I mean what the freak is my problem? **I hate how sugar is so addictive** and now I feel like a fat idiot. I could've controlled myself but I didn't! just because I wanted more..I went and got some. I know I shouldn't dwell on it now that the damage is done but I really wanted to get back on track. It seems that I keep screwing up, just when I'm doing good!

This is LIZABET's story:
hi, i am really overweight and i need help. i gain like 3 pounds in 1 day everyday, i am like

lawrence cause i am good at a spory but i cant do the runnin, i play hocky and i m 1 of the best players in the school at hittin but as i am real fat i cant run or if i do i get really out of breath quickly. **my current weight is around 560 pounds!!** that is so fat. i need help badly, i know i should eat less than i do and i know i should cut it in 1/2 but **i just cant seem to it. i eat aat mcdonalds everyday** and i always order the biggest thing in the shop and **i am adicttied** and **i cant stop goin and when i did i felt ill all the time** so plz can u give me sometips on how to lose all of my extra weight, thanxs:)

From hannah, Age 15 - 11/28/05
Ht. 5'3, Wt. 308 - Hi, i'm 15 i live in england and i am 22 stone!!! thats **308 pounds.** I have no friends, because people dont want to know anyone who is fat. I am so depressed that my school work is suffering. People laugh and stare at me when i go out.**I am addicted to food.I spend all my money on it-macdonalds,kfc,burgerking. I cant help myself.** Even my old friends are begining to get embarrassed I but i am disgusting. Does anyone know of a cheaper than usual wieght loss camp. Please help me. or just chat.

From chris , Age 13 - 4/24/08
Ht. 5'8", Start: 198 lb, Current: 199 lb, Goal: 170 lb - hi im really worried i weighed myselfto day and ive put on another pound im nearly over 200 pounds im 13 whats goin on **does anyone know how to get unhooked of fatty foods because im addicted to mcdonalds** (infact im goin there with my mates for dinner)and chocolate i love chocolate so much i use a least 1500 of my calories a day to chocolate some times i dont mind being fat because i have an excuse to eat loads but when i do swimming at school or go on holiday i dont feel right because i can feel my belly wobbling and everyone elses body is like WHOAH and all the girls go up to them and go look at his abs and when they see me they just think dont go near his fat might swallow us up i need help please reply

From Bianca, Age 13 - 7/10/06
Ht. 5'8, Wt. really big - I hate looking at myself and thinking that Im pretty and healthy when in reality i am not. **I am addicted to fatty and sweet foods. Especially pizza, ice cream, soda, and chocolate.** I dont have any exercise machines but yet i dont know what to do. I wan to be skinny for prom, or graduation, or my friends quincenera. I wanna be able to shop anywhere and I find the size that fits me. Please help me and I will help you too....i am desperate and I need to lose major weght!!!!! HELP ME!!!!!! (my weight problems sometimes led to suicide thoughts)

From Stephen, Age 15 - 5/22/07
Ht. 5'7", Start: 240 lb, Current: 233 lb, Goal: 125 lb - I am 15 years old. I don't know why I eat so much. I am trying to lose weight by eating three-four Lean Cuiseans a day with water and veggies. **I have an addiction and I don't know how to cut it.** My parents tell me eat more veggies. I ate an entire bag of salad without dressing and it didn't phase me at all, I just want more. What I am I to do? Please help. Steve

From Amanda, Age 14 - 10/09/09
Ht. 5'0", Start: 260 lb, Today: 304 lb, Goal: 100 lb - **I think I'm ADDICTED to FOOD,** ... I TRY to eat RIGHT but I go CRAZY until I eat stuff that TASTES GOOD!

From Michelle, Age 14 - 5/24/07
Ht. 5'7", Start: 182 lb, Current: 182 lb, Goal: 130 lb - Hi. I used to post here a lot, but I stopped for a while. Since not posting here, I've gained 32 pounds. Yeah.... Not good. I figure posting here will help bring it back down. **I have a candy addiction.** Don't have a problem with fast food, **candy is my Kryptonite.** I'm very active, on a swim team and other sports, it's just the startling amounts of sugar that does it.... Suggestions?

Even a 12 year old...

From lisa, Age 12 - 08/04/08
Ht. 5'11", Start: 200 lb, Current: 185 lb, Goal: 160 lb - eh i wanna lose weight but i **have a problem i drink starbucks everyday.. im adicted.** and i love cupe cakes i eat 2 or3 a week.. ugh i need help

Interestingly, Starbucks was described at the 2008 European Congress on Obesity as, "a candy bar in a cup."

From Jennifer, Age 16 - 08/05/09
Ht. 5'8", Start: 211 lb, Current: 228 lb, Goal: 140 lb - Hi. It's me again! Still no good news. I'm eating like mad. And I'm gaining. **It feels like I'm addicted to food.** I have to eat until I'm full. And then I eat again, perhaps an hour later. I'm getting so fat. It seems there's no way out.

And they may simply give up, as the teen above relates below...

From Jennifer, Age 16 - 08/07/09
Ht. 5'8", Start: 211 lb, Current: 229 lb, Goal: 140 lb - I've tried everything: Drinking water. Gym. Searching for (th)inspiration. Everything lasts only for a very short time. Sure, I drink water during the day, but in the evening I'm starving and eating nonstop. I'm getting fatter everyday. I gained around 20 lbs in only two month. **So I'm giving up and I eat what I want to. And how much I want to. At least I'm feeling good then when I eat.** And perhaps I'll get used to my bigger body some day...

Similar to quitting smoking

Kids compare the struggle of stopping overeating to that of quitting smoking.

This is Ashly's story:
I am 13 yrs old and I weigh 201 lbs! I get sick and tired of not being able to have a normal life. I have gone on a diet, but it is hard **i am so used to eating and its like smoking for me, I can't stop**.

From lisa, Age 15 - 01/29/09
Ht. 5'8", Start: 272 lb, Current: 258 lb, Goal: 120 lb - has anyone on here lost alot of weight?like 50 pounds??or 100?it seems like such a large task to lose 100+ pounds.ugh,i had been doing so well and then i gained back 10.now i cant stop,everyday is the same thing.**breakfast:none**.lunch:wrap w/ chips or chicken and fries.dinner:anything and everything-definatley my weak spot.I want to lose weight so bad....i dont know how to start back again....I dont think many people realize this when they make fun of us but what we have is a disease(obesity)..it kills..it should be considered just as fatal as cancer except we can stop it...but **its addictive,so i guess its more like smoking**.but the point is its not good and we need to fight it!!..

From Molly, Age 16 - 5/28/07 -
Ht. 5'7", Start: 198 lb, Current: 198 lb, Goal: 168 lb - so I am totally -annoyed and the fact that **I'm trying to detox my body- no sweets** is driving me crazyy and I am soo tempted to go get a cookie! BUT NO I promise myself I would do this! soo yeah thats basically what I did today-- I had soo much fruit during lunch! and part of me wonders **if it's this hard to stop over eating image how hard it is for someone who is trying to quite smokeing!**

The same teen below expresses the real meaning of being out of control (addiction?) - even though she is obese and knows that the food she is eating is harmful to her, she is unable to stop.

From Molly, Age 16 - 5/27/07 -
Ht. 5'7", Start: 198 lb, Current: 198 lb, Goal: 168 lb - so basiclly I want to lose about 30 pounds in about 2 and a half months. I seriously think that I can do it if I put my mind to it. BUT the problem is **I have a huge addiction to food! I can't stop eating even though I know the things I'm eating are bad for me.** My best friend is extremely skinny (it runs in her family.) She is so tiny compared to me and sometimes it makes me feel really bad about my image.

Love–hate relationship with food

Another teen expresses the love-hate relationship with food. She is drawn to the pleasure of food, but she hates what it does to her, again suggestive of an addictive quality or psychological substance dependence.

Reply from Claire, Age 19 - 7/20/08
I know **I just hate food now. I mean I love it but I hate it too you know?** we can do thisss just start over.

...and a teen who is drawn to binge but hates it.

From Ellie, Age 15 - 7/24/08
Ht. 5'4", Start: 164 lb, Current: 158 lb, Goal: 112 lb - **i hate binging**

The teen posting below believes that overeating is an addiction and needs to be treated like an addiction. She even notes that to break the addiction you have to cut out the addictive foods and fight through a period of cravings, which will subside after a couple of weeks This is similar to fighting through the cravings when coming off a drug (called 'withdrawal'), which typically subside after a couple of weeks.

Reply from Motivated, Age 19 - 7/17/08 -
sugar and over eating is an addiction, so, you need to treat it like an addiction- you need to stop the physical part by **dealing with the mentality behind the addiction.** work on your issues with food. meditate on it. **also, the addiction is physical-** your body is used to getting fed so many calories and so much sugar and processed foods. you need to cut back on all of the very sugary, processed foods and **fight through the cravings- they will subside after some time. even two weeks** of a strict, no processed-sugar diet will do wonders for not only your weight, but **your physical addiction to food,** and also build your self-confidence in your ability to take care of yourself and **get your life under control.** you can do this. you will do this. take it **one mouthful at a time,** remmebering that each bite counts, and you WILL succeed!

Tolerance and overeating

'Tolerance' is a characteristic of addictive-type behaviors. Tolerance means that the individual must engage in a behavior or use a substance more and more to get the same desired effect. Kids on the boards talk about eating "more and more," as below:

From big boy, Age 14 - 01/06/02 -
5'7" and weigh 180lb i had a lot of personal deaths and each of them was very special to me. and i think about them and **i'm always miserable and now i eat more and more**

From Tara, Age 13 - 07/21/05 -
Ht. 5' "2, Wt. 339 - ... im soo overweight and i get teased constantly and it never stops. i hate it. my life has been so cruel. ..when i was in 1st grade the **teasing** started....i got **teased** because i was alott bigger than everyone else.....so **i just ate more and more** and got fatter and fatter

From Adam, Age 16 - 04/07/04
Look guys i am **6 foot 3 and 300 pounds** ... I hate it. I have ot loads of sterch marks and when i am **bored** i eat even thou i feel full **i still eat more and more** and i don't know why.

From courtnie, Age 16 - 09/22/06 -
Ht. 5'7, Wt. not sure - ... **my depression** kicked back in. and **i started eating more and more**. .. i absolutely HATE it when my family brings up my weight because it makes me feel very self concious. cuz i know im not doing good. i know im killing myself by **eating more and more**.

Age 18, female, 5'2, 275 lbs - **before when i went out to eat i'd eat only a plate or two at a buffet and get stuffed. now i eat 3 and still feel hungry**

It's unclear whether the above kids are showing addictive-type tolerance. They may be in 'vicious cycles' (see Chapter 13). Vicious cycles are when kids eat more and more, because gaining weight makes them more unhappy or stressed, so they comfort eat more. Another possible factor is stomach 'stretching.' They may be able to eat more and more as their stomachs stretch over time, until they finally feel 'stuffed' (see "Overriding of satisfied feeling" on the following page).

We asked kids about this in a poll (http://www.blubberbuster.com/cgi/poll_new_90.cgi):

Do you think that you eat more now than when you first became overweight?

   YES: 62 votes (79%)

   NO: 16 votes (21%)

78 kids voted

Nearly 8 out of 10 kids voting say they eat more now than when they first became overweight. In the results on the following page, of those who eat more now, most feel it is because their stomach can hold more now, which implies stomach stretching.

158

If your answer is yes, why do you think you eat more now?

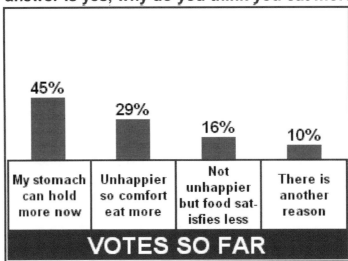

62 kids voted

But nearly 3 out of 10 of the kids feel that they eat more now because they are more unhappy and comfort eat more, which is likely a vicious cycle (see Chapter 13). About one out of 6 kids feel that they are not more unhappy but that food satisfies (comforts) less, which is suggestive of tolerance. Other reasons included "growing taller" and "i love food way to much and dont know when to stop."

If kids eat progressively more as they become more overweight, this would seem to be a contributing factor in obesity.

Overriding of satisfied feeling

Comfort eating seems to override the "satisfied" feeling that normally stops kids from further eating, so that they stop only when overfull, in other words when they feel "stuffed."

From Aaron, Age 13 - 09/10/01
Hi. I have a tendency to eat whole lot! I eat all kinds of junk food and overeat at regular meals. **I notice when I'm full, but I just keep eating and eating.** I know this is not healthy, and I really should stop, ... **stuffed** to your gill. I didn't use to do this, but I started at the begininng of the summer and I did gain some weight

From Jenny, Age 16 - 03/12/08
Ht. 5'2", Start: 190 lb, Current: 223 lb, Goal: 150 lb - I've been so much into eating the last half year that I've gained 33 lbs! I'm so disgusting fat. All my jeans are too tight now. But i can't stop eating. **I eat a full bag of potatoe chips and feel very full and stuffed afterwards.** But I cna't stop it. I'm always thinking "tomorow i'll stop eating so much crap", but then I do it again. In the last 2 weeks i've gained 5 lbs! that's too much. i

just need to eat and eat... my family is fat, too. my mother is buying all that stuff, and i can take it from the cupboard. there's always enough there. when i complain that i'm getting too fat she just says "you're right how you are". then i don't feel that fat anymore and i just eat some chocolate. what can i do?

From Jennifer, Age 16 - 09/16/05
Ht. 5'6, Wt. 280 - I feel embarrased writing this,but I have not been doing well on my diet,I keep saying ill do better tommorow,and I don't...I need to lose 90 pounds at the most hopefully 100... I pig out when I get home...**I feel stuffed when i'm done.**I'll get back on the right track very soon.Everyone else good luck and if anyone has tips for me REPLY please :)

From anastasia, Age 17 - 01/11/05
oooh boy do i hate myself now...i just had one of the worst binges of my life and feel sooo gross. ..**i'm so stuffed and miserable.** it's just terrifying the amount i ate!!! aaargh.....

They may continue to eat even after feeling stuffed.

From Emily, Age 13 - 12/11/05
Ht. 4' 10", Wt. 185 - Hey-Please reply to this message. Whenever theres plenty of good food to eat , **I eat eerything even if im completely stuffed.** What should I do? Please Help!

From cathy, Age 11 - 09/09/01
someone pleez come into the new chat room! im 11 and im way overweigh and i want to talk! **i weigh 205** and i just cant stop eating! **i will eat even if im stuffed** and my tummy is hard! if its sitting there i will eat it! ... i dont like exercise much either i dont even like to walk thats why im home schooled! so someone pleez come into the chatroom!

From Lucee, Age 17 - 08/12/08 -
Ht. 5'8", Start: 179 lb, Current: 154 lb, Goal: 150 lb - Aaagh i feel like crap! ...the thing is that im still hungry. Its completely psychological though as **my stomach feels full and bloated but my mind is telling me that im hungry so i should keep eating.** I hate this! ...this just shows that when i get there ill have to continue dieting or ill end up gaining all the weight back =/

From Alina, Age 15 - 3/16/07
Ht. 4'10", Start: 142 lb, Current: 142 lb, Goal: 120 lb - My problem is none of my clothes fit anymore, and I am getting really bad stretch marks on my skin (all over)! ... I need to know what type of food to avoid and **how do you stop eating before you are full?**

We asked kids in a poll what makes them stop eating.

160

(http://www.blubberbuster.com/cgi/poll_new_77.cgi)

When you are eating a meal, what makes you stop eating?

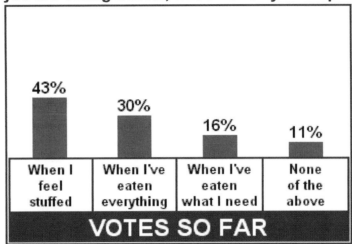

122 kids voted

Do you have a problem knowing when to stop eating?

YES: 70 votes (58%)

NO: 50 votes (42%)

Nearly half of the 122 kids responding indicate that feeling stuffed is what makes them stop eating, and nearly a third of the kids say they stop when they have eaten everything in front of them. Thus, in nearly three fourths of kids voting, it appears that normal "fullness" is overridden by the pleasure or comfort of eating - they eat either until they feel stuffed or until they've eaten everything in front of them.

Here are some of their comments:

Age 16, male, Ht. 5'9", Wt. 250 lbs - i always eat all the food in front of me. plus seconds and thirds. its hard to stop because i'm so fat, it takes tons of food to fill me up.

Age 12, female, Ht. 64", Wt. 181 lbs - Nothing usually makes me stop eating... unless someone tells me to stop.

Age 13, female, Ht. 5', Wt. 167 lbs - i eat everythihg in sight!! even when i am stuffed i can still hold a bag of chips!!!after i cant even sit up strait for at least an hour!!!

Age 16, female, Ht. 65in, Wt. 200 lbs - **when i get full, unless theres some left and i want to eat it all.**

Age 17, male, Ht. 6'0, Wt. 525 lbs - **i just love 2 eat and i dont when to stop**

Keeping track of fullness

So, what can kids do to stop eating when they are normally full but not stuffed?

From Rappy, Age 13 - 08/06/02
I have 1.5 lbs to go before I reach my goal for now! I may change it later, but this is how I did it. **Eat ONLY when you are hungry and stop when you arent anymore, not stuffed. If that is hard then cut in half what you would normally eat and save one half for later.**

Measuring

If the child or teen is accustomed to always eating until stuffed, they may have difficulty recognizing when they are normally full. It may help if he/she or the parent measures out a plate of normal size portions of food. The website, MyPyramid.gov gives photo examples of how much one serving size equates to in different food groups. Go to their "How Much Should You Eat?" page. The child or teen would eat only that measured amount on the plate, with no second helpings, even though they do not feel "full" or satisfied, until their body gets used to normal amounts of food. As the above teen suggests, cutting everything in half that he/she normally eats is also a useful method. Many overweight kids graze continuously throughout the day and may have never actually felt true hunger, but only emotional hunger. It may help if those kids eat only three measured plates of food a day, with only fruits for snacks in between, and no fast food or junk food. Emotionally, this is quite difficult to start with, but it gets easier, if the child or teen can just make it through the first few weeks of bad cravings and find non-food ways to cope with unpleasant emotions like stress, depression, or boredom.

Removing some pleasure from food

Another approach is to remove some of the pleasure from food, but leave the nutrition. Kids tend to overeat baked potatoes loaded with butter, sour cream, and bacon bits, or they may overeat toast smothered with cinnamon sugar and butter. They are unlikely to overeat plain baked potato or plain toast. Furthermore, if kids are truly hungry, they will eat even plain baked potato or plain toast. Thus, to break the comfort eating cycle, kids could be given mainly foods that have little added pleasure substances, such as sugar, salt, butter, or cream.

Eating slower

Eating more slowly also seems to help kids avoid eating until stuffed.

From amanda, Age 13 - 08/01/07
Ht. 5'7", Start: 200 lb, Current: 200 lb, Goal: 154 lb - hey ya'll well i have been doin sometin. well it isent a diet. when i put the name diet on something it sounds so harsh. i just realized how bad some stuff hurts my body, i mean we have always been taught not to do drugs cause it can kill us so can obessity! So on my health kick as i call it i just cut soda out completly.FAST FOOD gone! Water my new fave drink. Set bed times so you can be a bit routine. Eat breakfast, lunch, and dinner. You shouldnt skip meals cause then you binge eat which is the worse:(. **eat slower so your body has enough time to realize hey i just took a bite so you will know when you are full and not to over eat.** Sweets are not the enemy just limit yourself you dont have to eat the whole box. set a time line dont eat after 8pm. atleast that is my time. Cut it in half save some for later so you dont eat it all at one time this i found is easier then it sounds:). Do reaserch and find out what certain foods do to your health. Expeasily trans fat it causes your good chlestral to go done and you bad to go up that is bad:(trans fat=bad very bad. um, i will keep you posted on any more tips k, well if anyone wants to try it i think it will help well i sure do hope i was helpfull, bye k good luck erebody:

From rach, Age 13 - 04/06/07
Ht. 5'3", Start: 134 lb, Current: 134 lb, Goal: 120 lb - hey ya'll, **eat slow!! it givers ur brain time 2 relize that ur full!! it seriously works!!!** remember, YOU CAN DO IT :D

It takes 10-20 minutes for their bodies to recognize they are full, so kids could take a break halfway through meals to think about how much more they need!

Binge eating, which is typically brought on by severe stress (see following chapter), is helped by eating slowly.

From lola, Age 15 - 08/27/05
Ht. 5'3, Wt. 175 - ok I have a tip: **When your binging (because we all do it sometimes) just eat slowly and take in what your eating I mean really enjoy it.** Than hopefully you shouldnt eat as much :)

Eating more slowly probably also works by inducing relaxation and decreasing stress. Slowing down, relaxing, and taking deep breaths between bites helps to relieve stress that frequently results in overeating (see following Chapter 10).

When kids overeat until "stuffed" they are usually feeding emotional hunger rather than nutritional hunger. They may be stuffing their emotions by stuffing themselves with food.

Learning to express their emotions like "I'm sad", or "I'm angry" and finding other ways to deal with emotions that don't involve food will help avoid this.

When do kids overeat?

What times of the day and on which days do kids tend to overeat? What are they doing when they overeat? If kids can become conscious of their eating patterns, they are more likely to develop a plan to improve them.

We asked kids in a poll when they overeat:
(http://www.blubberbuster.com/cgi/poll_new_86.cgi)

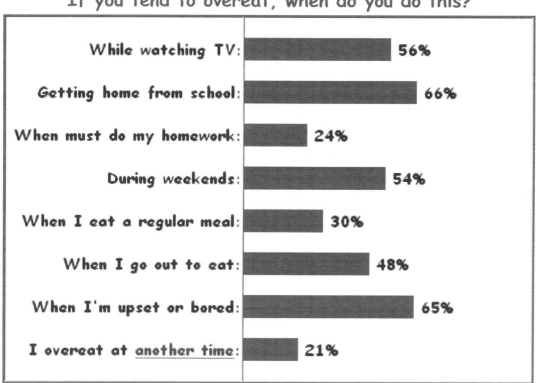

If you tend to overeat, when do you do this?

While watching TV:	56%
Getting home from school:	66%
When must do my homework:	24%
During weekends:	54%
When I eat a regular meal:	30%
When I go out to eat:	48%
When I'm upset or bored:	65%
I overeat at another time:	21%

104 kids voted

Nearly two thirds of 104 kids responding, indicate that they overeat when they arrive home from school, and nearly the same percentage overeat when upset or bored. More than half specified TV watching and weekends as times when they overeat. 'Another time' included: "When I go food shopping," " i was on vacation," " When I'm laying down before bed," "At family and friends houses," " when ever i am alone," " When I am with my dad, we overeat both," and "when i am mad or jelus."

After school eating

From the above results, arriving home from school appears to be the highest risk time for overeating in kids. When kids arrive home they are typically still "wired" from the educational stress and social challenges of school, and there may be no activities at home to relieve the stress. Plus, if there are family problems at home, the child or teen must deal with that stress as well. The result is that many kids head for the fridge or grab a bag of chips to cope.

From Claire, Age 18 - 05/08/07
Ht. 5'4", Start: 210 lb, Current: 159 lb, Goal: 130 lb - binging like crazy after school. We're all teenagers here, and I'm sure this is common. **I'm so stressed especially with college coming and all and I just find myself binging after school.**

From Kat, Age 16 - 11/20/07
Ht. 5'4", Start: 150 lb, Current: 149 lb, Goal: 135 lb - Can someone help me with **after school eating** plz?

From Kim, Age 17 - 7/24/08
Ht. 5'7", Start: 190 lb, Current: 170 lb, Goal: 145 lb - ... **I always seem to eat when I get home even if I'm not hungry.** Does anyone have a suggestion for me. **Like I walk in the door and eat and I don't even realize I'm doing it till I already ate.**

The below teen has insight as to why he/she overeats after school .

From someone, Age 17 - 10/27/05 -
Ht. 5'7, Wt. 178 - i think to loose weight u gotta deal with the issues i ur life. i know everyones always told this. but i noticed my habbits. for ex. **i eat too much every day afterschool to avoid hw and cuz the day made me upset.** i think im gunna... work on my life and see what ahppens. cuz i really think i ve tried everything else and i cant control myself enough to eat right. so i need to control my emotions

Here's a tip from one teen on dealing with after school eating.

Reply from ellie, Age 15 - 7/24/08
prepare a lunchbox of an allowed amount of healthy snacks **for you to graze on when you get home**

If both parents work, or it is a working single -parent family and no one is at home when the kids arrive from school, they may also experience loneliness or boredom. Many kids say they binge when alone at home, if there is pleasurable food in the house.

From Claire, Age 19 - 07/05/08
Ht. 5'4", Start: 210 lb, Current: 176 lb, Goal: 140 lb - UGH...I just had a very disgusting binge. I ate everything like--everything. **Usually this happens when no one is home,** so I hate it when someone leaves. When I'm alone I feel like I have so much more freedom and I can't control myself--and then I go off binging

Eating while watching TV

Kids spend many hours watching TV, and they typically eat while doing so. What do kids say about this?

From Claire, Age 17 - 7/21/08
Ht. 5'2", Start: 200 lb, Current: 200 lb, Goal: 100 lb -.. i got out of bed late .. so i didn't eat anything until like 5pm and that was pizza and waffles which is bad ..., **it's night time when i watch tv that i overeat ..**

From chloe, Age 12 - 09/04/07
Ht. 4'10", Start: 218 lb, Current: 218 lb, Goal: 110 lb - right ive always been a chubby kid. but now its kinda got out of hand im obese. i eat and eat and eat. .. **i just sit around in my room watching tv and eating.**

In the poll below, most of the 225 kids responding feel that TV causes them to gain weight because they eat while watching TV. More than a third think that TV causes them to gain weight because it keeps them from exercising. Less than one fifth of the kids feel that watching TV does <u>not</u> cause them to gain weight.
(http://www.blubberbuster.com/cgi/poll_new_9_percent.cgi)

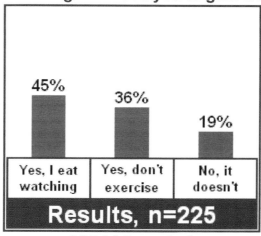

225 kids voted

Why do kids eat while watching TV? Could it be simply because there are so many food commercials? Or is it something else? Watching TV tends to be an escape from reality. Perhaps kids are jolted back to their painful reality at times, while they are absorbed with TV. Do they overeat to cope with these jolts back to reality? TV food commercials directed at children and teens may take advantage of kids' vulnerability to comfort eating and stress eating while watching TV.

What can be done to prevent kids from overeating while watching TV? Engaging in other activities while watching TV, such as knitting, putting together a puzzle, or even walking on a treadmill, may help to relieve stress, maintain a connection with reality and avoid TV comfort eating and stress eating.

Video games are frequently incriminated as a contributor to childhood obesity. Playing video games may also be an escape from painful reality by kids, and similar to watching TV, kids are intermittently jolted back to this reality. Thus, comfort eating and stress eating while playing video games may be another time kids overeat.

Parental divorce

The pain of parental divorce is an all too frequent cause of overeating in kids.

From Melissa, Age 15 - 5/15/05 -
Ht. 5'1", Wt. 175 - i had to go through a **really diffucult divocre** aroudn 7 grade which lead my kinda chubby body to ballon out because **i ate whenever i was unhappy.**

From Megan, Age 15 - 1/25/08
Ht. 5'2", Start: 195 lb, Current: 193 lb, Goal: 145 lb - **After my parents divorce several years ago, I coudn't find anything to do but eat.** After realizing how much weight that I gained, I realized that I needed to lose weight. This is almost impossible for me to do..and i truly need motivation. ... I want to be healthy, and im tired of being called fat everytime i turn around. I just dont know what to do.

From Kristen , Age 15 - 4/30/05 -
Ht. 5'4", Wt. 150 - I am really overweight and **the whole reason is because my mother got re married and I hate him and his kids and i just eat when im sad or mad** and that is why i started to get this big

From kate, Age 11 - 7/24/08
Ht. 4'8", Start: 110 lb, Current: 109 lb, Goal: 99 lb (BMI 95 %tile) - ...**I keep eating and eating,** I can't stop. I'm just so stressed out. **My mom and dad got divorced when I was 7. That was when I started getting bigger.** I live with my mom and **she has**

a **boyfriend that is a butt head,** and **he moved in** along with his tooth pick annoying daughters. I'm so messed up. I need a goog diet. and just someone to talk to.

Parental separation and divorce is obviously quite painful for kids. Hence, kids may seek comfort in the pleasure of food. What can separated parents do to prevent this? Talk with the child or teen. Encourage him/her to express what they are feeling, so that he/she doesn't deal with the painful emotions by stuffing themselves with food.

When a child or teen starts becoming overweight, the child's weight may upset one parent in particular, so that the child or teen may withdraw to the other parent. This may be a problem if the parents are living in different households and if one parent is enabling the overeating (e.g. feeling guilty, trying to please the child). If your child or teen's weight gain upsets you, try not to withdraw from him/her, as this may make him/her seek even more comfort from food, as well as food from the enabling parent. Talk to the child or teen and encourage him/her to express how they are feeling and explain this to the enabling parent.

Comfort eating tips

Here are two great tips from the Success Stories Board on dealing with comfort eating:

✴ From Isabella, Age 13 - 1/30/07; **GREAT MOTIVATIONAL POSTING:**
Ht. 5'5", Wt. 166 - (Was: 184, Now: 166 Goal: 145-150) - Hey peeps! I've.. learned to look at more positive things about your body and flaunt them! I realized that I have shiny hair, great calves, and muscular arms, so I work it out! And having hobbies and friends to support you really helps. Look for inner beauty as well. Focus on things, have big dreams, set goals, be a better student, learn something new, who knows! Remember: you're not just a number on the scale, a pant size, measurements, the number of zits on you face, a shirt size. You're a person with brains and feelings and talents. For real. **This might sound cheesy, but when you start to smile at yourself and be your own best friend, you'll be able to nurture your relationship with food as fuel, not a form of entertainment or comfort.** Look only at positive aspects of your life. YOU ROCK; NOW SHOW IT!!!! Love, Isabella (a.k.a. Izzy)

From Laura, Age 19 - 4/25/06
Ht. 5'6, Wt. 125 -.. In the past 2 years, I have lost a total of 45 pounds and plan to keep it off the rest of my life. **I was once overweight and know exactly how it feels to be the fat person. I know what it feels like to be emotionally addicted to food; but now food only means something nutritional that I need to put in my body.** I want to give you all the best of luck in making your lives healthier. You have to start somewhere...although it isn't easy... it is worth it in the end. I promise!

Further comfort eating posts and tips may be found at:

http://www.weigh2rock.com/emotional-eating

This chapter has presented the writings of kids who seek comfort in the pleasure of food when they are depressed, lonely, rejected, anxious, angry, and even happy, as the post below relates.

From unknown , Age 19 - 9/11/07 -
Ht. 5'10", Start: 238 lb, Current: 238 lb, Goal: 170 lb - i just started college after graduating this past may and im having the hardest time loseing weight... i hate being this way but **for some reason i cant stop eatting as hard as i try all i can do is eat. i eat when im sad, i eat when im mad, i eat when im scared, i eat when im happy..** i just dont know what to do anymore...

Why would kids seek comfort in food when happy? Similar to TV eating, kids may be anxious about the unhappiness that will soon come again.

Similar to comfort eating, kids on the boards say that they overeat to relieve stress. Kids are under more stress today than ever. In the next chapter we look at what kids say about stress eating.

10 | Stress Eating (Displacement Activity)

Overeating when stressed out

Along with comfort eating, stress eating appears to be a second major cause of overeating and overweight in the kids who post on our website. Comfort eating is typically a response to painful feelings such as sadness, loneliness, disappointment, rejection, or depression. Stress eating, on the other hand, occurs in response to life's challenges – school demands, family strife, money problems, peer pressure, moving, competition, and crowding, to name a few. Many overweight kids say that they overeat when under stress, for example:

From whitneyx<3, Age 14 - 11/15/05 - IP#: 68.191.24.xxx
Ht. 5'4, Wt. 280 - Hey.xx Well...apparently I'm on this board because I want to lose weight. **I have been eating a LOT for the past few days..and I think it's mostly because of stress...** Oh, oh--lookathowawful my weight is. Ugh....makesmesick.

From ShiningStar, Age 14 - 2/13/08
Ht. 5'6", Start: 184 lb, Current: 182 lb, Goal: 145 lb - Hi! This is my first post on Blubber Busters in...uh...gosh, it's been so many centuries I can't even remember! Anyway, I've returned because I am disgusted with my life. See, I started off at 184 lbs in Feb. of 2006. I bought The Diet for Teenagers Only, an amazing book, and began to turn my life around. I got as low as 164 lbs in May of 2007, but then **I had some really awful family tragedies during the summer, and my stress level skyrocketed. I started relying on food for comfort...**

Reply from Mikayla, Age 18 - 09/21/08
I totally know what you mean. I maintained 180 for two years. And then senior year, I worked out daily and had the same diet, **but with stress I ended up gaining 30 pounds even though nothing changed.** Stress is bad. ...

From mary, Age 14 - 12/18/06
Ht. 5'3", Wt. 153 - uhhhh!!!! Finals are next week and **i am really stressing out** over my biology final and **i am a stress eater** so i like ate a whole bunch of chocolate instead of eating lunch and my stomache hurts and i ate sooo many calories and im so frustrated!!! I

fully plan on getting back on track tomorrow i am going to give the rest of my chocolate to my friend. Hope everyone is doing better than me...

From megan, Age 14 - 06/05/05
Ht. 5'5", Wt. 168 - I'm trying my hardest to fight the **food cravings**.. I keep picking it up and putting it back down again.. **It's when I get sad or stressed that I eat** :(wish me luck

From Claire, Age 19 - 06/02/08
Ht. 5'4", Start: 210 lb, Current: 176 lb, Goal: 140 lb I used to weigh like freakin 159!...I should've cherished being 159 for the time being but I just screwed it up **by letting stress take over my life and turning to food once again.** I wish I weighed that much again and now getting there seems like such a hard thing to do! I wish I hadn't gained back in the first place. It makes me feel like a failure, really. :(

Most kids responding to the poll below say that they overeat when stressed out, and more than eight out of ten say their stress has increased over the past three years. (http://www.blubberbuster.com/cgi/poll_new_79.cgi)

Has stress in your life increased over the past 3 years?
YES: 54 votes (82%)
NO: 12 votes (18%)

66 kids voted

What kinds of stress are kids under these days?

Reply from Flower Fawn, Age 15 - 11/02/08
... I had gotten down to 163 last summer (2007) and then **some really, really, really bad things happened in my family -- parents always fighting, mom always working, money problems, stress. It was hell, and I was so upset all that time that I ate constantly** so by September 2007 I was back up to 178.

Reply from Motivated, Age 19 - 07/23/08
I know how you feel about both **gaining weight back because of family/other stress** AND having clothes that don't fit anymore. When i was in high school **i went from 175 to 140lbs, then i gained 75 lbs back because of family issues, financial issues, and school stress!** it's horrible.

Age 11, male, 4'10", 153 lbs - i eat when I feel nervous. whenever I have a big test at school, or whenever i have to get in front of the class and present something.

From Hali, Age 15 - 02/21/09
Ht. 5'4", Start: 181 lb, Current: 174 lb, Goal: 166 lb - So this morning I...found out that my dad is moving out... for a while at least. Its my fault, I wanted to go to this meeting thing so I pushed my mom to do it, who asked my dad to take me. Then when it was time to go he told my mom to take me, and she got really mad. I dont know what to do.Actually the reason im posting this on here is because all i can think to do is to eat. i need to stop but its the only thing i can think to do to forget what happened.

What exactly is stress?

What exactly is emotional stress? In 1936 Hans Selye first coined the term 'stress' to mean "the non-specific response of the body to any demand for change… demands which exceed the personal and social resources the individual is able to mobilize." [Selye 1936]. To put it simply, the person feels overwhelmed and is unable to cope with the demands of life. Stress may mean feeling unsure what to do, for instance not being able to face a situation which cannot be avoided. Stress, of course, means many things to many people, but it is an unpleasant emotion.

The above postings from kids reveal that they overeat when under stress. A recent research study found that living in a stressful household may raise a child's risk of becoming obese [Koch 2008]. Why does this happen? Some obesity researchers feel that hormones in the body, for example cortisol, which are released as a response to stress, cause increased appetite and overeating [Torres et al. 2007]. But is that really what is causing the above kids to overeat when stressed out and to become overweight? What about a thing called "displacement activity?"

Displacement Activity

The most common way of handling stress in humans, as well as animals, is "displacement activity." What is displacement activity? As the term implies, something is displaced or moved – in this case nervous energy and an unpleasant situation.

The one thing I remember about introductory psychology in college was a little fish in an aquarium bouncing on his head. The fish was a male, who was attracted to the female in the tank. When the male of that species mates with the female, the female then kills the male, so he won't eat the fry (babies). Thus, the male has a tremendously stressful conflict, wanting to mate but fearing being killed. To relieve the stress the male bounces on his head.

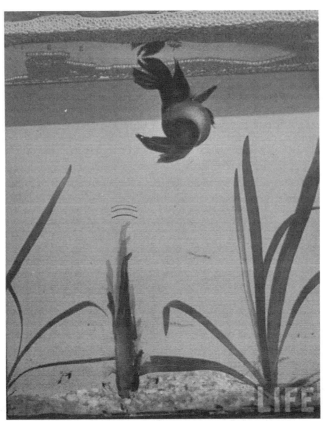

Fish displacement activity (head bouncing)

*Many animals show displacement activity when under stress, for example birds pecking at the ground when threatened by a predator, and **wildly eating anything**, e.g. grass, rocks. The Encyclopedia Britannica states: "Displacement activities often consist of comfort movements, such as grooming, scratching, drinking, or **eating**. In courtship, for example, an individual afraid of its mate may, instead of fleeing or courting, stand still and **feed** or groom itself."*

*Humans likewise show displacement activity when under stress, such as head scratching (unsure what to do), pacing back and forth, nail biting, hangnail picking, and **eating**. These behaviors use up nervous energy, distract from disagreeable occurrences, and relieve tension and stress. The McMillian Dictionary defines displacement activity as: "Something that you do in order to avoid dealing with an unpleasant situation." Hand-to-mouth movements, biting, chewing, tongue action, and swallowing use up nervous energy and distract from unpleasant situations when eating.*

Examples of human displacement activity are pictured on the following pages.

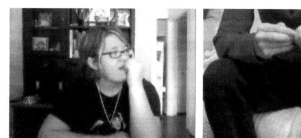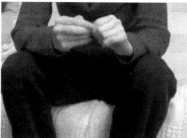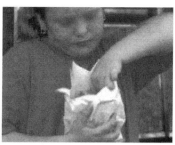

Human displacement activity: nail biting, hangnail picking, and eating

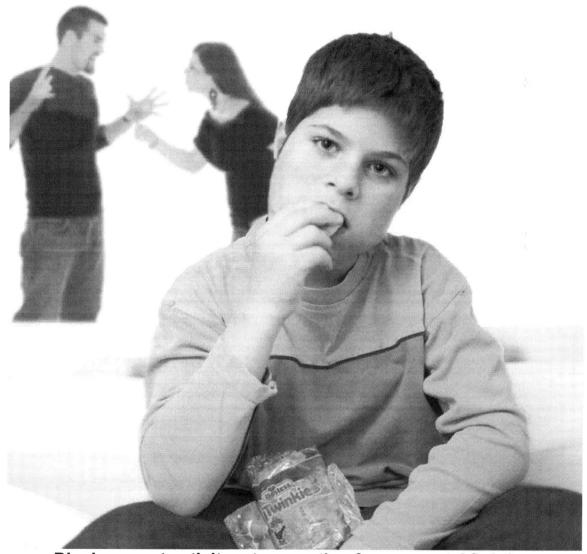

Displacement activity: stress eating from parental fighting

Nail biting and hangnail picking

Nail biting and picking at hangnails are displacement activities. Such behaviors have no purpose other than to use up nervous energy. Some kids bite their nails or pick at hangnails until bleeding and sore, as shown in the photos below:

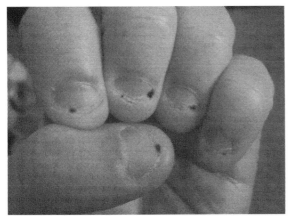

Severely bitten nails in a teen

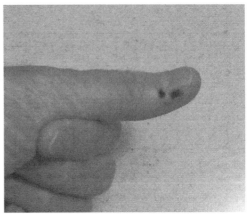

Picked at hangnail

In the poll below, more than three fourths of 106 kids responding say they think overeating is like nail biting, and most say they bite their nails:
(http://www.blubberbuster.com/cgi/poll_new_78.cgi)

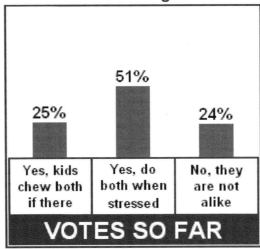

106 kids voted

Do you ever bite your nails?

YES: 66 votes (62%)
NO: 40 votes (38%)

Kids may mindlessly chew on food when stressed out, or if food is simply in front of them, the same way they mindlessly chew on their nails or pick at hangnails when stressed out. It's very difficult to resist these displacement activities when stress levels are high.

Here are comments from kids responding to the poll on the previous page:

Age 16, female, 5'6, 155 lbs - **Biting your nails is a nervous habit or something you do without realizing it...Nevermind. I really think is like overeating then.** - I sometimes bite my nails.

Age 15, female, 5 feet 8 inches, 153 lbs - **Overeating is like nail biting because it's a habit that you do when you're restless, bored, etc.** - I never bite my nails.

Age 14, female, 5'4, 230 lbs - **some kids do different things for being stressed out so they are very much alike** - I sometimes bite my nails.

Age 13, female, 5'2'', 158 lbs - **I bite my nails when I am nervous or stress. I also overeat then too.** - I sometimes bite my nails

Age 15, female, 5'0, 187 lbs - **I think they are the same cuz when im trying to lose weight and i eat less i start to bite my nails more.** - I sometimes bite my nails.

Age 12, female, 5'6", 185 lbs - **I bite my nails, and overeat so i can compare to this.** - I sometimes bite my nails.

Age 13, female, 5'5", 140 lbs - **They are both an addiction sort of thing. They both are like cravings. When you have a certain feeling, such as boredom and stress you bite your nails or eat something. They are almost exactly the same.** - I never bite my nails.

Age 16, female, 5'8, 178 lbs - **i bite my nails when i'm nervous or when their to big, but i think people eat food because it tastes good,and when their bored** - I sometimes bite my nails.

Mindless eating when under stress is, therefore, likely displacement activity.

From mary, Age 15 - 2/13/07 -
Ht. 5'3", Wt. 158 - My family is driving me crazy!! I am an emotional overeater, so when someone makes me mad, or if im sad, then i eat. **My mom made me soo made today that i ate like 10 hersheys kisses and 3 oreos. Im so stressed out right now.**

Binge Eating

Binge eating, which is eating large amounts of food very quickly, appears to be mainly displacement activity to relieve stress. Binge eating is generally associated with being quite stressed out, and quite suddenly. Large amounts of certain types of food are consumed very rapidly, without really enjoying the food, and frequently in secret, in a desperate attempt to relieve the stress. Binge eating is rare before adolescence, so it appears to be a learned behavior [Stice 1998].

From Lucee, Age 16 - 1/28/08 -
Ht. 5'8", Start: 171 lb, Current: 171 lb, Goal: 140 lb - Yesterday was soooo bad **i was stressing out big time about my exams which started today and.. i had the biggest binge ever**..okay well not ever ive had worse before but it was huuuge- a family size bag dorritos, pringles, 3 packets chips, 15 chocolate biscuits, 4 bits of caramel shortcake, 2 jam donuts and probably other stuff ive forgotten.

From Cat, Age 17 - 10/20/07 -
Ht. 4'11", Start: 171 lb, Current: 160 lb, Goal: 106 lb - Hey guys. I love coming to this site because its so inspirational, though this is the first time I've ever posted. I have a big problem. **I tend to binge, BIG TIME. And I've figured out that these binges happen when I'm alone, when I'm bored, or right after I get home from school.** Any tips on how to beat this? Thank you,

From Lauren, Age 14 - 01/28/09
Ht. 5'3", Start: 180 lb, Current: 175 lb, Goal: 135 lb - I've figured out my problem. **I'm a binge eater.** Seriously. **When I start eating, I can't stop.** I just eat eat eat eat eat untill my stomache can't tae it anymore. **I'm not even hungry when I do this.** Its a real problem. ..

From Claire, Age 18 - 05/07/07
Ht. 5'4", Start: 210 lb, Current: 159 lb, Goal: 130 lb - ... I've been doing veryyy bad :'(What do I do? I'm still on this plateu. I hate my stomach, seriously...my waist has gotten bigger. I used to be so good with this whole diet thing but lately **I've been so stressed and I just find myself binging all the time and I can't stop. It's all so hard and I'm just very stressed right now.** I feel like my goal is a million miles away and I'm just screwing everything up for myself.

From Lucee, Age 17 - 06/08/08
Ht. 5'8", Start: 179 lb, Current: 163 lb, Goal: 150 lb - .. **theres days like today when im in the house bored all day (because i had 2 stay in 2 study for a sociology exam on tuesday) and what do i end up doing? bingEING!!** Honestly i must have consumed at least 5000 calories today and i purged which im really mad about cos im in

recovery for bulimia which was going really well but **i have relapsed quite a few times in the past month which i think is down to exam stress...**

From Caty, Age 14 - 08/23/04
i was doing good on atkins cept i blew it yesterday. **there were some family problems nd i cried alot and i turned to food!** not onli that, alot of food..... with alot of carbs. i ate cinnamon rolls, hot pocket, donuts and other stuf. i cant blive i ate that much. **i was so full but i kept on stuffing myself** even tho i felt lyk throwing up.

Stress eating (displacement activity to get rid of nervous energy) and comfort eating (to soothe sadness or depression) may be mixed. Kids commonly say they are both stressed and depressed (as below), so they may stress eat and comfort eat at the same time. Hence, they may choose foods that are both soothing (often sweet, creamy textures) and also get rid of nervous energy (chewy, crunchy textures), such as caramel chocolate bars with nuts.

From paige, Age 14 - 11/17/07 -
Ht. 5'4", Start: 189 lb, Current: 187 lb, Goal: 145 lb - i only try to lose weight for myself not for anyone else but i have a problem **i eat when i am stressed out and depressed its soo hard for me** i mean like i feel fat and i want to lose weight so i try and it never works

Kids say they binge to combat boredom. Boredom, of course, is unpleasant and thus stressful. Are these kids stress eating because of boredom?

From Elizabeth, Age 13 - 06/30/06
Ht. 5'7, Wt. n/a - deep down i know the only way to lose weight is to eat right and excercise but this month i havn't been doing much beside going to the gym and swimming a bit. **my main problem is i binge when im bored.** its usually not that unhealthy but its extra calories i dont need and i sometimes aren't even hungry. so anyone got any suggestions? thanx =D

From Erica, Age 16 - 06/16/08
Ht. 5'4", Start: 148.9 lb, Current: 158 lb, Goal: 115 lb -
I can't stop binge eating. It's like I eat even when I'm bored...and it's a problem.....PLEAsE GIVE ME ADVICE IF YOU SUFFERED FROM IT AND KNOW HOW TO STOP:)

... and kids say they binge to comfort a rejection, which again is stressful.

From Whitney, Age 18 - 03/27/08
Ht. 5'9", Start: 200 lb, Current: 180 lb, Goal: 150 lb - Weighed in @ 180 today. I guess I'll take it a loss is a loss. Dont really know how I managed it. **I binged horribly last night cuz I found out the guy I was talking to is talking to some other girl too.** Sad

story but I'm over it and its actually working to my advantage cuz its motivating to do this for myself not that I was feeling pressure to do it for anyone else cuz I mean he "liked" or "likes" me now but I just need me time...

It doesn't seem to matter whether binged food is highly pleasurable or not. For example, a mother posted the following:

From Nicole, Child's Age 15 - 1/27/08 -
My child is teased all the time at school and has terrible self esteem issues. ...**We dont have any junk food around but she will stuff herself on apples and 100 calorie packages.** ...Shes **5'10 and weighs 250.**

Binge eating therefore appears to be using up stress energy (a huge amount of it), without much pleasure to the eating, in other words mainly displacement activity.

Controlling stress eating and binge eating

How do successful kids stop displacement activities such as stress eating and binge eating? The answer is that they learn to cope with stress without using food, as follows:

➤ Relaxation, meditation, and deep breathing

*Relaxation and meditation with slow deep breathing seems to help relieve stress, for example **yoga**.*

From Isabella, Age 13 - 12/23/06 -
Ht. 5'5", Wt. 167 - Hey guys well the last two days have been hell for me because I consumed so much crap, then this morning I woke up feeling lousy but I thought to myself, "If you feel lousy than make a change, get back on track and you'll feel better!" So I got up and did my 45 min. **weight loss with yoga** DVD, which I love because it has cardio and flexibility plus **meditation and relaxing music. Yoga has been proven to give young women better body images!** ... I feel better already. :0)

From Jenna, Age 16 - 12/25/00 -
... at the end of my 8th grade year I was **5'1" and I weighed 180 lbs.** And I wondered why I had never had a boyfriend. I was tired of being worn out after doing simple exercises. And I was so embarrassed of myself I would purposefully avoid swimming pools or anything that had to do with a swim suit...I was just plain and simple FAT... My friends would "tease" me, my grandma was always making comments about my weight in public and to her friends. It really hurt. I finally decided I had to do something... That June a friend of mine introduced me to **yoga**. I thought yeah right. This is so corny. How is this ever going to help me. But I was so surprised... It's very quick and healthy. You'll see results

within the first week u do it. Doctor's even perscribe it to their patients... u move into **meditation** by laying down somewhere quiet and **completely relaxing your body and clearing your mind**. You will feel much better after you have done this. I am now half way through my 11th grade year and I am **5'3" and weigh 123lbs**...

The slow inhale and exhale of cigarette smoking is similar to deep breathing relaxation exercises and may be one reason that smoking relieves stress. Of course, kids should not smoke to relieve stress, but they can do deep breathing exercises.

➤ *Take up a musical instrument*

How about taking up a musical instrument? Playing a musical instrument is actually a displacement activity and can relieve stress. Plus, it's fun!

From beth, Age 14 - 11/20/05
Ht. 5ft 9, Wt: 204 lb, Goal: 150/160 - i agree with mark, loose weight to be healthy, don't worry when you muck up, everyone does! **I founbd a way to stop you eating when you're not hungry, take up a musical instrument**. I come from a musical family anyway, but was never really interested untill i got into the indie scene, I started playing guitar a month ago. When you want to sound good,(because ppl are always not as good as they want to be when coming to things like that!!!!!!!) you practice more and more. it doesn;t have to be expensive, just one you always wanted to play..... once you get your hands on one and you REALLY want to sound good, the more you practice, the more you practice, the better you get, AND **the less unnecessary food you'll binge on when your bored**. it might not help you, but it has me, I havent lost that much weight, but it's working slowly but surely :D

➤ *Squeeze your hands together*

*Simply **squeezing their hands together** really tight also helps relieve stress and avoid stress eating, particularly when kids are stressed out and have cravings. Squeezing your hands tight is a displacement activity and uses up nervous energy.*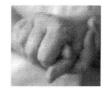

Reply from anne, Age 16 - 8/22/03
i read the blubberbuster advice for cravings and it said to **hold your hands together**. i was like yeah right! that is not going to work for me! but last night i watched my boyfriend eat a reeses sunday and i didn't have a single bite. **as simple as it sounds- it works**, hey- if you don't have your hands free then you won't grab and eat stuff. **also try to keep busy too-make it so you don't have time to binge**, whether it's mentally busy or physically busy...

➢ *Write down your problems*

*Kids **write down their problems** on a sheet of paper, and under each problem they write a plan (see pp. 287). It's the 'divide and conquer' approach. Then kids don't feel so overwhelmed.*

➢ *Exercise*

***Exercise, or any physical activity**, is actually a form of displacement activity. Exercise gets rid of nervous energy, and relieves tension and stress, as the post below describes:*

From Whitney, Age 19 - 01/03/09 - IP#: 67.142.161.xxx
Ht. 5'8", Start: 200 lb, Current: 185 lb, Goal: 145 lb - First off I am so excited there is a 18+ board! We are in a different place in our lives and now we can communicate with those who are on the same page. I've struggled with my weight since middle school, but now in college I need to take control of it. I have lost it before so I know I can do it again! ... My biggest obstacle is watching what I eat but being home from school I have really started paying attention. **I love to work out, its a great stress reliever and as long as I'm plugged into my ipod I'm good to go!** Well I will keep posting, especially when I know where I'm at, good luck everyone!

This may be why exercise helps so much to lose weight.

Even video games are a form of displacement activity and theoretically may help to relieve stress and avoid overeating, even though video games are often blamed as a cause of overweight in kids.

➢ *Out of sight out of mind*

How do kids stop biting their nails or stop picking at hangnails? They hide the nails with gloves or coat them with bitter paint. In the case of hangnails, they simply clip the hangnail before it is picked and keep further hangnails from forming by applying hand lotion or Vaseline.

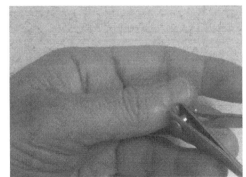

Hangnail clipping prevents picking

*Similarly, it helps to **hide junk food**, which kids mindlessly eat when it's in front of them. Put tempting food in a high, hard to reach cupboard, as shown at right. If it's out of sight, it's out of mind.*

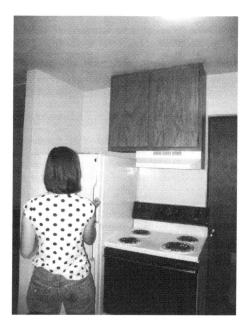

From Jenna, Age 16 - 05/13/06
Ht. 5'4", Wt. 175 - Hey everyone...we really don't need to post anymore "OMG! I'm fat! What can I do?!?!" ...We arent going to get ANYWHERE if all we do is complain. ... **I don't let my parents buy crappy food. If its tempting for me, I put it in the cabinet- if it is out of sight, its out of mind!**

*Comparable to hiding junk food, **removing food from the table**, before it's all eaten, also helps to avoid overeating.*

> ## Chewing gum

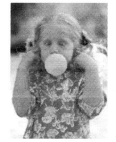

Chewing gum helps to reduce cravings.

A recent research study found that chewing gum before an afternoon snack helped reduce hunger, diminish cravings and promote fullness[Hetherington 2007]. The benefit of chewing gum is likely due to displacement activity, as the chewing muscle activity uses up nervous energy, similar to chewing on fingernails or on food. Of course, sugarless gum is the best choice.

Reply from Twitch, Age 14 - 07/27/09 -
I use to have the... problem with eating when i'm bored. Buy a gigantic box of gum from costco. And **when u get bored, just start chewing gum**. Change pieces everyonce in a while if it starts running out of flavor. Its definitely better to have 20 calories worth of gum then hundreds of calories worth of food.

Is stress eating like an addiction?

When kids use eating as a displacement activity to relieve stress and they become hooked on this behavior, is this like an addiction? We don't generally think of nail biting or hangnail picking as addictions, although they are difficult habits to break. Actually, the broad definition of addiction is: continuing a behavior even though the individual knows that the behavior causes problems in his/her life, as well as feeling out of control (http://www.faqs.org/health/Sick-V1/Addiction.html). Nail biting doesn't usually cause significant problems in kids' lives, even though the habit may result in bleeding, painful fingers, which can become infected; and nail biting is annoying to those around them. So, in the broad sense, nail biting is similar to addictive behaviors.

Nevertheless, calling a behavior an 'addiction' seems to be a matter of how much the behavior negatively impacts on the person's life. Stress eating, which appears similar to nail biting, does negatively affect kids' lives to a considerable degree, particularly bingeing. They may become overweight and obese because of it. And stress eating appears to be much harder to quit than nail biting.

'Tolerance' is a characteristic of addictive behaviors, as noted possibly in regard to comfort eating in Chapter 9. Again, tolerance means that the individual must engage in a behavior or use a substance more and more to get the same effect. Although some kids do post that they eat "more and more," as shown on pp. 156-157, it's unclear whether they are stress eating or comfort eating. Tolerance would not be expected to be a characteristic of stress eating, which is displacement activity, as displacement activity is simply muscle movement that uses up nervous energy. The same amount of muscle movement should always use up the same amount of nervous energy, so eating more and more to cope with stress should not be needed unless the stress level increases. Therefore, stress eating may not be an addictive-type behavior, which comfort eating may be. Of course, stress may worsen because of weight gain, so more stress eating may occur, in other words a vicious cycle (see Chapter 13).

Stress relief displacement activity foods

*In **Life is Hard, Food is Easy**, author Linda Spangle notes that if we eat when stressed, we seem to prefer foods that are chewy and crunchy, such as candy bars, chips, and nuts [Spangle 2003]. What she is actually describing is displacement activity. Foods, which are chewy and crunchy, such as candy bars, especially if they contain nuts, involve a lot muscle action of the jaw, tongue, cheeks, and throat to eat them, as well as hand-to-mouth movement. The muscle activity gets rid of nervous energy, similar to nail biting, pacing back and forth, or hangnail picking.*

Chocolate is the most craved food [Martin 2008]. Chocolate has a melting point just slightly lower than body temperature - "It melts in your mouth, not in your hands." Thus, chocolate may be licked, sucked, or chewed with a great deal of tongue and jaw action, in other words displacement activity, which relieves stress, and even more so if crunchy nuts are present. In addition, chocolate is sweet, creamy, and soothing - hence comfort food. Lastly, chocolate contains caffeine, an upper, but which may add to jitters and stress.

Smoking has displacement activity features. The cigarette gives the smoker something to do with his/her hands. Smoking thereby relieves stress in social situations. Eating likewise gives the person something to do with his/her hands and thereby relieves stress in social situations.

Mindless grazing

Mindless grazing on food is now thought to be a form of binge eating [Williamson 2008]. Mindless grazing is similar to mindless nail biting and is a way of dealing with constant stress. Both mindless grazing and binge eating appear to be displacement activities. The below post describes such mindless grazing.

From Megan, Age 19 - 12/31/08
Ht. 5'10", Start: 226 lb, Current: 226 lb, Goal: 180 lb - Hey everyone.. I went for a two mile walk yesterday and I'm feeling really good about loosing it this time.. **I actually realized most of my problem is I eat all the time.. I dont even notice it..** I just picked up a chocolate coved pretzel last night was was starting to put it in my mouth before I even realized it! so my goal for the next month is to only eat when I am hungry or well my 3 meals a day.. you know just not start picking up stuff cause its convinent... hopefully I'll start shedding soon!!! Hope everyone is doing well!!

Skipping breakfast

Several studies have shown that kids, who don't eat breakfast, are more likely to be overweight [Nicklas 2001]. What do kids say about this?

From Julie, Age 12 - 09/14/05
Ht. 5'4, Wt. 18- - im sad and depressed being overweight i had teachers come up 2 me telling me 2 lose weight.i lose all of my friends because im overweight.i try all i ca but i dont lose.my aunt even called me fat.ive been overweight since i was in kindergraden.i hardly eat and i still gain.people say im fat because **i eat 2 much when i dont eat lunch or breakfast**.i just started jr.high so i no its going 2 get harder.ive been teased more now then ever and i just want 2 lose it.so pealse be a friend a true friend 4 me.

From Ashley, Age 13 - 03/13/04
Hey, this is Ash again, I am trying to come up with different ways to lose weight!!! Like I said, **I skip breakfast and lunch and when I get home i pig out!!!** I know that isn't helping me any. Also when I am bored I eat, i feel like i have nothing better to do but eat!!! I am sooo fat and I even have stretch marks, how do u get rid of them and does anyone have any suggestions to help me with staying away from food. Thanks

Reply from Stacie, Age 13 - 03/14/04
Im the same way...**No breakfast, No lunch, and then wehn i come home i pig out and cant stop...**

Reply from Anon, Age 16 - 03/13/04
dont skip breakfast and lunch because then you will tend to binge eat the moment you get food.

Kids who skip breakfast say that they overeat or binge later in the day. Why would this happen? Hunger is an unpleasant feeling and is stressful. Kids who skip breakfast may thus overeat later to comfort and cope with the stress of hunger, as well as the normal hunger drive. Similarly, kids who go to bed late, get up late, and don't have time for breakfast before school, would have the double whammy of both fatigue and hunger, resulting in stress/comfort eating along with normal hunger eating later in the day (see sleep-obesity vicious cycles, pp. 216).

Combating stress in kids

We need to think up creative displacement activities for kids, as well as ways to reduce and help them manage their stress to begin with. The scientific term for this is "stress coping mechanisms." Kids today are lonelier and under more stress than ever, and food is more pleasurable, cheaper, and more available than ever. How can we reduce the stress level of kids so they don't turn to food?

➢ *After school activities such as non-competitive sports, dancing, and fun hobbies can help combat stress in kids.*

➢ *Parents should look at what factors could be elevating the stress levels of their kids and how these stressors could be reduced. For example, are initiatives such as "No Child Left Behind" and school testing really worth it, if kids are getting stressed out, and perhaps overeating because of this?*

➢ *Might a tutor or counseling help relieve school stress for your child? Free counseling for kids is available at most schools, as well as at community mental health centers. Tutors also are usually available through schools.*

➢ *Talk with your kids, help them work through stress, and find fun activities for them to do, or which you can do together. Monitor their TV and sleep time.*

Substituting low-fat foods?

Substituting low-calorie foods, even veggies or fruits, as displacement activity foods or comfort foods may not be a good idea, as using any food for that purpose may increase the likelihood of food psychological dependence. Rather, dealing directly with what's stressing or depressing kids and finding non-food ways for them to cope is a better approach.

Similar to stress eating, kids overeat for entertainment to relieve boredom. Boredom is especially hard for kids to deal with and is also extremely common among the overweight kids on our site. In the next chapter we look at what kids say about boredom and eating for entertainment.

11 | Boredom Eating

Boredom

Boredom is extremely common among the kids who use our bulletin boards and chat rooms. These kids say that they eat to relieve boredom.

From Macarena, Age 14 - 7/6/07 -
Ht. 5'4", Start: 153 lb, Current: 156 lb, Goal: 135 lb - hey... **i eat junk whenever I'm bored.** this is a problem. any ideas for stopping this. thank you!

From Nolie, Age 16 - 4/2/07 -
Ht. 5'9", Start: 212 lb, Current: 212 lb, Goal: 135 lb - Hey, im new and im soooooo ready to lose weight! I need tooooooo, to be healthy mentally and physically... ALSO, **im a majorrrrrr boredom eater** any tips on that?? in fact thats mostly my problem!

From Emily, Age 17 - 6/16/06
Ht. 5'10, Wt. 225 - HEY everyone...i figured somthing out today.....**i eat when i am bored**...it kinda weird but i just started my summer jon and i am so busy all the time that i dont even think about eating. I took a case of water and put it under my desk and some weight watchers food just in case....but i found out that usually i dont want to eat anything...so i guess **i am a boredom eater**...does this happen to any body else? if so **what do u do to avoid eating just out of boredom?**

Reply from beth, Age 17 - 6/17/06
haha it happens to me alot **i eat when im bored to and im not even hungry** its just a habit but were all learning to deal with it..

From panic at the disco junkie, Age 14 - 06/23/08
Ht. 5'5", Start: 183 lb, Current: 177 lb, Goal: 130 lb - ...i have 2 well maybe 3 huge problems 1. is that **i always eat when im bored, and i know its when im bored beacause i always say im hungrey and its when im not really doing anything so its out of bordum.**

Reply from cheryl, Age 16 - 6/17/06
I am the biggest boredom eater ever!!I just figured that out the other day and i've soo changed my life because of that.

From Leena, Age 14 - 4/1/06
Ht. 5'6, Wt. blah. - **I eat when I'm bored...like, really bad.** I'll be like, oh..theres nothing to do...let's go raid the fridge! Erg...any ideas?

From MaKayla, Age 9 - 03/23/06
Ht. 4ft 9in, Wt. 144 - hey waz ^ , my sister makes fun of me ,how can i make her stop .please put it on the board .and i have gained weight and **i can not stop eating when i am board**? help ME please. thank a lot

From sk8ergirl, Age 16 - 1/5/08 -
Ht. 5'2", Start: 215 lb, Current: 215 lb, Goal: 165 lb - ...**I eat cause I am depressed and bored most of the time.** That is the only reason why... I skateboard and everyone who saw me skate say I am really good and if I loose a lot of weight I could be a pro skater cause I am really good. Expecially for a fat girl...

In a poll we asked kids how often they feel bored.
(http://www.blubberbuster.com/cgi/poll_new_28.cgi)

How often do you feel bored?

45%	47%	8%
I am bored every day	Some days but not every day	I'm rarely bored, I do fun stuff

VOTES SO FAR

164 kids voted

Very few of the 164 kids responding indicate that they are rarely bored.

The following are some of their comments about this poll:

➔ Whenever im bored, i eat and eat, but even though i feel bad after i eat, i just eat more

➔ when ever i m bored i eat its cause i have nothin else to do or i'll be watchin tv and i eat i always eat i can't help it even if i m not hungry

➔ When i feel bored i usually eat a lot. I also usually eat a lot candy, icecream and chocolate when I am bored

➔ These days there is not much to do for teenagers

➔ I eat a lot when iam bored thats why iam so obese 9 years 9 m

➔ I eat when i get bored it is terrible. Also when something tastes good no matter if i am full or not i will eat it. That is what i need to fix!

In our chat rooms overweight kids frequently chat about being bored.

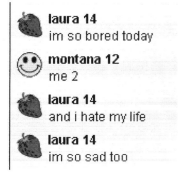

laura 14
im so bored today

montana 12
me 2

laura 14
and i hate my life

laura 14
im so sad too

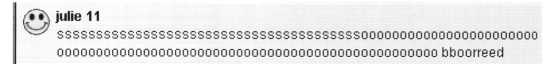

julie 11
ssssssssssssssssssssssssssssssssssssssssoooooooooooooooooooooooo
ooooooooooooooooooooooooooooooooooooooooooooooooooo bboorreed

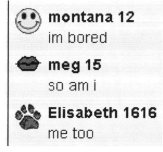

montana 12
im bored

meg 15
so am i

Elisabeth 1616
me too

190

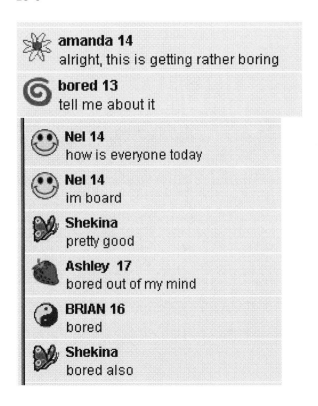

A teen actually remarked that the word 'bored' is one of the most spoken words in the chat room.

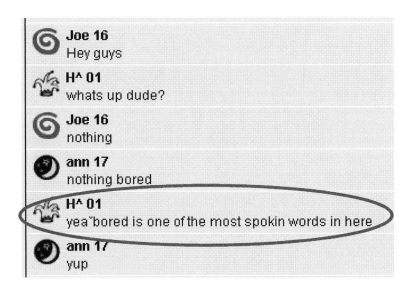

We ran a scan on our bulletin board database and chatroom transcripts and found that the kids were right. The word 'bored' or 'boredom' is used nearly as much as the word 'weight' (0.627:1 ratio.)

And kids in the chatrooms also frequently say that they eat to relieve boredom.

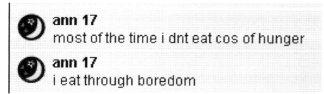

ann 17
most of the time i dnt eat cos of hunger

ann 17
i eat through boredom

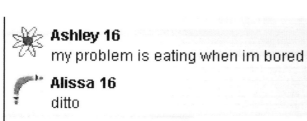

Ashley 16
my problem is eating when im bored

Alissa 16
ditto

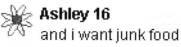

Ashley 16
and i want junk food

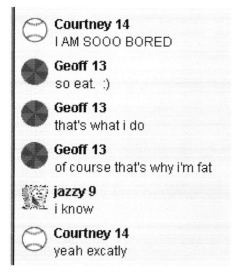

Courtney 14
I AM SOOO BORED

Geoff 13
so eat. :)

Geoff 13
that's what i do

Geoff 13
of course that's why i'm fat

jazzy 9
i know

Courtney 14
yeah excatly

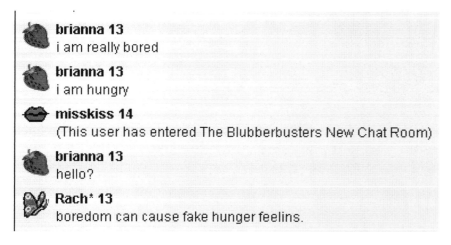

brianna 13
i am really bored

brianna 13
i am hungry

misskiss 14
(This user has entered The Blubberbusters New Chat Room)

brianna 13
hello?

Rach* 13
boredom can cause fake hunger feelins.

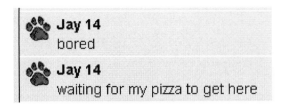

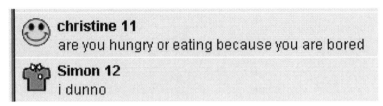

What is boredom?

Webster's dictionary defines boredom as, "the state of being weary and restless through lack of interest." Wikepedia defines it as, "an unpleasant feeling in which the individual feels a lack of interest or dullness."(http://en.wikipedia.org/wiki/Boredom). Lack of stimulation is a cause of boredom, but stimulation may not relieve it.

Boredom, depression, stress, and anxiety (nervousness) appear to go hand in hand with overweight kids. As a matter of fact, many kids say that they are bored when they may be actually depressed, stressed, lonely, or anxious. "I'm bored" is more socially acceptable than "I'm depressed." Many of the comfort eating and stress eating posts contain the word "bored," for example:

From ChElssEa, Age 13 - 04/03/05
I hate when I comfort eat but i do it alot and i just cant stop it that and **i eat when im bored I DONT KNOW HOW TO STOP ITS KILLING ME**

Age 11, female, 5", 140 lbs - i eat all day even whens thier nothing else to eat. i'll make an food out of no food at all **m not even hungry just bored and depresed**

This is ALYSSA's story:
I cant stop eating what do i do? **i eat when im bored and when im sad, im an emotional eater.** i really want to have a nice body! help me!

Reply from sk8ergirl16, Age 16 - 1/12/08 -
Ha **im so bored right now and i need to find something to do otherwise im going to eat. I eat for depression and boredness too.**

This is KAYLA's question:
Being overweight is hard. I am currently **235 pounds and 16 years old**. I am overweight by 100 pounds. Its hard when you go to school and all your friends are skinny and wearing belly shirts. The mall is the worst part because when my friends and I go to the mall, all this guys flirt with my friends, but ignore me. I get **depressed and sad. I eat when I am bored and have nothing to do.** I was diagnosed with depression a year ago … the reason is because I am overweight.

From Kat, Age 15 - 6/22/06 -
Ht. 5,8, Wt. 183 - Well,i keep trying to loose weight but it keeps finding me..lol. I try over and over again but i just cant stick to a diet!..**i get bored.or sad and then BANG there i am gettin food again even when i am well over full ugh**

Therefore, boredom eating in kids is likely mislabeled comfort eating or stress eating.

Boredom can also be described as lack of distraction. Distractions allow kids to avoid having to face the pain of their lives. This description suggests a "cure' for boredom: kids facing their problems head on, instead of seeking distractions such as TV, video games, or food. Writing down their problems, 1, 2, 3… can help greatly - anything in their lives that is bothering them. Underneath each problem they write a plan (see pp. 287).

In Chapter 13, a vicious cycle is described of detachment from life, resulting in boredom, eating to combat boredom, more pain, more detachment, and so on.

When do kids become bored and overeat?

While watching TV or using the computer...

From Madison, Age 12 - 6/19/06
Ht. 5'7, Wt. 174 - Hey guys .. just a quick question, i want to loose weight this summer, and usually im sort of active, but **when i watch tv, i get bored and eat like even when im not hungry!** it turns ill just have 2 cookies into ill only have 10 cookies, how do i stop this??

From Montana, Age 13 - 01/09/06
Ht. 5'1, Wt. Don't wanna say... - Alrightyy... Here iz my problem.. I think I do okay UNTILL I come home from school. I usally be lazy and sit on the computer all night and I usally eat junk and buy junk after school and I can't help it. I'm usally bored and nuttin to do so **I sit on the comp and eat or watch tv and eat** cauze I have nuttin else to do...

In the wintertime when they can't go outside...

From Sara, Age 16 - 3/3/08
Ht. 5'8", Start: 330 lb, Current: 283 lb, Goal: 150 lb - I know I have a lot to go, but every pound counts. I really haven't been working out. It is way to cold and I have been busy. I cannot wait for summer. I will be working and swimming, and doing etc. **I hate being stuck in the house during winter. I get bored and eat.** Not the best thing. Only 8 more pant sizes to go. Do you think I can do it?

Holidays from school...

From Lucee, Age 17 - 07/01/08
Ht. 5'8", Start: 179 lb, Current: 161 lb, Goal: 150 lb - **AAGH, i just cnt stand the holidays! Its only been one day and i am already bored out my head, all i ever want to do when im lazing about my house is eat**, thats probably why every single summer (except last year) i have gained weight when i have intended to lose some. ..

What helps?

What have kids found that helps them to avoid eating when bored?

From Whitney, Age 17 - 3/13/07 -
Ht. 5'8", Start: 200 lb, Current: 170 lb, Goal: 150 lb - Well I didn't weigh in again, I think i'm avoiding the scale...haha ... But lets see a lot of people were asking me how i lost all the weight and **i actually lost like 45 lbs** and was down to 155 but i kinda gained some of it back but really all i did was cut out the bad put in the good and exercise everyday. I mean i know it sounds incredibly easy but thats b/c it is, i mean **my main problem was fighting off to not just eat when i was bored so I just found stuff to occupy my time.**

Age 15, female, Ht. 5'8, Wt. 240 lbs,
i just zone out and not think about anything. ill sit there for hours just listening to my discman, and i wont eat, because im so abosorbed in the tunes.

Age 14, female, Ht. 5 '0, Wt. 105 lbs,
when ever i am board i think of somthing to do and stay away from the kitchen

Fun activities

Exercise and fun activities, especially with other kids, are the best ways for kids to avoid boredom and overeating.

⁕ From Lucee, Age 17 - 7/1/08
Ht. 5'8", Start: 179 lb, Current: 161 lb, Goal: 150 lb - ... yesterday before dinner i was reallllly bored with nothing to do (all my friends are on holiday/busy) so i went out on my bike for about 3miles and then later on in the evening i was beginning to get that bored hungry feeling ... so i did 30mins on my exercise bike. **Basically everytime im hungry (from boredom, not from real hunger) i am going to exercise!** In two weeks i will be working 9-5 monday to friday at a University on top of my usual weekend job so hopefully the weight will come off easily then cos ill be really busy and wont have time to boredom eat!

⁕ From Adrienne, Age 13, female - 4/20/02
... **i started only eating when i was hungry** and in 1 1/2 weeks i lost 7 lbs ... i drank a lot of water and **when i was bored i went outside and jumped on the trampolene or went out with my friends just 2 chill.**

⁕ From michelle, Age 13, female - 3/23/06
Over summer break **i tried not to be at home so much so i didn't get bored and eat. ..** and **i also joined a softball team.** At the end of the summer i had **lost 35 pounds.**

⁕ From Jane, Age 14, female - 2/16/02
I loved food and just couldnt stop overeating!!!**Whenever i'm bored, sad, happy, watching tv I crave food.** So i didnt worry **there was another way...excercise.** I jog every morning for 25 min and i dance for half an hour and in the day in school i play around with my friends and i joined alot of sport

So, kids have had to figure out for themselves that they are bored, depressed, or stressed and help themselves deal with that emotion. Eating to escape or eating for entertainment is unfortunately the way overweight kids (and parents) commonly seem to deal with these feelings, as commented on below:

Age 14, female, 5'6", 130 lbs - It seems like people live to eat these days...**its become like entertainment or something to go out and get food somewhere.** Well we need to all just eat to LIVE!!!!!!!!

What is the solution for so much boredom causing kids to overeat? If boredom is lack of distractions to cope with depression, loneliness, or stress, then fun activities, hobbies, musical instruments, and books can help. If kids are detaching from their lives, then facing their emotions and life difficulties head-on is the answer. But kids need help and support to do this, from their parents, teachers, and health professionals.

What's the health profession's view on emotional eating?

*In December 2007, I submitted a letter to the editor of the journal, Pediatrics, in regard to their special supplement on "Assessment of Child and Adolescent Overweight and Obesity." In my letter I noted that the supplement made no mention of the emotional reasons for overeating in children and teens. My letter was not published, with the following reason given by the supplement author: "Although the writer has a legitimate concern about the issue of emotional eating, esp in the context of boredom, but there is virtually no scientific literature on this in the context of obesity assessment, or more specifically, intervention trials in which emotional eating was treated, and outcome was change in BMI (or even energy intake)…One could expand on that answer, to be more respectful and to acknowledge the valid concern, but **all of that takes time that I don't necessarily think is justified**."*

Is time justified to investigate emotional eating when so many kids identify it as a reason for their overeating and overweight? Another researcher has stated, "I eat for comfort. Everyone does. That doesn't imply that it's causing obesity." [Hill 2006].

Per the post on the previous page from Jane, Age 14, exercise, or any physical activity, especially with other kids, is a wonderful way to combat boredom, as well as loneliness, depression, and stress, which are many times described as boredom. House chores also might be a way for kids to stay busy and combat boredom.

In the next chapter kids talk more about exercise…

12 | Exercise

Most weight management programs believe that exercise, or any physical activity, is essential for weight control. Exercise has many benefits, including:

➢ *Exercise burns calories.*
➢ *Exercise increases endorphins, natural chemicals in the body which improve mood.*
➢ *Exercise distracts from eating.*
➢ *Exercise is a form of 'displacement activity', which relieves stress and boredom, so that kids are less likely to overeat for those reasons.*
➢ *Exercise enhances the health of the heart, muscles, and bones and combats diseases such as diabetes and cholesterol elevation.*

We asked kids about exercise in a poll:
(http://www.blubberbuster.com/cgi/poll_new_15_percent.cgi)

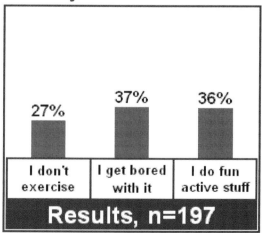

How do you feel about exercise?

| 27% | 37% | 36% |
| I don't exercise | I get bored with it | I do fun active stuff |

Results, n=197

197 kids voted

More than a third of kids voting say that they exercise, about a third say that they get bored and quit, and the rest don't exercise.

Comments from kids on this poll:

➜ I like to excercise but I often forget or loose interest!!!!

➜ even if i dont lose weight, it helps me feel better

➜ I think its great but sometimes it can be really rough

➜ I just think it is boring

We know that exercise enhances weight loss, but overweight kids have particular obstacles to exercise that need addressing.

Obstacles to exercise

Physical reasons

Unfortunately, significantly overweight kids may not be able to move much without easily getting out of breath or causing pain in their joints due to the burden of carrying around the extra weight.

From Sarah, Age 17 - 01/07/09
Ht. 5'2", Start: 315 lb, Current: 315 lb, Goal: 215 lb - Hi. I weighed myself today and I couldn't believe how much i was! I mean I knew I was VERY FAT but i had no idea I was over 300! Thats the first time I've weighed myself in about a year because I was always too scared to see how much I gained… this year Im going to try so hard to lose some weight. I really have no idea how though. **I can hardly exercise because I'v got so big!**

From Ben, Age 12 - 11/30/07
Ht. 5'5", Start: 220 lb, Current: 221 lb, Goal: 130 lb - I am always like the fattest in my age group.. even on blubberbusters. I've tried to lose weight before.. but it didn't work out. I am big, fat, I look fat. I am in 6th grade. **I can't exercise as much because of my foot.**

→ i get sick when i exercise.. sometimes i even trough up

→ I cant exercise because it is hard for me. Im so big that when i start exercising i break into a sweat. if i would get used to exercising i could do it but im big and fat

→ iam so fat i cannot run my legs rub it huerts

→ I cant run my thighs smash together really painful with every step my knees are bouncing my bely around......i'm 12 and 5 feet tall and 480 pounds

It is tragic that eating too much results in kids not being able to participate in sports, as the two posts below relate.

From Lisa, Age 11 - 6/27/08
Ht. 4'10", Start: 231 lb, Current: 231 lb, Goal: 150 lb - Hi! I'm **11 years old** and I'm really overweight. I weight **231 pounds** and I really need to loose weight. I just don#t know how. I have some trouble with walking. **I can only walk very short distances. So I don't know how I can do sports**....

This is MICHAEL's question:
i live in Mississippi.Down here sports i a really big thing. **i weigh 230 lbs and id like to try and lose some weight to become something better than a 4th string offensive lineman and maybe make the baseball team.** id like to try and lose 80 lbs.

Embarrassment

Overweight kids say they're embarrassed to exercise in front of others.

From Jennifer, Age 16 - 07/29/09
Ht. 5'8", Start: 211 lb, Current: 223 lb, Goal: 140 lb - I'm thinking about doing some sports to lose weight. I hate walking and going to the gym, but swimming could be a good idea. But I feel fat, fat, fat, when I put on my swimsuit (which is a tad tight, too). **Do you think I can go to a public pool if I look so fat? I'm afraid people would stare at me**....

From jim, Age 17, male - 1/19/02
When I went to high school my weight was at **13 stone (182 lb.)**, by the next year it was at **14 and a half**. My self confidence was low, people laughed and ignored me. **I refused to do sports in school because of my size.** Then there was the **bullying some kids pinched the fat till it bruised and then there was the Physical Education teacher who made life hell and one day gave me a 10 minute insulting in front of the class.** By this point i had started trying to mutilate myself cutting myself with knives, stubbing fags on my arms etc. **I got a job which involved a lot of hard physical work pushing, pulling, lifting, walking etc.** I continued to eat the same - which wasn't much having previously visited a dietician and made little difference to my weight. I make a lot of money and still go to school. Yet the biggest advantage is my weight is down to **11 stone (154 lb.)**.

Reply from Flower Fawn, Age 15 - 8/8/08
Ht. 5'5", Start: 184 lb, Current: 177 lb, Goal: 145 lb - **I know what you mean about embarrassment about exercise. I still can't use my new bike becuase I'm scared people will stare at me and point or snicker** and I'm just so self-conscious, so I use exercise DVDs.

From lorenda, Age 17 - 06/07/06
Ht. 5'3, Wt. 186 - ...i have just discovered that i weigh 186. this is the biggest i have ever been in my life. i just want the quickest way to lose weight. **im to ashamed to let anyone see me run because i feel so big.** i would really apprciate any who has any great ideals because im very desperate.

→ i don't like 2 excercise @ home b-cuz i get made fun of, my parents or brother will make comments like: o lookshes ACTUALLY trying 2 lose wait" and then they'll start laughing, so i become extremly discurraged and VERY embarrassed

Eating more after exercising

Exercise is a key part of losing weight, but unfortunately kids may eat more after exercising.

From Pam, Age 16 - 10/19/08
Ht. 5'5", Start: 170 lb, Current: 150 lb, Goal: 130 lb - OK... I swim for at least two hours for at least four days a week. But the thing is, **after I swim I can't stop eating. And usually, I use it as an excuse to eat more.** But I want to lose weight, and I don't know how to control my appetitite after practice.

→ **ITs hard to keep weight off after you exercise you tire yourself and then just makes you go for a snack!!**

→ **I don't really lose weight by playing sports. But now I know why because this site has helped me to learn why. The answer is I ate the same amount of food that I burned off so I have to eat less food!**

This is ADRIENNA's question:
... i decided to run track but **after i run im so hungry so i eat alot of food but i want to stop** and look great for the summer..but **how can i do this? Please Help Me!!!**

Fun Ways to Exercise

From Michelle, Age 14 - 7/19/08
Ht. 5'8", Start: 228 lb, Current: 194 lb, Goal: 150 lb - ok... **I got my skateboard and i lost another 4 pounds** thats 8 pounds for the whole summer ... i think that it has alot to do with **i found an exercise i like no i love (which is skateboarding of course)i can't help but go outside and ride it like every 2 hours** .. and its really helping.

Dance Dance Revolution

Kids say over and over again on the bulletin boards and in the chatrooms that DDR (Dance Dance Revolution) is the most fun way to exercise. DDR is a game you play with your computer. There is a floor plate or mat where you put your feet. The idea is to put your feet in the same spots as the dances on the computer screen show. DDR is played to music. Kids say when they play DDR, they don't even know they are exercising. And kids also may play against each other, as shown below:

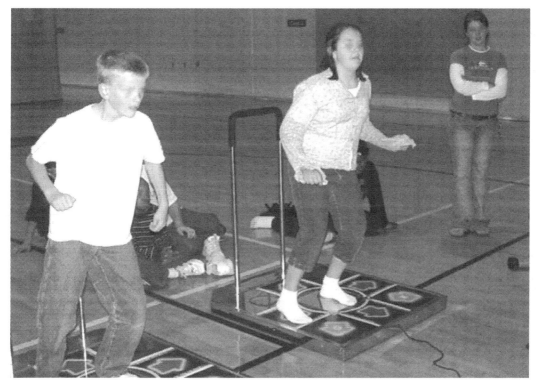

Kids playing Dance Dance Revolution

From Carli, Age 14, female - 1/14/05
Hey! I used to weigh 123 pounds and 4'7. For Christmas we got a **Dance dance revoultion game for the ps2. ive lost 10 pounds by playing it!** it makes me feel great that i can play ninentdo and still lose weight!

From Sara, Age 16 - 3/16/08
Ht. 5'9", Start: 330 lb, Current: 282 lb, Goal: 150 lb - So **I got DDR for my birthday. It is amazing.** It counts how many calories you lose and it tells you how much weight you lose. I lost 854 calories playing for four hours. I am hoping I can lose a lot on this. I hate going outside in the winter. It sucks...

From Julia, Age 16 - 1/30/07
Ht. 5'6", Wt. 176 - I just want everyone to know that **Dance Dance Revolution** makes for a great workout! It even has a workout mode where you put in your body info and it will calculate how many calories you burn in the songs! ♥

Reply from ella, Age 13 - 2/11/07
i got **ddr** for christmas and i use it everyday, **i get hooked on it** and can play for 2 hrs. staight. it's a really good exercise

Dancing

Dancing is great exercise, helps kids lose weight, and is s-o-o fun!

⭐ From Jennifer*, Age 14, female - 12/4/05
I am at 158 cuz i dance!

⭐ Reply from Claire, Age 19, Wt: 198 - 08/14/08
... **dancing is a greatt exercise! the only one I like anyway lol**...if my scale says that I gained a lb. I suggest we both have a bonfire and throw them in!

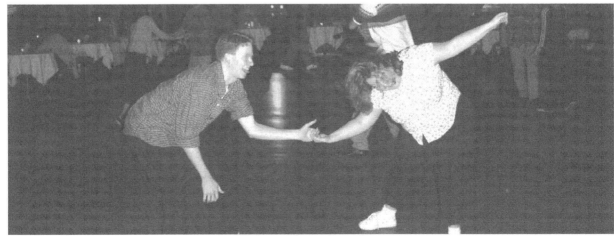

Kids swing dancing

⋆ From Autumn, Age 14, female - 6/7/03
wus-up everyone. I'm 14 yrs old,5'9 and now weigh **254lbs**. 2 weeks ago **i was 263**. I tried every diet... I was very depressed. Then as i was searching online i found this web site. you people really encouraged me and help me loose weight. **Now I don't eat out, eat junk food,or drink soda or juice**. I eat lots of fruits and veggies. I drink tons of water(a gallon a day). I also don't eat after 6 o'clock. **I exercise by dancing for 1hr or MORE! I love to dance**... OH YEAH, my weight goal is 160lbs.

Reply from Tricia, Age 16 - 07/10/03
I go dancin at the community center thing every Sunday. Im shy but **theres guys who are worse dancers than me**... lol.

Dancing in their rooms

Kids can just dance by themselves in their bedrooms or rec rooms.

Reply from Emily, Age 12 - 05/19/07   - IP#: 4.239.255.xxx
Dance! put on your favorite music and dance to it. It is a fun exercise that also burns alot of calories

⋆ From Jennifer, Age 13, female - 10/29/02
the best, easiest and funniest way to loose weight is to dance. at home put ur music loud and just dance to the beat. feel relaxed and tell yourself wow. trust me it works. i had curves and a flat stomach in within a few months...

Other fun exercise

What other fun ways do kids say they exercise?

Reply from Alexandra, Age 14 - 08/15/07
Well **for fun exercise I do a pilates** video by Kathy Smith for the abs and lower body its actually fun and relaxing. Not many reps too so its not really difficult. I bought it at tj max. haha.

This is SAL's story: i think maby you should the **rocky traning video** because that modavated me to lose some weight and it still does .

Reply from Miss K, Age 18 - 06/10/05
... just make sure you're active. **Ride a bike, go swimming, take a walk with the dog. fun exercise :)**.

Reply from Sean, Age 14 - 02/17/05
… go swimming because its the easiest and prob the most fun exercise you can do. :)

Reply from Tricia, Age 16 - 07/10/03
I got a dog. Hes wonderful. Hes my friend and we take walks together every day, even we jog some. That keeps me from heading for the fridge all the time and is fun exercise.

Like most of us, kids come up with excuses for avoiding exercise. Making it fun is the best way to motivate kids to exercise.

*In the next chapter we look at **Vicious Cycles,** which overweight kids fall into, including several involving exercise.*

13 | Vicious Cycles

Overweight kids seem to get stuck in many "vicious cycles," aka "vicious circles." Vicious cycles are situations where the situation contributes to the cause of the situation itself, thus making the situation continue. 'Vicious' means that the cycle is harmful. If the situation contributes significantly to the cause, then the situation may increase as a result, thus increasing the cause even more, and this may become a runaway situation, truly vicious. Overeating in kids frequently seems to be a vicious cycle.

Some types of overeating vicious cycles

Comfort eating vicious cycle

From cayla, Age 12 - 2/9/08 -
Ht. 5'3", Start: 145 lb, Current: 150 lb, Goal: 100 lb - I feel so fat. It is not healthy for a 12 year old to way 150.Sombody please reply.I started out the year waying 145 and now way I way 150. If I keep living like this I will be the only person one earth that ways 700 pounds! **I am unhappy because I eat Ieat cause I am unhappy.**

Kids seek comfort in food because they are unhappy, to make themselves feel better. But then they gain weight, which makes them feel more unhappy and rejected, so they eat more to make themselves feel better, gain even more weight, and so on, as illustrated at right. This can result in a runaway cycle where the overweight child is increasingly unhappy, grazes on food continually, and becomes obese.

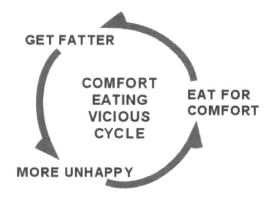

From Lilliie, Age 15 - 03/13/09
Ht. 5'2", Start: 155 lb, Current: 260 lb, Goal: 100 lb - Hi I'm Lillie and i'm new on here i'm really overweight and i cant seem to lose weight **people tease me because im fat which makes me eat more** since September i've gained 55 lbs

From Shan, Age 19 - 08/16/06 -
Ht. 5"3, Wt. Overweight - ...I just feel so alone. I feel like every day is a struggle because **I'm not sure whether I'm going to have that yucky feeling after eating so much.** I wish I could tell people so they could support me, but there's no one to tell. It's not that I'm worried about losing a lot of weight, even though I have to. Right now I'm worried about gaining a lot. **I'm in that vicious circle where I eat a lot then feel bad then eat more and more and my weight is shooting up.** I feel like I can't pull myself out of this alone. My whole day revolves around eating. I hate everyday lately:(Please help

From Sophia, Age 12 - 3/9/08 -
Ht. 5'7", Start: 187 lb, Current: 190 lb, Goal: 145 lb - I have been trying soo hard to move forward with everything that I deal with stress wise and just my life. Starting in about first grade I relized that some kids will put you down, **I didnt know how to handle that so I ate away my emotions. Now all of that eatting has made me feel worse and almost 200 pounds** at 12 years old.

Reply from lola, Age 15 - 04/30/05
... dont put yourself down so much else you'll never lose weight... remember the **vicious circle? u eat when ur depressed, u put on weight then u get sad so u eat to forget about ur depresion and so on...**

Parents see this in their kids, as well.

From Nicole, Child's Age 15 - 1/27/08
My child is teased all the time at school and has terrible self esteem issues. **When shes depressed she eats and when she eats she gets more depressed because the fact that she ate that, meant she put on more weight.** ... Shes 5'10 and weighs 250. Please help, I want to put an end to her depression.

What can a parent do about this vicious cycle? Loving the child in spite of feeling upset about the child's weight and talking with the child about the vicious cycle, in which the child is caught, helps more than anything. (see also parental vicious cycles, pp. 210-211).

Pleasurable food does comfort the pains of life, but only briefly. Once the food is eaten, the pains of life come back. The same is true if food is used for stress relief.

Stress eating vicious cycle

From Brianna, Age 14 - 5/2/07 -
Ht. 5'6", Start: 171 lb, Current: 171 lb, Goal: 120 lb - This is my first time here having to to write my wieght was very hard for I have very felt self confident until now I don't even like shopping any more. **Every time I'm stressed I eat and my weight is making me stressed...**

Eating to cope with stress can be a vicious cycle. Being obese is stressful itself, so the child may eat to relieve the stress of being obese, which worsens the problem. Also, when kids overeat as a way to cope with stress, they feel disappointed in themselves. This adds to their stress, which may cause them to overeat even more.

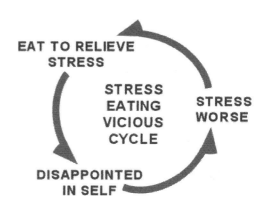

The below posts further describe this cycle:

From Flower Fawn, Age 15 - 8/8/08 -
Ht. 5'5", Start: 184 lb, Current: 177 lb, Goal: 145 lb - ... my life is very, very stressful sometimes. Let's just say that my family is going through a tough time tight now...that's one of the reasons it's so hard for me to loose weight. **When I'm stressed, my face breaks out and I overeat, and then I feel lousy and hate myself,** and it just starts this really **vicious cycle that's hard to break.** But in good news... I've slowly been weaning myself off desserts and second portions...

From Bianca, Age 14 - 10/27/07 -
Ht. 5'10", Start: 250 lb, Current: 249 lb, Goal: 140 lb - Well the past few days something personal has happened and I've been totally depressed. Due to that I've been binging every now and then. I know its bad but I didnt know what to do. **Now that I ate that I feel absolutely terrible.**

From Taryn, Age 18 - 12/28/08
Ht. 157 cm, Start: 86 kg, Current: 86 kg, Goal: 65 kg - ...I don't want to be the victom anymore and **I hate being teased because I just eat more on the sly then...** (Note: 157 cm, 86 kg is 5'2", 189 lb.)

Kids also overeat when other people comment about their weight or comment about their bodies.

BRITTANY's story:

i love to eat especially since **im stressed all the time** and **ppl all comment on my weight which makes me eat more.** plz help me to lose weight i weigh about 326 now

From Justin, Age 16 - 10/18/08

Ht. 5'7", Start: 298 lb, Current: 298 lb, Goal: 175 lb - can someone help me? people always make fun of me cauze i got man boobs that shake- it really sucks. What shoudl i say to them because **it really hurts me and then i eat more and get even fatter**

Age 13, male, 5'7, 185 lbs **i over eat** just like when im board but stress does effect some people **also when people tell me im fat**

Just weighing themselves can put kids into an overeating vicious cycle...

From Morgan, Age 15 - 8/26/06 -

Ht. 5'4", Wt. 201 - This morning I got on the scale and saw that it read "201", and I started crying. I'm still crying. **I saw my weight, got depressed, and started eating.** I really really need help. It scares me. I'm really scared right now. I need help.

From jenny, Age 12 - 06/13/05 - IP#: 24.124.120.xxx

i go on diets and it feels like i am losing weight but then **i get on the scale and i see i weight more and then i eat more and i feel bad..**

From Claire, Age 19 - 07/05/08

Ht. 5'4", Start: 210 lb, Current: 176 lb, Goal: 140 lb - ... **I usually eat a lot when something is boterhing me** (emotional eater,you guessed it)...but lately **what's been bothering me is the fact that I'M NOT LOSING WEIGHT.** DOes this make any sense? and then I jsut start eating

Exercise vicious cycles

*Overweight kids fall into vicious cycles with exercising, actually with **not** exercising. As noted in Chapter 12 on Exercise, quite heavy kids simply may not be able to move around, without becoming short of breath or experiencing joint pain. Lack of exercise contributes to further weight gain, which then makes it even harder to move, as shown in the Exercise Vicious Cycle 1 (right).*

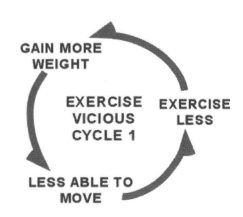

From Amanda, Age 13 - 01/16/09

Ht. 4'11", Start: 260 lb, Current: 267 lb, Goal: 100 lb - What do you HATE most about being OVERweight?? I hate getting called names but I REALLY hate being BIG and

REALLY REALLY HATE being TOO HEAVY!!! It's hard to fit in the desks at school and seats in a movie theater because I have so much FAT. It feels HORRIBLE to SQUEEZE into a seat that's TOO SMALL! **Being TOO HEAVY feels even worse because I get SO TIRED just walking.** Some days I HATE doing anything because I have to carry all the WEIGHT. **When I tried to jog and lose some weight it was TOO hard to jog being this HEAVY. That's so UNfair because the more you NEED to exercise the harder it IS to exercise!!! I could exercise if I WEIGHed less but I can't weigh LESS withOUT exercise!** I HATE being OVERweight!

From Jessica, Age 13 - 07/19/08
Ht. 5'3", Start: 362 lb, Current: 406 lb, Goal: 120 lb - I'm so sick of this...
I literally haven't a clue how to stop eating. My stomach hirts so bad right now, and yet I'm still eating. Why? I don't even know!... I hate the way I look and the way I feel. I look in the mirror and what stares back at me is huge, fat, bulgy, and gross. And **I can barely move because I'm so big. It's so hard... everything is so hard. And yet I keep eating...** Because no matter how big I get, or how bad it hurts, I CAN'T stop. **And I can't exercise, because I'm almost too big to move. Exercise is pretty much impossible.** I feel hopeless. ...

From Lisa, Age 11 - 6/27/08 -
Ht. 4'10", Start: 231 lb, Current: 231 lb, Goal: 150 lb - Hi! I'm 11 years old and I'm really overweight. I weight 231 pounds and I really need to loose weight. I just don#t know how. I have some trouble with walking. **I can only walk very short distances. So I don't know how I can do sports**....

Or they are embarrassed to exercise in front of others.

From Flower Fawn, Age 15 - 6/17/08 -
Ht. 5'5", Start: 184 lb, Current: 178 lb, Goal: 150 lb - Hi guys. For the first time in MONTHS I was actually pretty happy with how I did today.... I also did laps on my bike around the parking lot for about 10 min, tomorrow I hope to go for about 30min. How did I do? I hope to ride my bike a lot over the summer. :) **I've never rode the bike trails near my house before, but there are a lot of cute guys from neighboring schools and I'd like to check it out. The problem is...I feel REALLY self-conscious exercising while there are people around.** I know it's ridiculous and I can't hide forever, so how do you guys deal???

This may result in a second exercise vicious cycle of less exercise, more weight gain, more embarrassed to be seen, and so on (right). To break this vicious cycle there are ways kids can exercise by themselves, such as Dance Dance Revolution and simply dancing to music in their rooms.

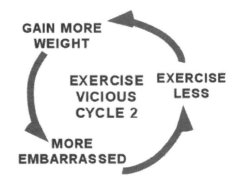

Depression and exercise vicious cycle

Depression itself can sap motivation to exercise. More weight gain then occurs, more depression, less energy, less exercise, more weight gain, etc. – another vicious cycle.

From Caitlin, Age 16 - 11/09/08
Ht. 5'4", Start: 145 lb, Current: 149 lb, Goal: 125 lb - so i have gained four pounds and it kinda sucks and yea. I have a giant lunch and **never exercised cause i just was too depressed**....what should i do??

This is ALLY's question:
How do you start to exercise if you have no energy?

Exercise discomfort vicious cycle

The discomfort of exercise may result in comfort eating, which results in further weight gain, less ability to exercise, etc., as the below post describes:

This is Teri's story:
My mom works at a gym and told me to **excersise**. at first **the pain was horrible it made me want to eat and eat and then eat again.**

Parental vicious cycles

Overweight kids may get stuck in two types of vicious cycles with their parents:

1) Parent being upset about the child's weight:

When a child or teen first becomes a bit overweight, this may upset one or both parents. As a result, the parent(s) may become critical and not as loving. The child or teen may then seek comfort in food, which

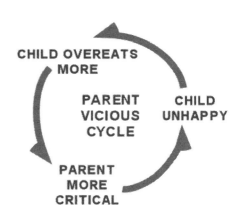

results in more weight gain, more parental criticism and withdrawal of love, and so on…

From Jaimie, Age 14 - 09/04/08 -
Ht. 6'0", Start: 174 lb, Current: 196 lb, Goal: 163 lb - My mom always critizes me she calls me fat and it does hurt… kuz i never was lyk this till i got in to the7th grade…i probably put on a few pounds that year but **she made it worse kuz that made me sad and i guess i wuld eat mor, and i still do**… im a good student but no **she cares about the looks** not the schoolwork…

Even if the parent is not critical, simply bringing up the subject of weight may upset the child, resulting in comfort eating, as one parent describes: **"I talked to him about his weight and told him it was only going to get worse if he continued to eat like he did but that only made him upset and when he's upset he turns to food."** *This is a tough situation. However, just asking the child what he/she feels and not warning that things will get worse with health risks, etc. may avoid resulting comfort eating.*

2) Parental food for love:

Parents may feed a child as a form of love, but they also want love and attention from the child. When the parent gives the child any food he or she wants, in order to receive love from the child, a vicious cycle may result. As the child learns how to manipulate the parent, the parent may feed the child more and more food to continue to get love from the child. As a result the child may become overweight or obese. This is also called parental 'enabling.' Wanting love also may be the reason that many pet owners overfeed their pets. Many dogs and cats are now overweight. Pets are like children to many people.

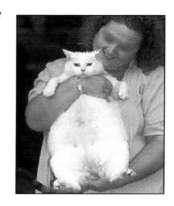

Dieting vicious cycle

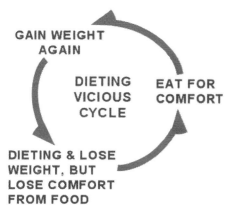

GAIN WEIGHT
AGAIN

DIETING
VICIOUS
CYCLE

EAT FOR
COMFORT

DIETING & LOSE
WEIGHT, BUT
LOSE COMFORT
FROM FOOD

The dieting vicious cycle is where the child or teen gains weight, goes on a diet, loses weight but also loses comfort from food, gets stressed or depressed from lack of comfort, starts overeating again, gains the weight back, goes back on a diet, and so on. This is also called 'yo-yo' dieting. Kids may become so discouraged in this cycle that they give up, which makes them feel like a failure resulting in more stress/comfort eating.

From Lucee, Age 17 - 07/27/08 -
Ht. 5'8", Start: 179 lb, Current: 157 lb, Goal: 150 lb - ...The thing is that i keep binging. I keep gaining a few lbs from weekend binges taking me to about 160 and then i spend the next week dieting so i get back to 157 by the next weekend but it keeps going on like that. **In the couple weeks i have gained and lost the same 3lbs numerous times...**

From michelle, Age 14 - 07/13/08 -
Ht. 5'8", Start: 228 lb, Current: 202 lb, Goal: 130 lb - I can no longer do this... **I've been dieting on and off sense i was 8 years old,** why because sense then my grandmother has always said something about my weight ....and **i can't just keep eating right one day and chips and cake the other**

From AShley, Age 15 - 01/23/08 -
Ht. 5'4", Start: 150 lb, Current: 150 lb, Goal: 130 lb - hellllp. i suck at dieting its week three **the first week i got to 144 but then i completely screwed up the other 2 and now im 150**

From Sade, Age 17 - 01/28/08
Ht. 4'10", Start: 165 lb, Current: 162 lb, Goal: 100 lb - ... I still can't believe I gained 3 pounds back. I'm really mad at myself **it feels like this overweight cycle is never going to end.**

To stop the dieting cycle, the child or teen must deal with the reasons that prompt them to overeat. Kids must learn to face their problems head on, instead of using food to escape from them. Here is where open, supportive discussions with parents or others can be helpful.

What is the child missing in his/her life? Does the child lack friends, parental support, school performance, or a stable home life? Write down what the child is missing and come up with a plan to deal with each item. For example, if the child is having academic problems, the school may be able to arrange tutoring help. Pets and hobbies can help supply comfort instead of food.

Willpower vicious cycle

There is the willpower vicious cycle. The child or teen desperately tries to resist a craving for junk food. Trying to resist is stressful, which results in even less ability to resist stress eating. So the child finally gives in and eats the junk food, feels disappointed which results in even more stress, craves for the stress relief of

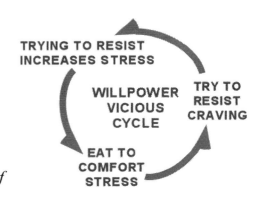

food, tries to resist, gets more stressed, gives in again and eats more, feels further stress, and so on…

From Amanda, Age 14 - 10/09/09 - IP#: 75.125.237.xxx
Ht. 5'0", Start: 260 lb, Today: 304 lb, Goal: 100 lb
…when I get a CRAVEing I have to have it and I go CRRRAZY until I do! I can't think about ANYthing else and **the LONGer I resist the more I PIG OUT once I get it!**

From Pecan, Age 15 - 01/22/06 -
Ht. 5'2", Wt. mmhmm - …our coaches decided to have a dinner from 7:30-9:30. the problem is that for girl scouts I also have a meeting where they were planning on eating dinner, AND drivers ed where we were planning to order pizza. **I am afraid I will loose control and willpower and eat three dinners**

Out of control vicious cycle

Similar to willpower difficulty, kids hate feeling out of control, which is stressful. As the teen below relates, every time she tells herself not to binge, she binges. Feeling out of control makes the need to numb feelings even greater, feeling more out of control – a vicious cycle.

From Claire, Age 19 - 07/19/08
Ht. 5'4", Start: 210 lb, Current: 176 lb, Goal: 140 lb - Ok so **my binging has gone out of control. Like completely out of control! I feel like I can't control myself.** My brain just switches off and I eat everything I see and thats why I hate it when people leave the house and leave me alone and I go to the fridge and just eat everything like a pig. I feel like if I don't stop this I'll be back to where I was and that's the last thing I want! I can't get back to something that horrid! **everytime I tell myself to not do it, I binge.** It's like I don't listen to myself. It just happens like a reflex and **I can't stop it**… that's whats made me gain the 18 lbs over the past year.

From angie, Age 15 - 10/02/05
Ht. 5'8, Wt. 160 - I really think i have a problem with binge eating, when i start to eat junk food **i think to myself like..ive eaten this much so i might as well eat more and its soo bad because i get out of control! and like the next morning i feel terrible about myself**:(i really dont know what to do!

Self-esteem vicious cycle

Overweight and obese kids tend to have low self-esteem and thus may not take pride in how they look. But which comes first, becoming overweight

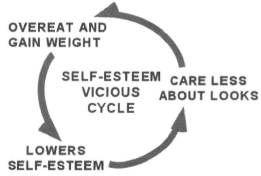

or losing self-esteem? Actually, they appear to feed on each other – another vicious cycle. Gaining weight lowers self-esteem, with less caring about keeping up appearance, more weight gain, and so on. Furthermore, low self-esteem adds to the comfort eating and stress eating vicious cycles, as described at the beginning of this chapter.

Age 13, female, 4 foot 11, 121 lbs - I am depressed and have a **terrible self-esteem.** Though being overweight is part of the reason why I hate myself so much, **I eat to try to make the pain go away. It never works, I just feel even uglier than before,** but I do it every day after school. **I can't stop.**

From Carly, Age 12 - 12/24/03
I lost 20lbs!!!Want to know how ...**I am 12,5'3,and 130lbs.In Early September I was 150.I lost 20 pounds**...I HATEDEVERYONE.I got stuck in the triangle... **when people called me "fat" I did what I knew solved problems...ATE.Pizza,Ice Cream,Cake,Whipped Cream,**No end in sight.What I changed~If you got stuck in the triangle,**chances are you lack self-esteem,(Like I Did)**..But,If you...~Eat ONLY 3 meals a day~Bike a half hour~Eat HALF of what you normally eat~Drink water instead of Pepsi...**You'll feel better.**

How do kids break the self-esteem vicious cycle? As the child above describes, if they are able to lose even a little weight, they feel better about themselves with improved self-esteem, start to care again, and are better able to resist further overeating. The post below also echoes that restored caring about appearance helps to break the low self-esteem overeating vicious cycle.

From jessica, Age 17 - 01/04/06
Ht. 5 5, Wt. 135 - ... I went to a diet when i was in feburary of my 10th grade year and **lost 30 pounds i used to weight 165** ...you have to put your mind to it and when you really think about it **when you eat that 5th candy bar your basically saying i wanna be fat and i dont care how I look just tell yourself that and you wont want to eat it thats what i did when temtation came...**

Enrolling in a charm school course for girls, or a body building course for guys, are ways to improve pride in their appearance.

Reply from Jackie, Age 17 - 11/20/05
I think becoming a **body builder** is a very realistic goal. Just start small and work your way up. I suggest checking out books from the library on body building...

From LeYaNiS, Age 13 - 12/27/03
heres a message to all GIRLS. i notice that sumtimes when girls r overweight they forget about being feminine and they feel really ungirly because of their weight. but fun ways to **keep u in touch with ur girly side** are these: belly dance...it feels great and is amazing to

watch no matter how u look..actually, any type of dancing that you'd never catch boys doing works!!!! another GREAT way to walk ur fat off is SHOPPING. take a trip to the mall for a whole day with ur best girls and go in like EVERY store. it doesnt matter what sizes the clothes are, just look at them and admire their variety. **go into accessory shops and sample perfume, or get your makeup done somewhere**... reward yourself with a manicure or pedicure!!! good luck and remember to stay a girl! ;)- LeYaNiSz

Bulimia vicious cycle

Bulimia may be a vicious cycle. Again, bulimia is defined as eating large amounts of food in a short period of time followed by extreme measures to prevent weight gain, which is called 'purging.' Purging typically consists of inducing vomiting by putting a finger or object in the back of the throat. Or purging may involve using laxatives, fasting from food (self-starvation), or extreme exercise. Dieting actually may be thought of as a form of purging.

Purging is stressful, so that the child or teen may then stress/comfort eat, feel guilty, purge more, followed by more distress from purging, more stress/comfort eating, and so on...

From britt, Age 14 - 06/12/08 - IP#: 209.240.206.xxx
Ht. 5'4", Start: 198 lb, Current: 154 lb, Goal: 125 lb - **i purged again anyone got any tips to stop this disgusting once a day habit???**

From Kristen, Age 16 - 03/19/08 - IP#: 76.83.230.xxx
Ht. 5'8", Start: 228 lb, Current: 178 lb, Goal: 160 lb - ... you ..pig out and eat a ton.. in a effect you feel incredibally guilty and then to feel better and feel like you didnt mess up, you make yourself throw up... But you know what... i realized that **it would only turn into a cycle** and that in order for me, in the future, to have a healthy lifestyle it was important for me to learn to not do this.

Note: We monitor the boards regarding bulimic postings and do not allow such on our site, unless the child or teen is requesting help. About 15% of overweight kids have bulimic behavior. Our site does contain information and resources for bulimics.

The child or teen may even gain weight from bulimia, as described below. This may be the vicious cycle of self-disgust from purging and further stress eating and comfort eating, such that not all the additional food is purged away.

From Sue, Age 16 - 07/14/03
hi guyz...like alot of you i need to lose some weight during the summer. i'm around 140 and am 5'3..i really need to lose 15 pounds because i feel disgusting right now so if you could please help that'd really be great. I was a bulimic and still am. **Being bulimic made me go**

from 114 to 140 and gaining. I'm not sure what to do or how to cure myself please help me!...

Boredom vicious cycle

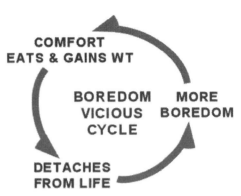

Boredom may be a vicious cycle. Kids may emotionally detach from life to escape from painful problems, stress, or sadness. Detachment may be described by the child or teen as, "I'm bored," as he/she has no interest in anything. But detachment itself tends to be unpleasant, perhaps because the child is periodically jolted back to reality. Kids say they use food to cope with boredom. As a result, they may become more overweight, which renders their life more painful, more detachment to escape, more boredom, more overeating, and so on. Examples of this vicious cycle are noted in the many postings by kids in Chapter 11 on using food to cope with boredom, similar to the below post:

From Rachel, Age 19 - 9/16/06 -
Ht. 5'0, Wt. 140 - hi guys. i'm so tired of overeating. it's been going on for several YEARS now. and i'm more than ever determined to stop this **vicious cycle of overeating**. could anyone post some tips that has actually worked very well for you to resist overeating and/or **eating out of boredom, stress, sadness** etc? Thank you very much.

Sleep - obesity vicious cycles

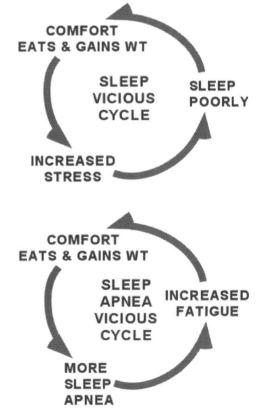

Research studies have revealed an association between insufficient or poor sleep and overweight/obesity in kids, including sleep apnea. [Landhuis 2008]. But does overweight cause poor sleep, or does poor sleep cause overweight? This may be a vicious cycle, where they cause each other. Insufficient or poor sleep causes fatigue, stress, and inability to handle stress. This may result in comfort/stress eating, more weight gain, more stress, which then further impairs the ability to sleep, and so on (upper cycle at right).

Sleep apnea (pauses in breathing during sleep) is associated with obesity in kids. These disruptions in breathing result in poor sleep and fatigue. Fatigue from sleep apnea might bring about comfort/stress eating, with more weight gain, more sleep apnea, more fatigue, more comfort/stress eating, etc.(lower cycle at right on previous page).

The post below describes eating when fatigued and stressed:

This is ANGEL's question: ... I also have the problem of eating way to much even when im nto hungry. **I eat when i am tired, stressed out..**

This is one reason that a complete history and physical by healthcare providers is important to determine underlying causes of overweight in children and teens.

Note: Vicious cycles are not always runaways that spiral out of control. The cycles may simply continue at the same level.

Other vicious cycles

Weight loss camps and centers vicious cycles

Weight loss camps and centers may be a potential vicious cycle. Most overweight kids are able to lose weight when they go to a weight loss camp. Unfortunately, after they return home, some start to gain the weight back, they thus feel disappointed in themselves, so they may comfort eat and gain even more weight. Some may even return to the weight loss camp the following season, lose weight again, go back home, gain the weight back again, and the cycle continues.

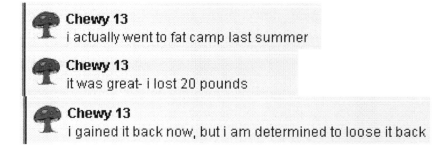

Chewy 13
i actually went to fat camp last summer

Chewy 13
it was great- i lost 20 pounds

Chewy 13
i gained it back now, but i am determined to loose it back

How can one avoid such a cycle problem with weight loss camps? Find a camp which teaches kids how to deal with the world of tempting food once they return home and further teaches them how to deal with emotions like stress and loneliness without seeking relief and comfort in food.

Home schooling vicious cycle

Home schooling may be a vicious cycle. Obese kids frequently are home schooled, in order to avoid teasing, problems fitting into desks, etc. But home schooling may produce more isolation and less activity, making the child's or teen's obesity problem worse, with more need for home schooling. The home school curriculum should therefore include physical activities and social outings with other kids.

From Megan, Age 11 - 11/26/05
Ht. 5'3, Wt. 185 - Please Help Me I am so fat I come from a fat family so please help me. **One problem is I am homeschooled and my mom lets me eat all day.**

From kate, Age 13 - 04/16/05
summer is coming up in 2 months for me. a little less actually. how much weight can i lose if i really worked hard? i bought a nice bike 2 days ago so im gonna try to get into the habbit to ride it alot... **ppl make fun of me and i dont really have any friends because im homeschooled. everytime i go to a party people just stare or point and start laughing. it hurts so bad**

From Ashley, Age 17 - 1/26/06
Ht. 5'6", Wt. 272 - ..I am 272 pounds. I wasn't always this big, but **2 years ago I started getting homeschooled and since I wasn't doing as much as I used to the weight just poured on.**

From Meg, Age 14 - 01/13/09
Ht. 5'5", Start: 210 lb, Current: 210 lb, Goal: 145 lb - I'm a homeschooled freshman and i really need to loose weight **its really hard when homeschooled cuz i dont have pe and stuff...**

From Halle, Age 13 - 11/11/03
..i fink i have the worst case on here im **13 6ft and 400 lbs!** i cnt walk dwn the stairs i have eough trouble walking 2 the bathroom **i comforteat** i have 2 i stay in bed all day **bored my mum homeschools me so i have no friends im all alone** never been kissed im ugly and fat .. **i cant exercise**

Health professional vicious cycle

Health professionals may place blame on an overweight child or teen for "not eating healthy, not exercising, or not trying hard enough to lose weight." Health professionals also may shame the child or scare him/her with health risks. This may

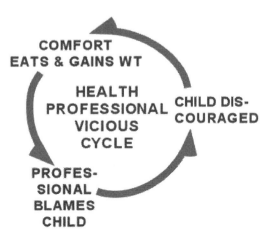

upset or discourage the child, resulting in more comfort/stress eating, more weight gain, more blame from the health professional, more comfort/stress eating and seeking less care by the child or teen – a vicious cycle.

From Dayna, Age 13 - 09/18/05
Ht. 5'3", Wt. 165 - im 13 and i REALLY want to lose weight....**my doctor also makes me feel bad about myself because he told me that it may take me 3 years to drop a mere 20 pounds**.but im continuing to try.

Grace O'Malley, a member of the European Childhood Obesity Group, states: "So many of these kids are in real pain - emotional, physical, and perhaps even spiritual. I often wonder about the iatrogenic [provider-caused] effects of their contact with health-care providers and obesity researchers, who have sub-optimal training or experience in this area. Such persons may play the blame-game without adequately utilizing a problem-solving approach to holistic management and support." [O'Malley 2008]

Slip up vicious cycle

If a child or teen gives in to eating a fattening food, they may feel, "Since I've blown my diet I might as well eat whatever I want now." This may result in bingeing, further self-disgust, and continuing to blow his/her diet - a vicious cycle.

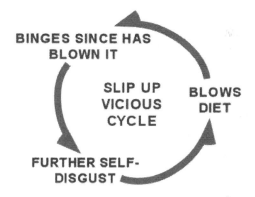

From Katherine, Age 14 - 07/28/04
i have a huge problem when i binge. lets say that i went over by 2 pieces of pizza, not that bad right??? well, for some reason i can't stop there, then i go on to eat ice cream and cake and chips. i keep telling my self i should have stopped at the pizza, but for some reason i can't. maybe its because **i think since i've already messed up, i might as well just forget the whole diet?????** can somebody pleasssssse help me so i won't do it again in the future!!!!

From angie, Age 15 - 10/02/05
Ht. 5'8, Wt. 160 - I really think i have a problem with binge eating, **when i start to eat junk food i think to myself like..ive eaten this much so i might as well eat more and its soo bad because i get out of control!** and like the next morning i feel terrible about myself:(i really dont know what to do!

From heather, Age 14 - 06/02/05
Okay well this is the story....**i like slip up and eat 1 bad thing..i just give up and eat bad things for like the rest of the day cuz i think it doesnt really matter and i might as well eat more**...can sum 1 plz help!!! i'm so un-modivated ugh!!

From Orcy, Age 15 - 11/10/06
Ht. 5'7, Wt. 172 - ahh i screwed up pretty bad today =(. I had a bagel in advisory today (so it was like a 2nd brekfast) and usually im good about not being like "**crap i screwed up, now i might as well screw up more**" but idk what happened. ahh this sucks.

Kids need to realize that one slip up doesn't ruin all their efforts. They should forgive themselves for slipping up today and prepare themselves to start fresh tomorrow, as the below post suggests:

From Kayla, Age 15 - 09/19/06
Ht. 5'7, Wt. :) - Just another fun little tip from your always dieting pal Kayla... **if you make a little slip up don't seat it**. What I'm trying to say here is that if you do happen to have that piece of cake or have cold pizza for breakfast **don't say "Oh man, my day is shot. might as well have whatever I want for the rest of day."** What I've discovered is if you just go on with your diet like usual you'll probably stay the same or you may still lose weight. If you eat whatever you want I've alway felt gross and gained like 3 pounds overnight. That weight takes a week or more to take off, but it only took one night to put on. Doesn't seem worth it to me. So **if you accidentally stray off your diet don't completely trash your day. You'll be better off in the long run.** Hope this helps!!! ...

Sitting on the sidelines vicious cycle

Overweight kids may sit on the sidelines and avoid things in life because of their weight. This keeps them from really enjoying life, so that they may turn more to food for happiness, again a vicious cycle.

From chelsea, Age 15 - 04/07/04
Ht: 5'1", Wt: 150 - I'm very depressed right now and actually crying. I don't know If I even want to live anymore. All I want In life is to lose this weight and I keep gaining. I'm 150.. was 145.. and the scale keeps going up. I'm homeschooled because I get embarrassed of myself in school and I never do anything with friends..**I always make up excuses because I feel fat...I always eat to numb the pain and I can't stop.** I try to exersize but it doesn't make up for the calories I consume. I just feel hopeless. **I'll miss out on so much waiting for the weight to come off.** I want to weigh 110 so it will take 20-40 weeks if I lose 1-2 pounds a week .. and that's just to damn long to wait. **I feel like I'm missing out..**

Overweight kids should try to do the things they enjoy, which will help them feel better and lose weight, instead of thinking negative things, which keeps them sitting on the sidelines. Life then won't pass them by while they're waiting to get to their goal weight. As John Lennon said, "Life is what happens while we're making plans for life."

Friend food vicious cycle

"Food is my friend" may be a vicious cycle. Using food as a friend, rather than having real friends, makes the child or teen more socially isolated, and in even more need for food as a friend.

From Mallory, Age 15 - 03/01/04
k im really upset ...and **know im going ona eat know think later food is my friend binnge** and i dont know what to do!

Overweight kids need to socialize with other kids as much as possible in order to develop social skills and avoid turning to food. Clubs, dancing lessons, non-competitive sports, hikes, or anything they enjoy, which involves other kids, can be helpful. Communities should help plan such activities for kids, e.g. after school, on weekends, and during summer breaks. Social activities and sports may be challenging for overweight kids, particularly if they are teased. Adult organizers therefore need to be alert to support overweight kids.

Breaking vicious cycles

In order to lose weight, overweight kids must break their vicious cycles. How do they do this?

Reply from Caragh, Age 17 - 10/19/09
Don't get too frustrated with yourself! ... **Whatever you do, don't give up and go pig out because you're depressed about not losing weight, break the vicious circle!** Even if you're not losing weight at the moment, the fact that you're making an effort to change your lifestyle and break the unhealthy habits is the important part. Stay on track, it's just too important not to!

Distracting activities (fun things)

From Vanessa, Age 14 - 07/01/07
Ht. 5'4", Start: 230 lb, Current: 227 lb, Goal: 205 lb - BEST IDEA EVER!!!!!!!!!! okay they always have the vicious eating circle on this site,eat more,unhappy, get fatter, well i finally figured out what one gets me!!!!!!!1 **itsssssssss answer B !!!!!UNHAPPYY!!!!**if im posting things on here im obviously bored and sad, i was just about to make cheese nachos, so **i called up a friend,** and she wasnt busy, were anging out!!!and im always really active with her, then if i'm happy when i come home i wont wanna eat the world!!!!**therefore i wont**

gain weight, there fore ill be happy, there fore i wont eat, i challenge every blubberbuster right now TO:call a friend, clean, go swimming, walk the dog, even , PLAY VIDEO GAMES!(if it makes you happy, ...

✯ From LAUREN, Age 16, female - 8/4/07 -
WELL I WOKE UP 1 DAY I NOTICE MY JEANS JUST WUDNT FIT ND **INSTEAD OF FEEDING MY SORROW IN CHOCLATE I DECIDED TO DO SOMETHING ABOUT IT I WALK EVERY DAY FOR A HOUR** AND I DO NOT EAT JUNK FOOD I ONLY DRINK WATER AND NOW AFTER A YEAR OF FOLLOWING THIS PATTERN OF HEALTY EATTING I AM A SIZE 10 I AM VERY PROUD OF MY SELF AND I HAVE BLUBBERBUSTERS TO THANK BECAUSE THEY OFFERED SUPPORT WHEN I NEEDED IT THE MOST THANK YOU LOVE LAUREN XXX

✯ From Daisy, Age 14, female - 5/1/06
I have recently **lost about 35 pounds**, I would say in about a month and a half (maybe two months) ...**I weighed about 175 pounds and was 5'7". Now I weight 150 and am the same height. .. I would not take up my time eating to make myself feel better because it will just lead to yourself feeling worse in the end** by you probably gaining weight! **I found other things to occupy my mind, to do, to think about and such that made me feel better without a bad reaction happening in the future.** ..I found out that finding new ways to think about it, and **not eating because I am sad and doing something else instead made it better**. Hopefully some people can try and find something to do instead, that one thing can really do alot!

Pets, counseling, dancing, volunteering

Reply from Tricia, Age 16 - 07/10/03
...Its tough to lose weight if your depressed because if your like me (225 lbs) you use food to treat your depression. But what I realised is that **its a vicious circle thing because when I overeat I get more overweight and I get more depressed so I eat even more to make myself feel better and gain even more weight, get more depressed and it just gets worse.** What I did to **break the vicious circle** was... **1) I got a dog.** Hes wonderful. Hes my friend and we take walks together every day, even we jog some. That keeps me from heading for the fridge all the time and is fun exercise. **2) I been going to counseling** at the mental health clinic. It doesnt cost much. My counselor talked about a antidepressent medication but I dont think I even need it now. **3) I go dancin** at the community center thing every Sunday. Im shy but theres guys who are worse dancers than me... lol.

Reply from Sandra - 04/03/09
Do you think she would be interested in some activities outside of school like a local

literacy program where she teaches others to read, or **volunteering** at a pet shelter? **Those types of things might help break the vicious cycle of feeling bad, eating, feeling worse, eating some more...** Volunteering might reduce how much she eats just because she's out of the house or "distracted" more and at the same time, might help raise her self-esteem.

Any fun activity with other kids seems to be the best way to break vicious cycles. Physical activity is actually a form of 'displacement activity' (see Chapter 10), which relieves tension and stress. And social activities are a wonderful source of comfort.

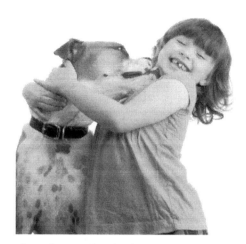 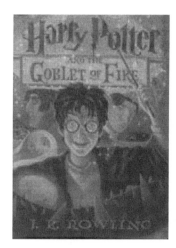 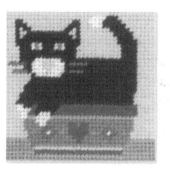

The idea is for kids to substitute other activities for the comfort and stress relief they seek from food, such as pets, hobbies, musical instruments, non-competitive sports, counseling, religion, volunteer work, and books. Books can be wonderful adventures. It has been said, "If you have a book, you are never alone."

The next chapter presents what overweight kids live for - **Success Stories!**

14 | Success Stories

Overweight kids live for the day when they can post their success stories.

From k- hunnie, Age 15 - 10/19/05
Ht. 5'7 1/2, Wt. 253 - ... let me tell you something i will no matter what have lost atleast 50 pounds before June 2006. i need to lose about 110//120.. **the next thing i wanna do is be leaving my success story on this site :)** xo Love Always ox k--hunnie! :)

From Vanessa, Age 14 - 07/01/07
Ht. 5'4", Start: 230 lb, Current: 227 lb, Goal: 205 lb - ... **i promised myself i will post my success story on the board at the end off the summer** and it will say, i went from 230 to 200!yay me!!!!!!!!!!

Kids post inspirational stories about their progress in their weight loss journeys.

What is the secret of successful weight loss?

Eating healthy and exercising is what some kids say is the secret to losing weight.

⭐ From Rosalyn, Age 20, female - 8/11/05
I'm so happy. I've only lost a few lbs but the change of lifestyle to healthy eating and exersizing has given me so much energy and confidence. It's like magic. **After 10 yrs of trying to lose weight I finally found the secret...Just eat healthy and exersice!!!**

⭐ From Melanie, Age 17, - 5/6/03
... i have lost 40 lbs and i am down to 120 lbs it is an awesome feeling getting into a size 5 instead of a 13... try to **eat right and exercise it really works...**

⭐ From Linda, Age 18, female - 6/11/03
I have battled with my weight for most of my life... by the time I was **16** I had topped out

at **195 lbs** and knew I had to do something. For me, every pound was extremely difficult. **I finally realized that there really is only one way to lose weight healthily: eat less and exercise more**. There's just no way around it.

Exercise

Some kids are able to lose weight mainly by exercising.

⭐ From Gabrielle, Age 13, female - 11/8/06 -
...when i was last on **i weighed around 260** but now i lost alot of weight i've go a tip for you guys firstly if you don't already at your shool **have a exercise club suggest to your gym teacher**. i spoke to my gym teacher about wanting to lose some weight a she was really nice about and said she would help me so **before school at lunch and after school i would go to her and she would give me exercises to do**, its been two years and **i have lossed over 160lbs** try my method it really works trust me

Reply from Bethany, Age 14 - 5/4/08
when i came on this site for the first time **i was THIRTEEN and i was 290**! i was even embarrased to put my weight on here with people with the same issues as me. **im 14 and 260 now** but **i didnt even change my eating habits all i did diff was take P.E** i plan to lose about 100 pounds more and my ultimate goal is to weigh about 135.

⭐ From Alexandra, Age 14, female - 8/17/07 -
Hi everyone I am so proud of you all for having the courage to open up to other people your age about your weight. The fact that we go on this site proves we want to take responsibility for oursellves and our habits. I was **165 pounds September 2006** and now it is **August 2007 and I am a healthy 116 lbs. I exercised 6 days a week** and ate 1400 calories a day. **I used the exercise bike, walking, pilates, and tennis** to make sure I was burning 600 calories on days I exercised.

⭐ From Renee, Age 19, female - 1/5/04
All you need to do is 20-30 min. on the tredmill 3 times a week! The tredmill is everything you need. **I was at 155 and using the tredmill for 4 months brought me to a healthy 135**. ?I look amazing!

⭐ From KRISTEN, Age 10, female - 8/1/07 -
BY DOING ALOT OF EXIRSE AND ACTIVES.

⭐ From erica, Age 26, female - 5/8/05
I have lost ten pounds just by eating only when I'm hungry, **walking, joining a walking**

club, and avoiding sweets. **I also purchased a portable cd player. You would be surprised how much your favorite music will help you forget your exercising...**

⭐ From Austin, Age 19, male - 10/11/02
...Weight has always been a big struggle for me in my life...I eventually tipped the scales at **218**.... So, I went from doing no exercise to doing about 15 minutes a day... After graduation I was able to spend more time **exercising (about 30-40 minutes a day)** .. **I am now at 167**. I have **lost 51 pounds** in the course of 8 months and I feel really good about myself for the first time that I can remember. The only diet changes that I made were **cutting out all sodas and limiting sweets**...

Exercise definitely helps, but it should be fun.

⭐ From grace, Age 13, female - 3/21/02
hello. i am 5-4, and **i used 2 weigh 153 pounds. but now i weigh 145 pounds**, and the funny thing is, (now i know this isn't good, but listen). when i lost my 8 pounds, i didn't reduce my food to a minimum at all. i just ate normally... the thing is, i kept FORCING my self to walk 30 minutes a day... but you know what the moral of this whole story is? **dont force yourself to do some kind of work out you hate.** i found that out the hard way. because when u force yourself to do an exercize you hate, yeah, you do lose weight, but its just not fun to think of it as, if i keep doing this, im gonna lose weight. **do an exercize you like. you will enjoy it more,** and if you do it longer than that other exercize you used to do, u may see results quicker. trust me.

Walking works!

⭐ From mercedez, Age 17, female - 9/7/06
Ht. 5'5, Wt. before- 205, now- 145 lbs - whats up every1...i came to this site like a few years ago wanting to lose weight really bad, but just never had the will power in doing so. so last year when i was **16** i decided that it was time to lose weight...so all **i did was eat my breakfast,dinner,supper in smaller portions with water with every meal** and i **walked about 4 times a week for like 40 mins**,and **never ate after 8 oclock**...i was 205 lbs and now i am 145 lbs...so i lost 60 lbs in 7 months....i know it may be hard but i also **tried to not eat junk food** while i was on my diet and sumtimes i did but i learned that its ok to have that piece of cake on ur bday and stuff...just dont make it a habbit of always eating it..cuz it aint good for u at all lol....on my whole journey to losing weight **i did not do any kind of exercise...only walking alot...trust me...walking works**..............i hope this helps all u ppl out there who r trying to lose weight cuz i kno its SOOO hard,but trust me, do what i did and i will guarentee that u WILL lose weight....maybe not at 1st but u will start noticing in a month believe me............

Kids say that exercise alone is generally not enough to lose weight. They say that changing eating habits is usually necessary, as well.

⭐ **From Jade, Age 16, female - 11/30/03**

For the person who said "do not go on a diet" i have to completely disagree with you. **Although you might have succeeded with just exercise, this most likely will not work for most people here.** Here's an example. I was 160lbs, and i joined cross country and **ran at least 4 miles per day, and when i didn't change my eating habits i lost practically nothing.** .. because **most people get fat due to excess eating instead of lack of exercise,** ..

Exercise seems to be key for maintaining a healthy weight, especially fun activities. And exercise can be many types of fun activities.

⭐ **From Sara, Age 13, female - 7/5/02**

Hey people! I have not lost weight, but I have done something that I am very proud of. **I have maintained my weight of 118 lbs. for the past 2 years.** I didnt diet, and I didnt excercise every second of the day. I would still eat a chocolate sundae fir desert, but with every meal (except brreakfast) I would make sure that I had a veggie, a fruit, and milk. **I excercised every day, but every day, it was different. One day a walk, one day rollerblading, sometimes dancing, and sometimes jogging.** Also, make sure you have a positive attitude. Being negative makes u negative. Have a great day!!!!

How do successful kids actually do it?

Eating right and exercising seems simple, but as illustrated in Chapter 8, most kids struggle to lose weight and maintain it. How do successful kids actually do it?

Some kids lose weight just by cutting out junk food.

⭐ **From amor, Age 12, female - 6/27/05**

I use to weigh 160 and now i weigh 133. i am not exactly at my goal weight but it was one heck of a job losing that weight. **I didnt exercise to lose it** all i did was eat way healthier.i **cut out all the junk food(candy,chips,icecream,etc.)**

⭐ **From Camille, Age 17, female - 3/2/05**

I have been on a diet since January 10th, 2005. I am **5'8**, and when I started I was **175 pounds**. Now, almost two months later, I am at **153 pounds!** This is how I did it. First, I talked to my mom about how I wanted to lose weight. Together, **we took all the junk food out of the house and filled it with healthy and tasty food.** She is my weight loss buddy, and it helps so much to have someone dieting with you and supporting you. I eliminated juices and high calorie drinks from my diet and started **drinking lots of water.** I fought cravings and only had one small snack in the afternoon. I ate a good sized meal at supper but NEVER ate anything between supper and bedtime. These are all good eating habits that helped me and will certainly help you! Good luck to all!

⭑ From Marie, Age 13 - 02/25/06
Ht. 5', Wt. 139 - hey guys! ...**i was 164 and now im 139!! i lost it in about 6 and a half weeks**... trust me once you go threw **not eating junk food, and also dont drink pop! thats wat i did** it was really easy **just dont look in the frige for somthing to drink!** also **DONT look in the chip cabinet and the sweets cabinet cuz once you see it then yuou want to eat it but if you dont no its there then u dont want it!!**

*Kids have **many** clever tips.*

⭑ From ~*Kaylee*~, Age 14, female - 7/23/06 -
To lose weight you have to use more calories that you eat. That means eat less, move more. Things you can do to help that is eat a healthy breakfast to start your day. Eat lowfat/fatfree dairy (yogurt,milk,cheese) **Brush your teeth righ after dinner so you will pass on desert. Chew gum when your not hungry but want to eat. DRINK LOTS OF WATER!! Get up and move when ever you can.** Shopping, cleaing, yardwork, running, the gym, hula hooping, swimming, b-ball, soccer, weights, walking the dog, anything that gets you moving is great!! You can do it!! **I was once 5'1 and 150 lbs and nOw I'm 5'3 and 128** so it's 100% doable!!

⭑ From Ana, Age 15, female - 10/9/01
...**I want to speak to all of u who are very unhappy about their wieght, your not going to lose any pounds whatsoever if you don't work on the inside first, because thats where losing wieght starts.** First be happy with who and what you are, be content, then work to make changes in you and your body that will help you become a better person than you already are...

⭑ From Holly, Age 17, female - 12/2/05
Hi! I started out at 217 pounds a year ago and **lost 55 pounds** so now I weigh 160 pounds and feel better than I ever have. **One thing I would suggest is printing out a calendar every month and track not only your exercise but also the progess you've made in losing pounds and inches. Whenever you need a boost, just look at that** and it should help you to continue. Good luck!

⭑ From Erika, Age 13, female - 8/19/02
Well...i have **lost 21 pounds**... i am vvery happy, I started at 170, and now im on 149... i eat normally just not alot, **If you eat a lil and chew alot it works**..also i go to the gym everyday to burn off the calories..I love the gym its Awesome!

✭ From eric, Age 24, male - 4/3/05

...i weighed in at **255 pounds at 5'7**... Fast food three times a day, and nothing but soda & juice. **I simply cut those out completely and ate those green foods most people avoid.... Switched to only water... I went from 255 to 195 exactely.** My energy levels sored to the point where i didnt want to live my old seditary depressing life style...

✭ From Shannon, Age 14, female - 6/11/03

...It's really great talking to someone who is just like you and can help each other the way you would want to be. **Eating healthy is what's hard for me but I had to do it I mean some of the hardest things in the world are to tough to but as long as you try your already succeeding. I was 200lbs but now I'm 112lbs!** "WOW". I feel great and you will too if you **just try!!**

✭ From stacy, Age 15, female - 4/9/02

I lost weight by not eating after 7:o'clock. I... lost two stones you should try it!!! the only thing you can have after 7 is water nothing else!!!!

✭ From Mary, Age 17, female - 12/7/02

When I was about 13, I started to get really fat, and by the time I was in 8th grade I was about **189 pounds**. I felt disgusting and I hated myself.... It's really sad that I got this way cause I used to be so active and skinny when I was little. So I got fed up with being fat and when I was 14 we got a dog.... and so **I walked my dog every day for 30 to 40 minutes. Within a year or two I had gone from 189 pounds to 143 pounds**...(I am 5'9")... Believe in yourself, be patient and never ever give up!

✭ From ashley, Age 14, female - 6/12/03

This site is very helpful and its been on my faves list for about 5 months. i am 5'4" and i used to be 170lbs... i am now 150lb's...i did it all natural...**I also heard somewhere when you chew the food more it makes you feel fuller so try that it works for me and i no longer feel like food is my life anymore!!!**

✭ From roxie, Age 15, female - 6/21/02

...i have lost ten pounds i went from **165 to 155** and im sooo happy !!! all i am doing is **drinking tonnnssss of wated** (if u dont like palin water try the flavored kinds)... **when i get hungry i sing or dance ar ride my bike i also chew gum and that helps alot** ps im 5'7.

Dealing with Parents

Kids ask their parents to stop buying tempting, fattening foods, which they can't resist, or hide junk food, so they don't see it in front of them.

⭐ From Ashley, Age 14, female - 3/28/05
I found that if I just stay away from the chocolate and keep moving I lose weight. And it also helps it your parents help. **Like my mom helped by keeping candy and sugars out of the house.** And I really cut back on the soda too. Just next time when you go to the grocery store **ask your parents if they can stop buying certain foods for you.** It helps out alot when you have others around you that are willing to help you.

⭐ From renee, Age 13, female - 1/31/02
hi guys, i have **lost 18 pounds** in 3 months, i still have a long way to go. i weighed 207 now i am 189. i stopped drinking regular soda and now only drink diet soda. **my mom quit buying junk food and that has helped the most because if it were here i would eat it.** i also only have one helping at meals, no seconds...so if you follow what my doc says, no soda, no junk fod, eat fruit when you crave sweets, walk (which i dont do) and portion control, one plate of food at meals, take what you can fit on that plate and no more! but i **think the biggest thing is support from people who care about you!**

⭐ From Sammy, Age 12, female - 5/7/05
I have lost close to **10 pounds** now. All I did was exercise everyday but Saturdays and cut out most junk food... I talked to my mom, and **when she buys junk food, she hides it in a place I don't know or wouldn't look when reaching for a snack. This has also helped because I forget very easily that we even have junk food in the house...**

⭐ From Liv, Age 13, female - 12/26/03
I lost 13 ibs...Try to keep sweets as far away as possible. Ask your Mom to either hide them or stop buying them... Low-fat and Sugar-free foods help a ton. Great snacks are pretzels, or baked chips. Good luck!

Dealing with cravings

Cravings worsen considerably when the child or teen attempts to lose weight by cutting down or completely stopping pleasurable foods, which is similar to stopping cigarettes or coming off a drug.

How do kids successfully deal with cravings?

⭐ From Leah, Age 20, female - 4/11/05
I was fat my whole life. By the time I turned 18 **I weighed 195, and I am 5'5"**...some

tips that worked for me: DON'T EAT WHEN YOU'RE NOT HUNGRY. IF THAT'S TOO HARD, THEN EAT SOMETHING LIKE CELERY WHICH HAS ALMOST NO CALORIES. *OR* YOU CAN TRY THIS: CUT UP LIKE AN APPLE OR SOMETHING INTO REALLY SMALL PEICES AND EAT IT REALLY SLOWLY WITH A FORK. (THAT WAS ONE OF THE BIGGEST HELPERS FOR ME.)... AND **IF YOU'RE HAVING A REALLY BAD CRAVING FOR SOMETHING, JUST EAT TWO BITES OF IT *SLOWLY*. IT HELPS TO CURB CRAVINGS.** DON'T EAT A WHOLE PEICE OF PIE, **TAKE 2 BITES AND THROW IT AWAY AND DON'T LOOK BACK.** *ONCE YOU LOSE THAT FIRST FIVE LBS, IT WILL BECOME EASIER TO LOSE THE NEXT FIVE...

★ From Brian, Age 15, male - 8/30/04

Hey **I used to be 207 pounds but now I'm down to 159.** For years I have been failing at every 'diet' I tried. But than I just relized it's a matter of not sitting in front of the tv and computer all day and eating junk food... **One thing that I found helped was if I was having a craving and was ready to jump for the doritos. I would immediatlly go down to the kitchen and grab some fruit.** Because if I just sat there I would keep thinking about the craving and eventually just give in, thats how I always failed my 'dieting.' So just grab something healthy to eat so you don't do something dumb and dive for the doritos. If your feeling unmotivated just think of all the times people called you fat, or you didn't want to go somewhere (i.e. a party) because you were to self concious about what people would think of your weight problem. That should get you off your couch and start excercising. also, I made smoothies with my blender all the time which were awesome. Just add your favorite fruits a couple ice cubes and BAM you got an awesome healthy filling drink. And I know this is getting kind of long but one other thing I did to motivate myself was **booby trap my house. Get pictures of take pictures and put them on your fridge, on your computer desktop, anywhere you think laziness and junk food might take place.** I also took pictures of myself every 2 weeks to see my progress, its awesome seeing the before and after after 4 months :). Trust me, the life is a LOT better in the 'after' picture.

★ From Rina, Age 15, female - 6/1/05

Hey Everyone! I just wanted to thank you for all the support you've given me! I've lost 99 pounds as of today! one more pound to go. If I can loose weight anyone can. It's taken me almost a year on the dot, but it's so worth it in the long run! don't give up and remember to stick to it. **Even if you think you want that bowl of Ice Cream or those couple of cookies, wait a little bit and see if the craving goes away, it really worked for me.**

★ From Dana, Age 10, female - 12/11/03

Hi. I used to be **twenty to thirty pounds overweight** but with my dad's healthy eating program, **I lost most of it.** I just wanted to say that anyone who is overweight **I have a simple solution for you: If you want candy or bread, go exersize instead.**

⭐ From Jeanie, Age 17, female - 5/15/03

When I was 12 years old I was a size 20 and I weighed **215lbs**. I felt disgusting and never wanted to leave the house. Finally I had had enough and decided to start my very own diet... I have kept the weight off for four years and **now weigh 125lbs**, am a size 7... **When you start to lose weight you will find that it is truely more satisfying than eating junk food.**

⭐ From Thin, Age 15, female - 8/23/02

...I was **2 inches shorter and 40 pounds heavier**. I am now 5ft 2in 15 7/12 years old, and only 114 pounds!.. Anyway, number one don't look at the scale, weight is always flucuating **if you keep checking the scale everyday you will get depressed and comfort eat**, not because you are getting fatter but because your weight always changes little changes that don't mean anything but that can make you depressed. So ...try to hold it back to once every two weeks...Next, **just eat when your hungry**, just maybe a strong word. But when your hungry turn on some music because the sensation you feel when you eat is the same as when you listen to music (I read it in a womans mag.) then you won't feel like consuming calories, and hey maybe you'll even feel like **dancing** and then youll burn off even more calories.Lastly, **cravings only last about 10 min.** (I didn't make this up) so **when you get a craving try to busy your self with something (and not tv) for 10 min. and hopefully your craving will be gone.**good luck everyone!

⭐ From shena, Age 16, female - 7/11/03

After learning the importance of a healthy lifestyle last year,i realized that it was time for me to change my habits. Last year i weighed **190lbs** by slowly begining to excercise and consume less food, i slowly began losing weight. As the first few pounds of my weightloss shed off my body i realized i could do it. **I soon gained an amazing will power and became able to resist junk foods. I only ate what i felt would benefit me.**My excercise turned into a nightly jog for 20min and sit ups and leg excercises to follow it. I now weigh **148lbs** and am still losing weight, i fell alot better about myself and i am much more dtermined than ever.

⭐ From Tori, Age 15 - 07/04/04

When i vist friends, parties, barbeques and other places where junk and unhealthy choices are avaibale, I'm usually faced with the descidon to eat or well, not to eat. Some say only have just a slice of that cake, or only have one piece of pizza, but **my problem is that if i have that one slice of cake, next thing i know im having another one, and another one and yet another one. If your like me and feel that once you've had the junk food you might as well have more-** lsiten to this. There are two types of feelings when it comes to food- craving the food and then the inital guilt that comes after overindulging. Now both feelings are uncomfotable and hard to deal with, but you have to think about which one is more positive, obvisouly the craving. I learned that if I just stay away from the junk food completely, it won't put me on the track to the non stop junk eating road, and that I can

234

sit thruogh the activity craving the food (id rather have the craving feelings then the feeling of guilt) My two main points here are if once you start eating junk food you eat alot more then just that "one slice"...stay away from it completely! **Its better to do all your activies with that craving for a peice of cake in your head then the feeling of guilt and the extra calories and fat your body in turn needs to burn off.** Thanks...I hope this helped!

⭐ From Michelle, Age 17 - 02/25/09
Ht. 5'9", Start: 227 lb, Current: 173 lb, Goal: 150 lb - **every single time you are going to put food in your mouth.. think: how will this make me feel? cravings go away in 20 minutes..** all you have to do is last 20 minutes. Call a friend, draw a picture, take your mind off of it. i know it's hard.. and it's a lifelong battle.. you have to consciously choose to make this life your own. You are worth more than that one bite of food!... prove it to yourself!

Kids say that squeezing their hands tight together helps them to resist cravings.

Reply from JANEAL, Age 15 - 10/17/05
... MY DOCTOR GAVE ME THE FUNNIEST TIP EVER IT WORKS **SQUEEZE UR HANDS TOGETHER 10 TIMES** WATCH IT WORKS

⭐ From anne, Age 16 - 9/24/03
- i know you're not going to take this seriously- but just **squeeze your hands together** like this website says after you've already had half of your regular meal and when you're not suppose to eat so your hands aren't free and think of something else...

Comfort eating and stress eating

How do kids stop comfort eating and stress eating, which some kids say is addictive?

⭐ Age 16, female, 5'4, 156 lbs - I've lost **157** pounds! **Food was always a comfort to me but I learned that food is just energy you need to survive.** I don't deprive myself of the food I love, I just have them every once in a while. I love cookies and ice cream, I'll a have a cookie or a little bit of ice cream, but I won't pile my plate high with them. It really helps me get my cravings out of the way without feeling guilty. - My eating is not out of control.

⭐ From Colleen, Age 13 - 10/13/09
Ht. 5'5", Start: 163 lb, Today: 138 lb, Goal: 125 lb ...I had to get down to a healthy weight. I didn't snack, ate balanced meals, and **exercised when I was bored, instead of**

eating... I am also the happiest I've ever been because **when I was upset about something, I would eat. Now, though, I talk to someone about what's upsetting me, and I feel better.**

⁎ Reply from Veronica, Age 16 - 08/14/09
Ht. 5'6", Start: 191 lb, Today: 138 lb, Goal: 110 lb - I started my diet on Easter hollydays.Before,I ate horribly.Potato chips,french fries,juice and coke,and thats about it LOL,no wonder I was fat.Well ...**We have to have a skinny person mentallity.They arent opsessed about food and calories like we are.We need to look at food like a fuel,not comfort.I have plenty of hobbies so it takes my mind of food.**So,thats about it :D

⁎ From Hannah, Age 13, female - 8/20/03
Hey! ... I came to this website at **150 lb. now i am 130** ...i jusst cut down on all the junk food and when i went grocery shopping **i always walked bye the candy aisle and i was addicted i did not know whjat to do** so i went more to the fruit and veggie areas and picked out stuff i enjoyes eating and liked. just STICK with it and youll loose a lot of weight

Physical activity really helps...

⁎ From Mary Kate, Age 16, female - 3/24/02
As a kid I was always quite overweight. I was made fun of a lot in school. I must say my self esteem was very low. In about 7th grade I decided to start dieting. It didn't work. I could never stick with it. **I really did have a food addiction...** I had reached **220 lbs** at the end of my freshman year. The following fall in 10th grade **my mom got me some help with a personal trianer.** Since October I have been working out 4 times a week and following a strict diet. I am down to **140 lbs!!!!!!!!**

⁎ From kat, Age 17, female - 8/11/02
At first I realized what I was doing to myself. **273 lbs, high blood pressure, testing for diabetes, couldnt even walk around** the county fair without huffing. So one day sitting before the TV, I looked down at the **dog and said, let's go for a walk.** Did this everyday for a week. Second week came, and when I got home the dog wouldnt leave me alone. Everytime I moved, he jumped up and ran for the door barking. I realized he wanted to go for a walk. Started feeling guilty about not taking him, so everyday I came home and went walking right away. Began to feel awesome. **Pulled out my bike** one day and decided to ride it around my 3mile walk route. Barely made one mile, and so sore. But it was getting to be summer and too hot to take a long haired dog out. Now a year later, **I'm down 107lbs,** still riding, up to 20 miles a day, takes about 1 hr 20 min to do, but I love it. And water people, lots of water. I drink about a gallon a day. Hard at first, but now never far from a bottle.

Hobbies help, like needle point, electronics, art, collecting shells – just look online.

✳ From Kels., Age 15, female - 4/13/02

... I told my self I couldn't enter highschool fat, I couldn't. That summer I lost 20 pounds! This school year I have lost 10 pounds! (I started out 150 some pounds and only 5 ft tall, now I am 5ft2in and 123) Sure exercise, but the biggest thing is don't snack. Eat your three meals a day, skip desert and **don't snack unless you are actually hungry. Every time you are going to eat something ask your self why? If it's hunger go ahead but if not skip it and start doing one of your hobbies to get your mind off food.**

✳ From Kelsey, Age 14.9, female - 11/17/01

I am not quite there yet, but so far I have lost **20 pounds** and I have been eating plenty. What I have been doing is not snacking as much. I made a rule: No eating while watching Tv. Also when I snack I try to eat healthy things and than at meals have what ever I want because my problem has been snaking to much. Alot of times I wasn't hungry, and I didn't even like wehat I was eating but I just had to eat someting, **I thought couldn't help it cause I was an emotional eater (when ever I had any feelings I stuffed my face with food). Well now I just busy myself with things and so I am not thinking about food. Or if I feel like eating when I am not hungry I look into this website or a weightloss book** and that sets my mind in a mood of "you can do it".

✳ From Brittany, Age 14, female - 3/31/08

I have always struggled with my weight and i guess it was in my genes. My dad always says how big he was when he was young but when i look at old pictures of him i wanna cry. **I really was huge.** I am not proud to call myself **an emotional eater but i know i am** in one year after my best friend moved away i went from the 150's (even though i was already overweight) to over 190 at only like 5 2 i knew i needed to make a change so i thought you're 14 and you can barely run a 1/2 mile you need to make a change plus you really wanna get that hot body so i did it and since last september **i have gotten down from 198 to 166** and i know that i have a long way to go but i know that **all i have to say is wwasgd (what would a skinny girl do)** lol good luck

✳ From daniel, Age 15, male - 1/12/04

i used to be **220 pounds** but then i started eating right and exercising and i am **now 169 pounds** i am very proud of myself and i am not going to lie to you if you are barelly starting there will be some tough times ahead but just go through them and **whenever your tempted to eat something not good for you just think of how you will feel after** you feel empty inside and ugly and jsut imagine all those kids you make fun of you.prove them wrong instead of fast food eat veggies and fruits and good stuff like that **weight loss is not all about exercising it is even more in your head than anything else** so keep at it and stay happy.

⋆ From Belinda, Age 16, female - 9/6/04
ADVICE and SUCCESS!:) My peak weight was 106kg. The numbers still flash in my head. I always think "How can u let urself go like that?" Now i'm down to 62kg... **I don't feel the need for chocolate when i'm upset and i have realised that half the stuff i used to eat, i don't really like that much! My boyfriend would sit there eating chocolate and i would be like "don't eat it in front of me please!" but then i learned to join in. have a square or two... not the whole block like i used to!**

⋆ From Monica, Age 16, female - 10/1/05
I used to weigh 245lbs but now I lost 21pounds in like 21/2 months...**think about what u would look like if you hit your goal when you feel tempted. Dancing is always fun** and it burns calories.

Kids say that staying busy also helps avoid snacking on junk food.

From Ashley, Age 17, female - 6/5/06
I was always a chunky gal. When I went into high school **as a freshmen I was 239 pounds,** some would call me names and I never wore what other girls wore... I had a **black ring around my neck for being almost diabetic** I was determined to loose weight. I stopped drinking pop and exercised a little bit at a time. I couldn't run for nothing... It was hard to run a lap around the track. **Now I'm a senior of class 2007 and I am 148 lbs** ...I drank water all the time, I gave up pop altogether, some people find this hard but if you really want to be healthy is the best choice for you. I exercised everyday at least for 20 minutes Just walk, Run Play a game be active. **Keeping your self-busy leaves no time for you to snack on junk.** ...I love ice cream so I always get a Baby cone or Cup when I go to 31 flavors. I lost 87 lbs and so can you! ... Go to the park and walk, go skating with a friend Buddy up if you have to don't be afraid to succeed it's the greatest feeling ever!

⋆ From ams, Age 13, male - 5/24/06
Hey I have lost weight by exercising regularly(**gym,dog walking and bike riding**). And also cutting out the junk which is hard. so far I have only lost around 5 pounds but I am really chuffed with myself.

Meditation

Meditation and relaxation help.

⋆ From kayla, Age 18, female - 2/15/05
i used to wight 170 ibs and now i wight 119 ibs**I lost 52 ibs** just in tree month can you belived,and i am 5.7 inch tall. I feel so happy with my new body. what i did was I eat health

food. I woked out everyday. I want to the gym I jog, **i did yoga and i did medtation. it will woked.**

★ From Ros, Age 19, female - 1/3/06
I lost weight recently by getting rid of all food that is instant. **I had a problem with binging and everytime I felt out of control I'd grab anything right away,**so now without anything quick, **by having to wait for the food to cook, it made me calm down from my feeling out of control and eat normally.** I'm going to continue like this for a while and then I'll start to work on my behavior and see if I can be around food and not binge on impulse anymore. I feel very proud of myself lately. I feel like a normal person who eats regular meals when I used to be someone to stick my hand in a cereal box and without realizing it I'd finish the whole thing!

Eating only when hungry

These kids say they ate only when hungry, not for pleasure or entertainment…

★ From Tara, Age 12, female - 8/4/05
I used to be 160 pounds... Then I decided to lose weight... **I only ate when I was hungry**...Now I weight about 145 or 146.

★ From Jamie, Age 14, female - 1/31/03
I went to Florida on vacation for a week. Every day I walked at least five hours... **I only ate when I was hungery.** I drank only water or diet pepsi the whole time. I lost about five pounds in that one week, I went down to a size seven in jeans (I started at 10s & 11s)... I've started to get more and more confident around people at school, now that I've lost some weight. I am 5'3" and I am now 135lbs. **Ten less then I started**, all in one month.

★ From Paige, Age 13, female - 6/26/05
...I ate smaller meals, skipped desserts (most of the time :) - I've found it's okay to treat yourself now and then), and learned to love salad. **I also learned to eat for the sole purpose of satisfying hunger, not for pleasure or entertainment. My motivation was that I'd felt fat for as long as I could remember and I was just sick of it.** I was just like, enough already.

★ From Lucy, Age 11, female - 6/17/05
...**I ask myself if I am really hungry and ask if I really want to eat ice cream and have pleasure for a few minutes or not eat it and have the pleasure of losing some pounds forever.** I lost 15 lbs and I feel a lot better!!

⁂ From John, Age 17, male - 7/25/05

I lost 60 pounds, and went from a pants size of 40 to a size 30. When I was 16, I weighed 200 pounds and I hated the way I looked, so I began eating small, healthier meals and the weight came off, gradually...it's been easy to maintain my weight, because **I've reached a point where eating little is just a part of my life and I can ignore cravings.**

⁂ From sara, Age 13 - 7/27/08

Ht. 5'2", Start: 160 lb, Current: 148 lb, Goal: 130 lb - wow ok i started trying to lost weight over the summer. it's been a little over a month and i've lost about twelve pounds. it's been really hard, and really tiring, but i feel like i accomplished alot... its kinda weird though, because **ive learned alot about myself while losing weight, i really had to look at myself and see why the reasons i eat and it was mainly because i felt bad about myself.** i had to see who and what happened so that i felt this way. another thing is that i **had to find outlits instead, wheni felt that way, instead of eating.** its helped alot and i feel alot better.

⁂ From Kaia, Age 13, female - 12/14/02

... I have lost weight just by being realy active and forgetting about eating. So **I just eat when it is mealtime and I hardly ever think about food because I am studying or doing stuff with my friends. Food is not a hobby it is just a partof every day that I have to do to be healthy.** And I lost all my extra weight and now everyone keeps saying how slim I am.

⁂ From *A Success Story*, Age 18, female - 1/20/04

... Well I've been struggling with weight loss for many years and **now I am at size 2.** (I'm 5'2) Im proud of myself. **I used to be size 8.** All I ever heard was "eat right, exercise more" but I didn't have time to exercise everyday and its hard to always eat right. So I posted pictures of skinny models on my walls to push me to stop eating junk and eating more healthy. Whenever I would go to the fridge, I would see a thin body and then feel guilty and not eat. **I found that most of the time, I didn't even need to eat, that I was just eating b/c I felt bored or b/c I had a craving.** Now I watch every bite that goes into my mouth even though I have many slip ups...

Fun activities with other kids

Kids say that fun activities with other kids is the **best** *way to distract from overeating and cure boredom, as well as burn calories.*

⁂ From Jahzonae, Age 12, female - 4/20/08

Yes i did it!! **i went from a 160 to a 138** i am so happy **i started doing cheerleading last summer and the pounds and fat just shedded off like that.**I still want to lose more to be a healthier 118 by just doing cheerleading again and i will be a new happier me for the new school year[and by that everything will be changed a whole new ME!!!!!!]

⭐ From Ana, Age 17, female - 1/6/06

...one day, **I wanted to buy rollerblades(i wasnt planning on loseing weight) but after i got them, I did everything on them** from going to school, to just going to the park with my friend. I would rollerblade all day after school. **I noticed I was getting skinnier, And that inspired me to eat less.**

⭐ From Marina, Age 14, female - 7/10/02

Hey! I've gone from **137lbs, down to 128** ... It was hard work, eating smaller meals, getting more exercise & **doing fun activities.** SO FOR EVERYONE WHO THINKS THEY CAN'T DO IT, **JUST GET INVOLVED IN THE ACTIVITIES U LOVE MOST!! I've done volleyball camp for 2 weeks, soccer, & running with my dog!** its a lot more fun when you're doign what u like

⭐ From Caz, Age 15, female - 09/30/08

Basically from a young age i was bullied about my weight and then i decided to do something about it...**I started rowing club and it was sooo much fun! this got me into other sports which lead to more exercise** and also im a vegetarian well have been for 2 years and **I've lost like 2 stone (28 pounds) in the last 2 years** and i feel better than ever and i thank blubberbusters for the support =)

Volunteering

Many kids find that volunteering to help others actually helps themselves and helps to lose weight.

⭐ From Jon, Age 20, male - 10/4/02

..When I was only 13, I weighed 140, and in high school, I jumped over into the **200s.** I had such a hard time, because **people around me would make fun of me or tease me.** ...Since then, I've **been able to lose 30 pounds** and now weight 195... **I just started volunteering at a local YMCA to help kids, teens, and adults who were just like me and want to feel better about themselves and control their weight and self-image.**

Portion control - Just Say No!

Learning to control portion size is very effective for weight control, if kids can just do it. Remember that portion sizes at restaurants are set by people who want to sell food. As the child below says, it's not what you eat, it's how much you eat that counts. Just feeding a

child or teen the same foods they are accustomed to, but simply adjusting the amount of the food up or down, will keep the child's or teen's weight in a fairly narrow range.

☀ From Rina, Age 16, female - 8/10/06

... I was overweight from the time I was 3 or 4 til 14. .., **I ended up weighing 313 pounds when I was 14, now I'm 16 and 130 pounds**, I'm so happy. I didn't have surgery, no special diet, no pills... **I learned to exersise and eat moderately**. If you want a cookie or a little ice cream, have some! just don't sit there and eat 5 cookies or a pint of ice cream, it's all just common sense! remember, **it's not what you eat, it's how much you eat** that counts!

The final section of Rina's weight chart is shown below. The lower area is her goal weight.

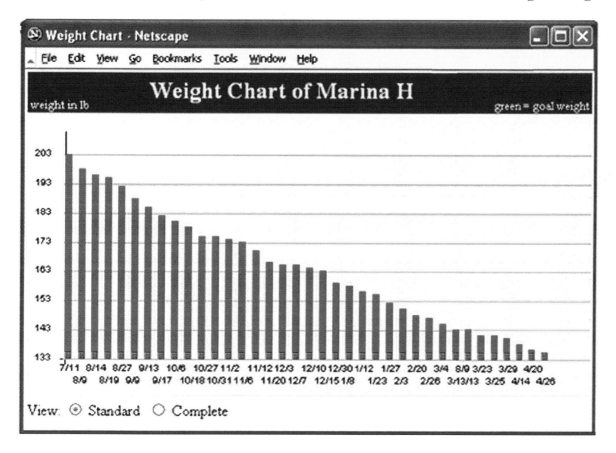

☀ From Ashley, Age 15, female - 10/10/05

I just wanted to tell everyone out there that **what you think is impossible, isnt.** I once weighed **185 pounds that was about 2 years ago, since then, ive lost nearly 50 pounds,** and im still working on it. Someday, I aspire to be a model. There is hope for everyone. **The one thing that really kept me going was that there are more important things than food out there, like relationships, intelligence, wisdom and just plain out having fun.** Everytime you go to grab that candy bar or snack just think how much work you will have to do to work it off, but how easy it is to eat it. Its not fair. **Just chose not to eat it**, its hard but the more you think that youre not on a diet, just eating healthy the easier it is, because then you dont have to think " not to think about food" when you actually are as you think that. remember, **eat what you want, just dont eat a lot of it** (minimal amounts) and dont forget to exercise :) running can be good, just think about how good youll feel afterwards. Good luck to everyone and all of my love

★ From Melissa, Age 14, female - 2/9/06
LAST year around this time I **was 5'3 150lbs**..Eventually I got tired of everyone making fun of me so over the summer **i worked really hard and cut down on portions**. Now Less than a year l8er i weigh **124lbs**..Im so HAPPY and proud of myself...

★ From Stacie, Age 15, female - 1/1/05
Two years ago I weighed 175 pounds. I tried weight watchers and exercising and other fad diets. I lost weight but always put it back on. Finally, I made a new years resolution and **I lost almost 45 pounds**. I weighed 130. **I found the best way to do it was to cut portion size...**

★ From Demetria , Age 14, female - 7/25/04
...Instead of changing my diet completely, **I found it to be helpful just by cutting porportions down**. I was **up to a 13/14 and now I wear a 9 in pants and a 7/8 in dress!** And it feels good!

★ From anoymous, Age 17, female - 3/4/03
i went on my first diet when i was five...one day i fianlly saw the light i stopped searching for a miracle the one diet that was going to make me then froever you know the diet where you can still eat mashed potatoes and ice cream and lose weight without exercise this time i tried the one thing i had heard medical experts reccomend but diddn't believe actually worked i began to exercise cut calories by a moderate amount i ate six meals a day and still i ate ice cream **the key is portion conrol and moderation... i went from 143 to 122**

Measuring everything they eat helps some kids to control portions.

★ Reply from misty, Age 28 - 4/17/08
I'm a personal trainer, reson for this is because **I was a overwieght child who got teased from 3rd-8th grade** and decided to change my lifestyle **I weighed 170 at the height of 5'4". I just ended up with cutting back on food and measuring everything from tsp-1cup serving sizes**. Also walked or road bike and ran up and down my steps at home. It's not easy but, just keep thinking of how good you will feel when you get your goal weight. As a trainer you need to know muscle wieghs more than fat .
I am now 28yrs old and have 2 kids of my own, also **I weigh 135 lbs** 15% body fat and have kept it off for 16 yrs because **I never let my gaurd down meaning you will always have**

to workout daily and watch what you eat , but dont get carried away. I also have bad genetics my mom has always been overwieght and always will stay that way , that does not mean you can't fight this on your own.

Religion

Religious faith helps many kids lose weight.

⋆ From James , Age 15, male - 10/4/05
Well guess what everybody in the past 2 weeks I have **been able to go down ten pounds...I just went to bed early so I could not get hungary. I prayed to God everyday to help me lose** some weight and I know that without him I could not have done this.

⋆ From Carol, Age 14, female - 5/2/04
Hey you guys keep up the good work. you know the most common new years resolution is to lose weight . i wanted to do the same thing. since jan. **i've lost 15 lbs.** so i'm 157. maybe it might not seem very much but i'm really proud that ive gotten this far. and i have gotten to some places where i just didn't want to on but **i prayed and God gave me the strength to press on**. just wanted to give you guys some words of encouragement :)

Musical Instruments

Some kids have found that learning to play a musical instrument, like a keyboard, helps to prevent boredom and takes their mind off of food.

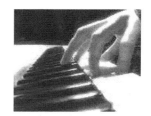

⋆ From Shan, Age 19, female - 5/14/06
Hey! I lost 20lbs so far... It took me only about 1.5 months to lose 20lbs. And the way I eat I have a lot of energy all day so I feel like being active. Even when I'm with friends, instead of staying in, I always suggest we go somewhere biking or rollerblading, or play soccer or basketball outside. **I also just got a guitar which takes my mind off food.** I hope this helps and good luck everyone!

⋆ From Brenden, Age 15, male - 1/9/03
well i'm not at my goal weight yet, but **i hav lost 70 pounds**. When i was 14 I weighed **230 pounds,** and over the summer and till yesterday 1-9-02 i weighed in at 160 pounds... My whole life i was being made fun of and during the summer i made a goal to lose some weight. I hung out with all the "cool kids" and stuff, but **the girls didn't like me. I was being made fun of** so i started listenin to music. PUNK music, and it inspired me to lose

weight, **i started playing guitar and singing in a band,** we practiced a lot, and a lot of singing. with all that i got sweaty and burned calories i guess. **I didn't eat as much because i was too busy and my mind was on music and girls.** hehe. yeh the whole summer i lost 50 pounds, and at the end of the summer until now i had lost 20 more pounds. **I found something to inspire me and keep my mind off food.** being a punk you dont want help from anyone so in my mind asking my mom for a ride was asking for help to go somewhere, so instead i WALKED. I walked everywhere, to my friends house, to knotts berryfarm (theme park) and i had a pass to knotts, so i walked inside too. ..SO if i can do it anyone can. Find something to inspire you to lose weight, alright peace out, fight and unite!!!

✭ From beth , Age 14 - 11/20/05 -
Ht. 5ft 9, Wt. 204 Goal 150/160 - i agree.. loose weight to be healthy, don't worry when you muck up, everyone does! **I founbd a way to stop you eating when you're not hungry, take up a musical instrument.** I come from a musical family anyway, but was never really interested untill i got into the indie scene, I started playing guitar a month ago. When you want to sound good,(because ppl are always not as good as they want to be when coming to things like that!!!!!!!) you practice more and more. it doesn;t have to be expensive, just one you always wanted to play..... once you get your hands on one and you REALLY want to sound good, the more you practice, the more you practice, the better you get, **AND the less unnecessary food you'll binge on when your bored.** it might not help you, but it has me, I havent lost that much weight, but it's working slowly but surely :D

Support network

Support people are key to successful weight loss, such as friends, kids on this site, family, PE teachers, counselors, and the child or teen's doctor. Support people help kids to resist cravings and to cope with problems without seeking comfort in food.

✭ From chris, Age 16, male - 5/19/07 -
i was only ten away from hitting **300 pounds** and i was really BIG at only **5'11".** but i had thought that it was ok because i was on the footbal team and that almost all of the guys in my family are big too. i had finally realized it wasnt when **i went to the doctors for an injury and he told me that i was morbidly obese. it hit me** and i couldnt understand why it didnt before. i mean i was wearng a size 42 pants and 2xl shirts. so i decided to take control of my weight. **in 6 months time, i have lost an amazing 78 pounds and i am down to 212 pounds!** one of the reasons that i was so successful was because i made **my dad go on the diet with me... it is easier if you have someone losing with you and is supporting all the way through.**

⁂ From Kassandra, Age 12, female - 3/17/06

..Well i used to weight **210 pounds** and everybody used to make fun of me and i was so hurt then i decied it was time to do something so i tried exercise and a diet but no matter how hard i tried i could not do it.so **i had to have a little encourgement from my family and friend and once i got that i started loseing weight blubber busters also helped me with that i talked with people that shared the same stories with me** and then after i lost all the weight i found out that i had a diese and could have died from it if i havent of lost all that weight.

What helps kids get through the bad cravings?

A little bit of pleasure

Kids say that having a little bit of pleasure in their food helps to get them through the bad cravings and antsy feelings, when they try to cut out the foods they are hooked on. Thus, kids can gradually get unhooked from the high pleasure foods. This may be somewhat similar to coming off a drug, by using a less addictive drug (such as using methadone in lieu of heroin).

⁂ From Christine, Age 15, female - 10/8/01

HEY There! My names Christine and i reached my goal of **128lbs from 166lbs**. It took me a little over 3 months to do...**I think my diet worked for me because the food i was eating still had a little fat in it. I liked the foods i was eating so i was not starving my cravings...**

Hang in there - it gets easier

Kids say that the bad cravings and antsy feelings get better soon, like within a week or two, if they can just keep going in their weight loss efforts. Support people can help kids get through the bad cravings period.

⁂ From randi, Age 15 - 8/17/07 -
Ht. 5'10", Start: 211 lb, Current: 209 lb, Goal: 150 lb
- just to tell everyone **if u can have enough self control and stay off the sugar for two weeks you stop craving sugar completly** and some sugar free sweets that you might not have liked before taste really good

⁂ From Melissa, Age 16, female - 9/6/06 -
Ht. 5'2.25, Wt. before- 175 now- 141 - well i have officaly **lost 35 pounds** this summer.. no one from school has seen me except my close friends im so excitied to go back tomorrow and show everyone i look fantstic.. and i know that with another 10 or 15 pounds i shall have the body of my dreams.. im almost there and i can't believe i finally did it .. and i

did it the heathly way.. i am so proud of myself.. i would liek to thank evryone for their encourgament and help and also i would like to encourage those who feel like they have no hope.. there is always hope... **after a week all your cravign go away especially if you are eatign really heathly with no refined carbs like chocolate** keep it up everyone if i could do it you can too you jsut need to really want it.. **have control over your body dont let your body have control over you**

⭐ From Dave, Age 18, male - 4/16/03
Just wanted to say I **lost 50 pounds** so far. Just eating better and excersizing at least 45 minutes a day...I'm about 6'2 and I know weigh about 188 pounds... The hardest part of any diet is the start....the transition from no excersize to moderate excersize, and the cutting down of food can be tough. **After about 3 weeks though of really keeping at it, your body will kick-start into weight loss mode. It will be easier to eat less, easier to excersize...** After that, it's just keeping up your diet and watching the pounds go away...

⭐ From Heather, Age 15, female - 4/11/06 -
well..... i was 14 years old,like 5'6 and 222 pounds. in 8 months i lost 70 pounds. i still cant believe it. **after the first three days** of cutting calories and meal portions **your stomach will be adjusted** so its really not all that hard as we all think it is.

⭐ From alex, Age 16, female - 7/8/04
I'm **5'2"** and 7 months ago **I weighed roughly 140.** I cut calories dramatically by eating smaller portions and only drinking water (lots), tea, or coffee. Today I have surpassed my goal weight of 120 and am now a **healthy 110. Dieting is hard at first, but you get used to it.**

⭐ From Jose, Age 16, male - 12/24/05
I remember i was in 7th grade and i was 5'2 about 145-150.. You just have to really stay motivated, **it is hard for the first week or so. But then your body adapts to it, and it isn't as tough anymore.** I am going to keep dieting for another 2 to 3 weeks i want to be down to 127-128 by New Years. Just keep working hard at it.

⭐ From claire, Age 19, female - 4/17/07 -
...i lost 35lbs in three months and have kept it off six months. **its hard at first but then it gets easier.** youve just got to believe in yourself. good luck everyone x x x x x x x x x x

⭐ From Jenina, Age 15, female - 5/27/01
I just want to share with you my storey about how hard it is losing weight, and trying to keep it off. I stared putting on my weight since I was about 4 years old now i am 15, and weighing **265 pounds.** I just started my diet... I never though it would be so hard. **During this pass week I have been tempted so many time to eat food that was not good for me, but I stuck it out and made it through.** I have been eating a lot of fruits and salads

and also i have been excirsing, but the most important thing i have been doing is drinking alot of water and very pround to say i have lost 1 pound. When i lost that pound it made me feel very good about my self, and **showed me that i can lose weight and that its going to be hard but i can do it.**

⭐ From Patricia, Age 20, female - 1/16/03
Hi! I... I ended up at **5'5" and 165 pounds**.... What I did was restrict all snacks. I used to eat cubes of cheese and drink milk in the afternoon... no more. **Whenever Mom came home with Little Debbie cakes, I took one but stored it in the freezer instead of eating it. That way I felt like I wasn't missing out.** I ate 3 meals a day, but never had seconds. I also never ever ate desserts or sweet things, except for fruits. **The longer you go without cake and ice cream, the less you will want to eat them.** Well, I lost 20 pounds in one summer, without exercizing, ... Later on when I got older, I lost 20 more pounds, and **now I weigh a slim 120**...

⭐ From PRESHUS, female - 1/28/06
It was about a month ago I was at my highest wieght of **190 pounds**, I could breath properly and my enery was really low. So the first thing I did was changed the way I was thinking...**The body needs everything but in MODERATION**.....so I started just exercising twice a week and increase my fruits and vegetables. **I know It's usually hard the first couple of weeks because the body is not use to such a dramatic change...but I stuck with it** and now it's been a month and a half and **I lost 15 pouds**. HEY... stick to it, YOU will feel better in the long run...DON"T GIVE UP....when your down think of all the good things you want to achieve...AND **FIND SUPPORTERS TO HELP ENCOURAGE NOT DISCOURAGE YOU...MOST AF ALL HAVE FAITH AND BELIEVE IN YOURSELF**

⭐ From Nora, Age 17, female - 6/7/02
... **once i stopped pigging out on things that made me gain weight, i didn't feel like i needed them anymore! not to mention, now when i go to pig out on things i used to love, they make me feel sick** b/c i've gotten used to eating healthier!

⭐ From Karry M., Age 15, female - 6/7/02
It really stinks being overweight for many different reasons but one big thing is not having a boyfriend, but someday i will. Right now i wear about an **16 to 18 in jeans** and i plan to get to a 10 or 12... when i get down and am about ready to give up i think of getting into that size ten or twelve pair of jeans, I also want to lose the weight to show people that it is possible and to be a role model for people my age to lose weight and show them that's **it's not easy especially the first few weeks but it does get alot easier** when you see your results.

☀ From Mike, Age 14, male - 1/8/06

hey guys my name is mike ... im **14** and im in 9th grade at the beginning of 8th grade i **weighed 186 pounds**.... thats right at age 13 i weighed as much as an asult should and it was embarressing.. **i never took off my shirt** ... im now 14 and **have lost 46 pounds** and i am now currently at 140 pounds and proud. My excuses were o ill start my diet next week or im nto fat im juss big boned... not true at all FOR EVERYONE OUT THERE WHO WANTS TO LOSE WEIGHT I PROMISE YOU THAT IF U REALLY WANT TO HELP YOURSELF AND FEEL BETTER YOU CAN DO IT. **EATING RIGHT IS NOT HARD AFTER YOU HAVE GOT PAST THE FIRST WEEK**.... remember when you wanna take a mouthful of some ice cream "NOTHING TASTES BETTER THAN THIN"

☀ From Ashley, Age 15, female - 4/18/04

I weighted **140 lbs**. Not much huh? But **I am 5'3''**... It was so hard to loose the weight though. **I would get so many chocolate temptations, but after a while I didnt**... I finally got to my goal of 120! When ever I got a craving for something I'd say to myself, "It will taste good for a few seconds, then once its done it won't." And that actuily worked and helped me put down a lot of food!

☀ From Megan, Age 17, female - 3/31/02

I had always been overweight for as long as I can remember,... I procrastinated constantly, saying "I'll go on a diet tomorrow..." and other things to that effect. **I was a compulsive overeater**, and very ashamed of the way I looked. By my sophomore year of high school, I weighed almost **270 pounds**, and I probably wore about a size 24 (I am 5'9" tall). ..**a month before my 16th birthday, something hit me and I decided I didn't want to be fat anymore.** I started slowly... trying to cut out most sweets. I would still have a piece of cake or something once or twice a week, but **was eventually able to cut sweets out almost altogether.** I gradually stopped eating fried foods completely, and **now just the thought of them grosses me out.** I'll occasionally have a cookie or a little bit of ice cream, but usually the guilt I feel afterwards makes it not even worth it. ..right now I weigh 130 pounds, for a **total weight loss of 140 pounds!** ...

☀ From John, Age 14, male - 6/7/03

I am a very short person...as of last year that people were calling me chubby... I ...watched what I ate,... **I gave up ALL sweets**. I never thought I could do it, but I did... After a few weeks, my 5' 1'' body was down from 132 to 125... **after a while, your body will stop craving sweets.** *...! *CUT OUT SWEETS! *Love yourself!

☀ From Katherine, Age 14, female - 4/22/03

... I am eating healthy and excercising and, you know what? I like it. **I dont really want the unhealthy food anymore and can refuse it when it is offered**... I had a **lot of problems at first** but just tell yourself that although being lazy or **eating that cake will make you feel good now, you will hate yourself later**...

249

⁎ From jeff, Age 14, male - 1/24/03

In about two weeks i have lost 6 lbs ... **It is kinda hard the first couple days but once you get through its really easy** ...i eat like a light breakfast like cereal and lunch fat free foods that are good like pudding and lays chips. I drink water all of the time and sometimes diet coke u get used to it quick. I eat what ever is for dinner and i dont snack on junk food. I also run every night... i do crunches and push ups. I want to lose like 6 more...

⁎ From Katie, Age teen, female - 11/3/02

I've **lost 22 lbs**... don't eat as much sugar, or unhealthy stuff. Eat morefruit. **Don't go cold turkey with sugar... Start to eat less, then when your stomach adjusts to that, you can reduce your food intake a little more.**

Here is a great reply to another teen, who was struggling to lose weight and resist cravings...

⁎ Reply from Motivated, Age 19 - 7/17/08

 sugar and over eating is an addiction, so, you need to treat it like an addiction- you need to stop the physical part by dealing with the mentality behind the addiction. work on your issues with food. meditate on it. also, the addiction is physical- your body is used to getting fed so many calories and so much sugar and processed foods. **you need to cut back on all of the very sugary, processed foods and fight through the cravings- they will subside after some time. even two weeks** of a strict, no processed-sugar diet will do wonders for not only your weight, but your physical addiction to food, and also build your self-confidence in your ability to take care of yourself and get your life under control. you can do this. you will do this. take it one mouthful at a time, remmebering that each bite counts, and you WILL succeed!

*And one teen says frankly that food was **like a drug** for her. She says giving up the large portions and junk food was hard at first. But she did it in small steps, she stuck to it, and it got easier.*

⁎ From elle, Age 14, female - 10/25/08

...one year ago i decied to stop being in denial about my weight and change my life for the better. It was hard but looking back on all the hard times it was the best decision i have ever made and most likely will ever make in my life....the biggest shock came when my friend told me i used to be morbidley obese. The biggest girl in the entire school. I was so hurt, i knew i was big, but i had no idea. I don't know what made me finally decide to lose weight. I think it was a variety of things, there was no final click. **I got sick of being looked at in disgust and not being able to fit into any fashionable clothes.** I remember seeing myself in the mirror and not recognising myself. I had stretchmarks everywhere and a double chin. **My thighs were so big that when i didn't wear bikeshorts underneath my clothing they would rub together so much they would bleed... I now weigh fifty seven kilos (125 lb.) and am 166cm (5'6") tall. I lost about 35kg (77 lb.) maybe more** in just one year. **I thought i would be fat for the rest of my life, i wanted to die.** I proved to myself that anything is possible.

I used to eat not only a lot of junk food but also large portions and just binge even when i wasn't hungry. Food was like a drug for me. Combine that with little education for whats good for you and little or no exercise and you have me...

i started running and walking and exercising and eating well. **it was hard at first.** and i **didn't do it all at once, i eased into it.** i never denied myself i just tried harder and it made all the difference in the world. I joined a gym that had a swimming pool and went swimming three times a week.

A few weeks later the weight just started dropping off.

...IT IS POSSIBLE, IF YOU SET YOUR MIND TO IT YOU CAN DO IT! DO NOT GIVE UP! **buy a diet book, eat less junkfood, smaller portions, start a sport, get a friend to help you.** i'm rooting for you babes, elle.

After school eating

After school overeating is the most common time that kids say they overeat (See poll, pp. 163). Kids may be still keyed up and stressed from school when they arrive home and thus tend to head for the fridge or grab a bag of chips to cope. How do successful kids deal with the problem of after school eating?

✮ From Alissa, Age 12, female - 2/28/07 -
Hey, my name is Alissa and during the year 2006 I was really overweight. Around my birthday, August, I decided I was tired of being made fun of, feeling depressed, and being picked on by my doctor. I started eating less: going outside and **playing basketball to keep me from eating after school,** and doing more chores around the house. I stopped eating foods like fries and cheeseburgers, and started eating fruits and veges. I am so happy with myself and I wish you all luck in losing weight.

✮ From Ana, Age 17 - 01/06/06
...I would rollerblade all day after school. I noticed I was getting skinnier, And that inspired me to eat less.. Well **I lost about 30 pounds..**

✮ From Hollie, Age 13 - 07/26/05
i was always told to exercise and i never had the energy to do so.
So i started eating vegitables and fruit and saled and it gave me energy to exercise. every moring i ran a mile and **after school i ran a mile. eventually i lost 40 pounds.** now i look and feel like i never had before.

Change your lifestyle

Weight loss professionals frequently proclaim to kids who want to lose weight: "Change your lifestyle." What the heck does that mean??? Simply put, the kids chose to eat healthier and exercise more, and they learn to deal with sadness, stress, and boredom without using food. Small changes are all it takes. **Remember, a big change is nothing but a bunch of small changes put together.**

✶ From Jasmine, Age 16, female - 11/22/06 -
At the beginning of my freshman year in high school, I weighed **249 pounds**. I hated getting dressed in the morning more than anything else, because it reminded me of how bad I was going to look the rest of the day. I wanted to fall asleep one night and just dissappear, and never have to face the world in my ill-fitting clothes. But I soon came to realize that just sulking and being consumed by my misery was doing nothing for me, so **I made some changes in my lifestyle. I started walking to and from school, and trying to get in a half hour of walking on top of that, every day. I quit drinking soda pop (and haven't had any since then, and I don't miss it at all!!) and stopped going to fastfood places. I started eating more veggies and fruits, and replaced the all the starchy foods in my house with whole grain foods. Today, I weigh 198 pounds**, and look pretty good in clothes. Clothes fit how they should, and I have never been happier!! Now I'm looking forward to wearing a bikini by next summer!! I am still trying to lose weight, but **I have hit that plateau that every person comes to when changing their lifestyle.** But I haven't given up my healthy habbits and I will soon be at my goal weight. **All it takes to lose weight is small changes.** Just taking soda pop and starchy foods out of your diet ALONE should improve anyones health. I also suggest seasoning your foods with herbs and natural juices instead of salt, it works wonders!! And walking is AMAZING!! **Just get out and walk, you won't be sorry.** GOOD LUCK TO ALL!!

✶ From mo, Age 12, male - 9/10/06 -
ok look losing weight isnt as hard as u think i lost 30 pounds **i went from 155 to 130 ... all u really have to do is walk and eat 3 meals a day no snack!!!** i didnt plan to lose weight i just made new friends and **we walked alot around parks talking and we played sports also.** u can do any easy sport **its just somethin to do instead of eating** ...

✶ From jane, Age 17, female - 7/5/06
I haven't always been overweight...Everything changed when I was 8 years old and moved clear across America. Without any friends, and both my parents always at work **I fell into a depression and used sugary foods, soda, and the television to comfort myself. Little Debbie Snacks, and Coke became my best friend since I had no real ones,** and by the time I hit school no one would talk to me due to the weight I gained and the fact that I

stuck out like a sore eye in my new school due to my apperance. I was also harrased like there was no tomorrow in every way feasable. The absense of friends, overabundance of the cruelty of my peers, and lack of activity continued to spiral and **turn me to my comfort food more and more** up until I **nearly commited suicide** at the age of 10 (I kid you not, the neighbor caught me and told my parents and I was thrust into counciling). Quickly my parents pulled me from the school and into another one which was just as bad. This processed continued, as well as moving 4 more times and 3 more new schools, until I had swelled up to a grand total of **240 lbs** when I entered my freshman year of high school. Once again, the teasing, harrasment, and pure agony inflicted on me by my peers was unbelievable (I've suffered every single type of harrasment at school and it pushed me into several fights). I didn't stay at that school for very long, and eventually my family moved again clear across the United States. It was at that point, and at another new school that I began thinking **"if I lost the weight then maybe school will be bearable"**. That was near the end of my freshman year. I've always been enamoured by music and it has always been a prominent part of my life, so for the next year **I signed up for marcing band**. In my sophomore year I lost around 20 lbs just from the practices and exercise from marching band; I dropped from 240 to 220 (I am **5'5"** and a medium frame). I also finally began making friends, and they became the best friends I have had my entire life. ..
I also began cutting out junkfood, soda, and along with my mom restocked the entire kitchen with fruits, veggies, whole grain breads and lean cuts of meat. I also became nutritionally informed on what the average person should take in caloriclly to sustain their weight and what I needed to lose. ...Some people absolutely abhorred the process of exercising in the weight loss process, but I relished the sweat coming off my forehead and **the exercise high became my best friend again.** It took nearly a year but eventually **I lost 100 lbs** and now I am at a very healthy and muscular **142 lbs**. ...As I began to become closer and closer to my goal weight I began to eat normally again; treat myself to a dessert once a week, or allow myself my favorite homemade pumpkin bread. Now I am eleated with how I appear and I will never ever go back to the way I was before. **I never realized this, but I was never really happy just doing nothing and shoveling food down my throat.** But one of my biggest hobbies now is when I exercise (Billy Blanks is my idol; I have at least 10 different Tae-Bo workouts). Even now I have just started a new job at Starbucks and part of the training is coffee tasting and pastry tasting; I can eat a pastry without worrying that I am going to gain weight. Eating right is still a must: very little of no red meat (last time I had it was two-three months ago), lots of fruits and vegetables, healthy whole-wheat breads or rye breads (white bread is nasty, I can't even fathoming eating it anymore), and when I am yearning for sugar I grab a yogurt out of the frige. I am so happy with how I look and just my general outlook on **life has changed** drastically. My personality has changed and this entire process of change, discovery and realization that I can do anything I would never take back or change for anything. For everyone out there who wants to lose weight, it begins with you. You CAN do it, and you WILL do it if you want to,. **Changing your life to a healthy style is the key**: not fad dieting, not crazy 500 calorie a day diets, not diet pills (which are nothing more then chemically processed

steroids). I will end with a qoute from Billy Blanks who in his workouts and through his passion for life has helped me to change in so many ways "Where I am today is where my mind put me; and where I'll be tomorrow is where my mind put me. So don't give up"

Cutting food in half

Kids find that cutting in half what they are about to eat, and saving half for later, is a great way to cut down on portions. They can save half for the next day, so they don't really lose the food they love, and, of course, this spreads out the calories.

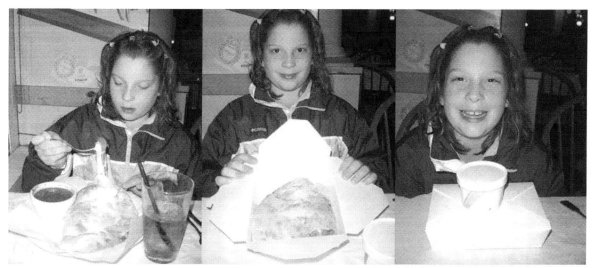

Cut whatever you are eating in half

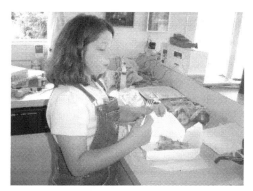

Save half of the meal for lunch the next day

✭ From krista, Age 12, female - 5/19/06 -
ok so far i **lost 56 lbs i went from 300 to 244** i went from a size 26 to a n 18 in womens... i got **a tip cut ur normal food in half then put it away and eqat it tommowor that is wat i do**

Reply from wierd, Age 12 - 4/5/02

...so exercise and **cut everything in half like wen u get a cookie break it in half and save the rest tomarrow same with pizza.** good luck

⭐ From Lynn, Age --, female - 3/14/01

I teach teenagers about health and nutrition. Your **advice about cutting the food in half is excellent.** That is something that a teenager (or anyone, for that fact) can do easily without giving much thought to planning or preparation. A person can eat the same things that others are eating and not be embarrassed about eating "diet" food or feel left out by not eating at all. Soon, new habits are formed and a person doesn't even miss the extra food(calories). I know this is true, because **this is exactly the way that I have lost about 20 pounds.**

⭐ From kiarra, Age 14, female - 3/29/04

o.k. i started to look fat at age 5 or 6, i never exersised and i ate every thing in site, at around **age 10, i was 175 lbs, at age 13 i was 203,and when i turned 14 i was 254 lbs,** my mom was lighter then me, she's 44 and she was only 180 lbs. i needed to loose weight, and my aunt dee sent me this program, and i lost 15 lbs in a week,i am now 239, i know it's still not healthy, but **i lost a bunch of weight in a short time, just by cuting every thing i ate in half,** not eating more than 3 meals a day, i got the splinda surgare, it's sweet no calories, no fat sugare, diet soda and and water only, and exersise every day for at least 30 minnits,i went 7 or 8 years hating my self and feeling bad about my self. just try it you can do it, it's easyer then it looks and sounds.

⭐ From Alicia, Age 15, female - 3/14/04

Hi my name is Alicia and I would like to share my weight loss sucess story **I used to weigh 290 pounds** I WAS MISERABLE well one day I got up off of my rear end and said to myself I CANT TAKE IT ANYMORE I was sooo sick of being obese my goal was 145 now I am 145 it took me 1 year on a steady diet ok this is what I did I guzzeld water every chance i got I even took bottles to school for brekfast I usualy ate 2 scrambled eggs and I didnt use grease in the skillet I used PAM that is very important pam is not fatty **for lunch I ate whatever the school served but i cut it in half** and i had a salad but I brought a Crystal Light drink for dinner... and I always treated myself i did my treat on Fridays I would buy a quart of ice cream and i would eat 1 scoop and 1 scoop only every friday REMEMBER YOU CAN ALWAYS HAVE A LITTLE TEMPTATION... you have to put forth the effort and try try try You will succeed if u try... remember if you try you will defiantely SUCCEED

⭐ From Hannah, Age 13, female - 7/22/03

My name is Hannah, when I first came to this site I weighed 145lbs, **(13lbs.overweight).** I started posting on the message board, and boy did it help. ...When it was time to eat and my mom served me my food **at dinnertime I would cut every portion in half and eat one** half. **Then I would cover the rest with plastic wrap and pop it in the refrigerator. The next day I would eat it for lunch.** I had been doing this for about a month when I weighed myself . I had already lost ten pounds, I just needed to loose ten more. I continued my "diet" and excercised and in another five weeks I weighed in at 124lbs.

⭐ From Jme, Age 15, female - 7/2/03

...I got from **over 200 lbs. last year to 124 now** here's how I did it: Firstly, I totally cut out all drinks from my diet besides water (& 1 glass of skim milk for health reasons)... Secondly: I found time every day to exersize in some way for no less than one hour... Working out should be something that you don't dread doing...It should be fun. As far as diets go: DON'T DIET!!! Diet is an evil word made by someone who wanted money. If you diet, you will lose wieght. But when you're done, you will gain it back. Instead you're making a total change in your life. You can't think: If I just lose 20 more lbs. then I can eat all the cookies and chips I want: It doesn't work that way. having a little junk now and then won't kill you, but if you start your old eating habits once you've lost the weight you wanted you will gain it back. Also: **cutting what you eat in half does help, but isn't the best method.** If you live on pizza and burgers, cutting them in half **will cut calories, but won't make you any healthier.** It's better to eat a huge salad than half a burger...

From Leslie, Age 17, female - 7/20/02

I haven't reached my goal yet but I have lost 2 lbs. in the past 2 days and I'm very happy. I did by swimming 30 minutes each day and **cutting back my foods in 1/2. It works! ;)**

⭐ From Rappy, Age 13, female - 8/6/02

I have 1.5 lbs to go before I reach my goal for now! I may change it later, but this is how I did it. **Eat ONLY when you are hungry and stop when you arent anymore, not stuffed.** If that is hard then **cut in half what you would normally eat and save one half for later.** Exercise alot also. Good luck!

⭐ From Zach N., Age 15 - 7/24/08

Ht. 5'6", Start: 300 lb, Current: 300 lb, Goal: 285 lb - ... today i had 2 waffles for breakfast. Wheat waffles with sugar free syrup. Yeah i kno, still unhealthy but a lil better. For lunch i had 2 slices of pizza, along with half a can of pineapple. MMMMMMMMM. Dinner i had chili dogs, with no bread, and **cut the hot-dag in half to make two. So kinda tricking my body, to think that i hate two hot-dogs when i only ate one.**

⭐ From Camille, Age 14, female - 7/21/02

I'm **5'5 and weighed 145 pounds**... First, **I thought that if I just cut all my meals in half, it'd do the trick...WRONG,** so I instead ate healthier- no more hamburgers, **instead of 4 slcies of pizza - only 1 slice,** friuts and veggies for snacks. Well that did help me.. **lose 10 pounds** in only two weeks! Then, I realized I had been forgetting the most important thing of all: **EXERCISE.** ... I ran/jogged for 25 minutes everyday on my mom's treadmill and after that did 3 sets of 10 crunches. Beleive me, that was the key, after about a month my stomach was actually flatter and I was down to **125**!

Eating in moderation

Kids find that eating in moderation is key to losing weight. This is really a combination of portion control and eating slowly. They eat only two cookies and not the whole bag.

⋇ From Daisy, Age 14, female - 5/1/06
Ht. 5'7, Wt. 150 -I have recently **lost about 35 pounds,** I would say in about a month and a half (maybe two months) ...**I weighed about 175 pounds and was 5'7". Now I weight 150 and am the same height.** ...**I realized how much moderation in foods does count.**

⋇ From Sabrina, Age 16, female - 4/27/06
Ht. 5'5, Wt. 135 - Hey guys... i want to tell yall how **i lost 80 pounds.**First off.. you have to be realistic...are you going to eat tofu and plain baked potaoes all your life? probably not so let me tell you my secret! I ate pretty much everything i ate before i decided to change my life, except sweets but i didnt cut them out completley. If i wanted a candy bar i had one but that was few and far between, **i learned to never deprive myself because it only made me want it more.** so if i wanted a hamburger i had me a hamburger but only 1. **it's all about moderation you can have just about anything in moderation.** i cut back and **dranks tons of water** and diet tea. At first **i excersised everyday for at least 30 minutes** a day(everyone has 30 mins) billy blanks, richard simmons, walking,and of course DDR thats awesome because **you can actually have a little fun and forget your excersisng!** Once a week i would weigh but no more than that(remember you didnt gain it over night so you wont lose it overnight)then i would eat ONE thing that i truley wanted whether it was a candy bar or a couple of tacos,but remember dont go overbored and dont fall off your diet! Anyways i lost the weight by doind what i just told you and i wasnt in agony and miserable because i didnt feel deprived. Whatever you do dont do the grainbars and apples and tofu "diet"unless you really like it becaue you have to be realistic and ask yourself...am i going to eat this way for the rest of my life? we like REAL FOOD!! anyways **i have kept it off for a year now**...i still exercise but only 3 times a week...and **i have found that my stomach can only handle that one hamburger , not 2 ham and fries like it use to**..i still **weight once a week and if i gain 3 pounds then i immediatley up my excercise and cut back** and then the next week i'm fine again and this is how i have maitained. hang in there the wieght will come off and **with every pound you will have more and mope confidence and that will give you the desire to follow threw.** One more thing i did was i would get one outfit(that didnt fit me) and hang it in my closet and when i was a size 20(yes i said 20 ladies) i would get a size 18 and every month i would try it on till it would fit me then a size 16...until eventually it was a

size 7! just remember you can do this and you truley dont have to be miserable doing it...i'm living proof...

Motivation

Here are kids' motivations for success:

☆ From Elizabeth, Age 14, female - 12/3/05
In the 5th grade I was a heavy kid. I weighed 230 pounds and was 5'6. I got picked on a lot and never had a boyfriend... **I'm down a total of 55 pounds**. I weigh 170 pounds and I'm 5'8 inches tall. .. I didn't change my way of eating or dieting to get a boyfriend if that's what you think. **I changed cause I wanted to have a good future and life.** I didn't see being 230 pounds at the time, giving me a good future. **If you want to diet and have your doubts just think on your future** and how good it will feel when you reach your weight goals. It's a awesome feeling!

☆ From Taya, Age 13, female - 3/24/05
in september i weighed a whopping (sp?) **200+ pounds** (i don't know how many stones that is, sorry)! i was at the worst i'd ever been. i think **a certain thing "clicked" in me and i just couldn't stand all the fat anymore.** i didn't have a terrible life, in fact, my life was going pretty great. i don't know what happened, but i think there is a certain point in being obese, that i just couldn't take it anymore...**i have lost a little over 50 pounds!**

☆ From Kristie, Age 16, female - 7/1/04
Hey. Since i was about 9 years old i was incredibly obese when i was **almost 15 i weighed 260 pounds**. Eventually **I got up to 300lbs**. I never was teased. Lucky for me i have the greatest friends and go to teh best school so i never was bugged about my weight. That was a problem for me though because i **never really got any motivation because i thought people accepted me for me**. I even had a boyfriend... anyways one day **my mom got really mad** with me and said somethings that no mother should have but it did change my life. **She called me some nasty names and said any hope in marriage for me can be forgotten** so at first i was depressed but then i turned tht into extreme anger and motivation. I got a pass to the gym walked everyday for 30 minutes ate no junk food. My friends strated to work with me because some of them too were obese... Now I am almost 17 in a lil over 1.5 years **i have lost 157 pounds**. I have always been a happy person and didnt think icould get much happier. Everyday my boyfriend kisses me and calls me gorgeous and i know hes proud of me and I showed my mom that i can do anything i want and be anything i want. I just want everyone to know thoough whether your 100 lbs or 500lbs your beautiful. Its ur personality that captivates people. Dont let others bring u down . Use their negative remarks to bring urself up... u guys all rock luv ya!~

✮ From Ryne, Age 14, male - 7/22/03

Most of my life, I have been overweight.....until now. I have always had so many friends, but when I started middle school, there were people I didn't know giving me rude remarks. Well, It had gotten out of control and I weighed about **250 pounds. So, one day, I got up and told myself I WAS going to lose weight, and I WASN'T going to be overweight again.** Now, I have been eating healthy and excersing ever since. **I have lost more than 80 pounds** and it feels great. I am 5' 10" and I have a large frame size. I weigh in between 165-170... I have even done this without giving up what I love eating. I eat what I want one or two days a week.

✮ From Andrew, Age 18, male - 5/1/04

all my life i was the fat kid getting teased. i have a twin sister, lizzy, who has been model since we were about thirteen. lizzy was the part of the popular crowd and i was , well, a loaner. **i remember having a crush on one of her friends** in the 8th grade and **knowing there was no way she would ever go out with me.** when i was 17 i went to one of my sister's runway shows and i heard one of the other models say "THAT is you brother,hes so.. big" after that we went home and i went to the bathroom and weighed myself i was shocked when the scale went **past 300 up to 318. I decided that day i wasnt going to be "the fat guy" anymore** so i decided to try the atkins diet the first week i lost 8 pounds and was so amazed. after the i lost the first 50 pounds people really started to notice and it felt really good. after a year and 2 months **i lost 132 pounds.** now i am 6'2" and 186 pounds. lizzy and i actually do look like twins now. i just recently went to another one of lizzy's runway shows but i heard a model say " your brother is so hot!!" something i never thought someone would say about me. stick to your diets!! you can do it!

✮ From mikayla, Age 13, female - 3/17/04

I used to be **175 pounds.** Then **I got teased and finally cared about what I looked like. I got down to 155 pounds** by cutting calories and working extra hard in P.E. classes

✮ From mandy, Age 18, female - 11/11/05

hi, just thought id share my story as well.. since i was about 10 to 16 i weight **178 lbs!** at a **size 18 im 5'5"** ... i have **gone from a size 16 to a size 3! and currently weight 118** ..never tell yourself you cant do something, its just another easy way out. **get a buddy and motivate eachother.**

✮ From Marina, Age 16, female - 1/29/04

I've lost ten pounds. Most Importantly, there is no magic secret to weight loss... I've been eating 3 meals a day, sometimes with healthy snacks in between. I've been drinking a TON of water and going to the gym about 5 days a week. I've pretty much cut out junk food completely as well. **The most important key to weight loss is motivation. I'm not sure where all of mine came from. I went to the gym with my sister one day and all**

of a sudden a burst of motivation came out of no-where & has stuck since... Just give it a shot!

⁎ From Elizabeth, Age 21, female - 1/20/04   ...my weight has gone up and down for the last 10 years...but take the weight off now...it gets much harder as you get older. Remember, that now **it seems so important to be thin because you want to look pretty and hansome, but there is a much bigger issue you have to consider: your health. What you do at 12, 16 and older does effect you life in the future.** Take control now so you can really enjoy the rest of your life!!! **I have lost 60 lbs** since august going to the gym and eating less refined sugar (candy, ice cream, that sorta stuff)and also going to the gym at least 4 times a week. All of you keep going and just imagine the possibilites you have when you are healthy and feel good about yourself...those thoughts are what inspire me everyday!

⁎ From Stacy, Age 14, female - 7/12/03
I **wieghed 180 to about 190 pounds**... the kids would really pick on me... at first i didnt see my self as overweight... i was in denile... then **i saw a modivation to loose weight... and that was my sister. She would always get the cute guys to look at her. And well i got the ugly glares.** So i cut back on a lot of my income, of food. I would swim almost everyday. **I lost about 20 pounds that summer. And a total of 10 pounds through out the year.** i still have some ways to go... my goal is about 127-132. Looking good makes me feel better. And to all you poeple who are stuck at the weight your at, and are disgusted, dont stop trying. You just need to find a motivation... Good luck!

⁎ From Mike, Age 20, male - 6/6/03
First I would like to say that this is a good site to share the stories of our weight loss experiences. I was always overweight most of my life but after i graduated high school..**I was 5-8 and 240lbs. I felt so embarassed and just hated the way I look.** I decided to go on a diet on Jan 2001 as my new years resoultion. Basically I stopped eating fast food and cut down on my meals. Also I was working a physical job so that helped too with the exercise. .. Now its June 2003 and **I have lost a total of 90lbs. I am 150lbs now** and I am very happy I lost the weight... Its a shame though how society judges heavy people. **I did it for health reasons and also social reasons.**

⁎ From randy, Age 13, male - 6/8/01
When i was around 11 years old i started gaining more weight. Before i knew it i was 13 years old was about **5'4 1/2 and weighed 140. I had always been trying to lose weight but never fully accomplished my goals. Then one night i realized what im doing to my body and that it's not healthy to be overweight.** I barely got picked on because most kids in my class weigh over 150. When i started to go on a diet it was tough, but i kept myself motivated. I road a stationary bike in my basement for an hour or two a day. I

stopped drinking pop with lots of calories and watched my intake of food. **Two months later i weight 115** and have never felt better...

⭐ From Rob, Age 17, male - 5/28/07
Hey about a year and a half ago I was **5 foot 6 inches and I weighed over 230 lbs. Then I realized that thats not healthy.** I ate less and I did more activities. Now I am on the football team, and a starter I may add. **I am 6' tall and 200 lbs.** That may still be overweight but I am proud of myself. I think that losing weight is healthy for overweight people. On a side not dont let people teasing you bother you. I know it is hard but in the end if you ignore them they will most likely go away. **If you dont like how you look, change it.** Thanks

⭐ From Michelle, Age teen - 7/26/08
Ht. ??, Start: 228 lb, Current: 197 lb, Goal: 127 lb - ok so i've been doing this sense i was 8 years old and i'm just now finding out how to stay on a diet **u have to have a reason for losing weigh not just want to be thin u have to have a real reason** i started at 228 pounds i'm now 197 i still have 70 pounds to lose but **i lost the 31 pounds by having a reason my reason is if i don't do this i'll never be happy** and i know that but anyway how did i lose the weight i did easy just sticking with what i started...

Make a plan

Kids say that making a plan for losing weight definitely helps.

⭐ From Tara, Age 14, female - 8/29/04
I have been to the site so many times, and everytime i look at it **i say i wanna loose wight and everytime i mess up or quit..** But **this one time i had maid a plan** out of what to do each day at the beginning of sumeer. walk 1 mile, then play ddrmax, its a game that u hit steps to win, then 10 sit ups morning and night..at the beginning og summer i **was 140 at 5'4..now at the end im 125 at 5'4..**so u can all do it..yes i cheated so many times but keep with it..i know its so hard I LOVE FOOD TO but if u work through it ull be impressed...**eat and drink what u want just not as much and exercise**...Tara gl

⭐ From Miranda, Age 13, female - 5/19/03
hey! if you make yourself up a **simple diet plan**, like no junk food, veggies, fruits lots of water and excersie, it does work. When I started 2 1/2 - 3 weeks ago i weighed **182 pounds, now i'm 170 pounds**...

Therefore, if weight is regained, they can go right back to their plan.

✴ From Tasha, Age 15, female - 4/28/02

On New Year's I vowed to loose 70lbs by the summer. I was 220 lbs, and I excersized for at least 40 mins everyday, followed a strict diet, and **lost 10 lbs** in a month. I was so excited! I kept going and lost another 5lbs until disaster struck . . . I became heavily depressed for various reasons. **I began eating out of depression and I gained ALL my weight back, if not more.** Recently I decided it wasn't worth it. **I went back to my plan** and I lost 10 lbs in 2 weeks, and I'm on my way again. I'm happier now, too. You just have to remember that nothing's worth making yourself feel even worse. Don't get careless and have fun while you're doing it, otherwise you won't see results.

But who helps kids develop such a plan? Parents and health professionals can help kids find other ways to cope without seeking comfort or stress relief in food.

Some successful kids say that they write down how they feel in a journal, diary, or notebook.

*Writing down how they feel **before, during, and after** they eat something really helps them to see where and why they overeat and what they can do about it. Keeping a chart of their weight can help kids see their progress.*

✴ From Cirene, Age 17, female - 4/3/04

In april 2003 i weighed 348 lbs today April 2004 i weigh 288 lbs exercise and healthy eating is how i did it and **writing down my feeling leaving spaces to come back and write later on on how sticking it out helped me out**

Eating a lot of fruit worked for one teen.

✴ From rutha, Age 18, female - 12/11/02

I would constantly eat so much even though i was full. it was like my mouth wanted it, just to taste it and my stomach didn't. I got tired of saying i would lose wieght... **I ate fruits everyday.** I started to think of fat food as an enemy. I then realized that it was workng. **I was 170 then i went down to 140** in 3 months...I ffeel so good. i'm 5'9... so what im saying is everyone can do it like i did! Just believe in yourself...

Other benefits

When kids are able to lose weight, it can even resolve type 2 diabetes.

✴ From Chantal, Age 17, female - 3/31/01

...i was overweight my whole lifein 1998 **i was diagnosed with diabetes type 2 because i was big! i weighed 198...** so i knew i had to do something with my weight ...i joined softball stopped watching lots of tv... i watched what i ate .. drank lots of water.. and now **3 yrs later i weigh 135!** ...so i am very happy.. **and i bet the diabetes!! :)**

Searching for tips

*Kids may view and search all the past 133,0000 messages from other kids – more than 40,000 archived posts and 93,000 replies at this printing - at **www.weigh2rock.com**. They may search on keywords like "tips." There are also many posts and replies considered especially helpful by the website moderators, which are placed in the Kids Helping Kids Area under various categories, such as "Teasing" or "Exercise," for each age group. Kids may view the messages in a category.*

Reply from Michelle, Age 14 - 4/6/02
..I have been on this sight for about 2 years. I am currently **148 pounds** and **5'2"** (I was **175 pounds** when I first came to this sight). **My best advice for you is to read into the archives of this board because there's tons of great advice.** Good luck.

Fast food and junk food

Kids say that resisting fast food and junk food is important for losing weight.

✱ From Rachel, Age 16, female - 2/8/03
...all i did was **cut down on junk food and other fatty food** and exerise 15 minutes a day and built up to 20 minutes. well, guess what? my pants that used to be really tight on me r already a bit loose!! i hope my story helped :)

✱ From Monica, Age 16, female - 2/27/06
I lost 14lbs in a month and a half. By drinking water only, no junk food, and cutting down my portions. good luck ya'll. and eating lots of fruits

✱ From kate, Age 18, female - 2/21/06
LOTS of exercise, LOTS of water, **ONLY food that is good for you (WE ALL know what foods those are)** I at one point went **from 150 to 108 doing this**. It did NOT take long!

✱ From Patrick, Age 21, male - 5/18/03
I weighed in at a total of **358lbs** on August 24th, 2002. Now almost 9 months later, I am **down to 245lbs, standing at 6'3"**. Ive tried everything I could think of since junior high... **Simple change of eating habits, cutting out fast food, deep fried food, pizza, pop, and simply hitting the gym.** It wasnt easy, and wont be, but is way worth it...

Kids want successful losers to say <u>how</u> they lost the weight.

⭐ **From Usha (pronounced oo-sha), Age 15, female - 2/18/06 -**
Ok, if anyones going to post a sucess story **PLEASE PLEASE PLEASE don't just say that you lost, that dosn't help, post HOW you lost**, otherwise whats the point? Thanks!

⭐ **From Deseray, Age 13, female - 6/26/02**
...i need to comment on sumthin i'm not tryin to be rude but most of u that r tellin **these storys arent tellin how u did loose they weight i mean ur just sayin i watched what i ate and excercised** i mean it helps but not much like what type of foods did u eat and what excercises/ how many did u do, ya know cuz almost everyone on here wants to loose weight and well we need advice thanx for ur tyme

⭐ **From Marshall, Age 12, male - 11/15/03**
Hi I just wnated to say to **everyone who has a success story to write what they did exectly to lose the weight** so other people can get ideas on how to lose the weight. This is to the people who are just posting how much they lost.
HOW YOU LOST IT AS WELL

⭐ **From moll, Age 10, female - 10/10/03**
hey, people who say their success story well i think u should say how you lost weight. Thanx for the peeps who did. But **America has a lot of obese people so mabey if u say how u lost it it could work for other people**. Thnx

Other books and programs

In regard to other books and programs, kids recommend one book in particular, and one program.

⭐ From Isabella, Age 14 - 3/12/07
Ht. 5'5", Start: 184 lb, Current: 164 lb, Goal: 150 lb - Hey guys! I don't know if any of you remember me but I've been on and off for a year now. I've posted many success stories and I am the Isabella on the My Story Page. I feel amazing now having lost 20lbs since Feb. of last year! I preach the **Diet For Teenagers Only**, which is a fabulous lifelong healthy-eating-plan book based on teenagers' nutritional needs that you can follow forever. It's healthy, real, not gimmicky, and produces great results!

⭐ From Chantel, Age 14 - 7/27/07
Ht. 5'4", Start: 160 lb, Current: 139 lb, Goal: 120 lb - Hey guys im back on track and weight 135 now. I got this great book today, **The Diet for Teenagers Only** by Carrie

Wiatt and Barbara Schroeder. Gives you great advice and even gives you a 7 day meal plan and some exercise routines! Recommend it.

★ Reply from Lucy, Age 14 - 8/1/06
oh my gosh!!! i love the **diet for teenagers only!!!** it is such a good book!!! the stuff u learn in it it wicked good!! like what it says about high fructose corn syrup and artificial sugars and everything!! its a real eye opener and it gives u excersise tips too!!!

★ From Flower Fawn, Age 15 - 09/30/08
Ht. 5'5", Start: 184 lb, Current: 179 lb, Goal: 145 lb - Hey guys! I just had my first official weigh-in with **WeightWatchers and I lost 3 lbs this week!! I am so happy right now! ;)** I haven't been in the 170s in a while. I really really hope I can be 170 by New Year's Eve! Lol. Anyways, you know what's really good to kick a chocolate milk craving? Chocolate soy milk! It may sound gross or weird, but trust me it's relaly good.

Reply from Jocelyn, Age 17 - 09/14/08
I've had success on Weight Watchers. I started in the middle of january at 157 pounds and now I just got to my goal of 125 pounds.
Weight Watchers is good because it teaches you a healthy lifestyle and it is not one of those fad diets that actually hurt your body. Just remember that weight loss takes a long time and it can't be fixed in like a month. It may take a long time to reach your goal, but slow and steady wins the race!

Reply from Jessica, Age 23 - 09/15/08
Yep, I'm down 26lbs since the end of May. **Weight Watchers works!**

But any program still requires that the kids stick with it.

★ From Steph, Age 18 - 08/04/08
Ht. 5'8", Start: 220 lb, Current: 191 lb, Goal: 130 lb - Hey I'm Steph and I'm from NZ. I've struggled with being overweight since form 2 (12 years old) when I first started to get bullied by the girls in my class. It lasted 5yrs, and I finally got some closure after joining a church and youth group where I made alot of friends and had the chance to share what happened to me infront of 400 people. **I have been trying to lose weight alone after joining weight watchers but finding it hard to stick to.**

Accountability

It helps to be accountable to someone when trying to lose weight. Not wanting to disappoint the person to whom they are accountable gives kids the motivation to make it through the worst cravings at the beginning of weight loss and keep going. Even after weight loss is successful, kids need to still be accountable to someone in order to avoid a relapse.

★ From Amy , Age 15, female - 11/28/05

Hey! 2 years ago when i was in the 7th grade- i went from about **184lbs to 160lbs...when u r tempted to eat something** like pie or something fatening, just **think of how much work it'll take to burn it**- its not worth eating it! its all in ur head- stop look'n at it and just walk away! (thats what i do) **pick someone in your family or friends that you care a lot bout and say ur gunna loose weight for them AND 4YOURSELF**- if u haven't seen someone in a long time- just think if you lost weight now then by the next time you see that person, then they would be shocked and surprised of how great you look! Then you would feel really good bout yourself

Testimonials

There are many testimonials about kids helping each other on the site.

★ From Saruca, Age 13, female - 10/31/05

I just want everyone to know how much I love this site, I've been a lurker for **almost a year** now. I **started out at 245 pounds, and now I'm down to 108!** I'm so proud of myself, and I want everyone to know that **I owe it all to tips and hints that I recieved from this site,** and I love you guys so so much. I still want to spot reduce on my arms a little bit, but I am so happy with my weight now. Thank you to EVERYONE

★ From Maureen, Age 17, female - 10/14/05

I want to say that it's not impossible to achieve weight loss....**i weighed a whopping amount about 2 years ago**, and **i followed all the rules and facts on blubberbusters and it helped me!** i am now feeling gorgeos and confident....you are beautiful and you can all achieve what you want! Just believe in yourself! ...xxx..X..xxx...

★ From Stephanie, Age 12, female - 8/2/03

Hey!I started a "diet" thing .... that meant for me: **no going out to dinner 24/7, no fastfood, riding my bike every spare minute i had, swimming laps in my local pool, eating when i was TRULY hungry and stopping when i was full,** hula hooping LOL, jump roping, playing games like basketball and volleyball, and doing crunchies and push ups every night. it was REALLY REALLY hard, but it was SOOOOO worth it! **i went from 197 pounds, to 96 pounds** ... pretty awesome huh??? i went from a 12 to a 7 jr.! i am so happy with myself! thanks blubberbuster!

Even if only a couple of pounds are lost, there is pride and thrills.

⭐ From anne, Age 16, female - 9/29/03
just for a quick update- i'm not 155 becasue **i lost two pounds las week. yaaaay!** i like coming here to brag because i don't like telling my friends at chool who are either not overweight and are thinking so what? or my friends who are and are thinking- oh great thanks for rubbing it in! so yeah- this site is awesome...

⭐ From Ki, Age 17 - 02/05/09
Ht. 5'4", Start: 180 lb, Current: 177 lb, Goal: 135 lb - YAY! **The first 3 pounds have come off!** I know it doesn't seem like such a big deal, but **when I looked at the scale I started jumping up and down because as many times as I have tried to lose weight, I have NEVER lost a pound. Wow. It's such a great feeling.** And it took a week.

The key to the kids' successes seems to be that they first examine themselves and decide to do something about their weight. They tap into their emotions, so they can see why they overeat and whether they seek comfort and stress relief from food. They may be embarrassed to ask for help from their parents or their health professionals. Or, such help just isn't there. So, they decide to do something about it themselves.

Become a helper

The final goal of losing weight is similar to the 12th step of Alcoholics Anonymous, to become a helper and mentor for those just starting out:

This is BRYAN's question:
i was obese once. i hated it. people would laugh at me, make jokes and tease me to no end. Dr.Kramer gave me this site to kind of alleviate my stress and give me the piece of mind that i wasn't alone in this fight. that other people were trying. other people were trying and winning the war. the seemingly impossible war. **with extreme dedication, effort, and this website was i able to win the war.** i come here to ask a favor. **i want to help out other people** i want to be able to tell them its okay and that im by their side to help them by ALL MEANS NECESSARY!!!! please be in contact with me i would like to help this website and give back for all its done for me   -sincerely Bryan

⭐ From anne, Age 16 - 12/21/03
 ... helping others helps me put things into perspective that i need to work on also.

Becoming a helper is a win-win situation. Teaching someone else how to achieve a healthy weight solidifies the knowledge and changes in the helper.

And most important, successful kids don't give up...

✴ Rickie, Age 10, Ht. 5'1.5", Goal 148.0 lb, Start 169.4 lb, Today 168.0 lb
1/10/07 - **Its very hard job, but i go on continuing**

15 | Where Do We Go From Here?

The most frequent post by kids on our bulletin boards is, "How do I lose weight?" The answer is pretty simple: eat in moderation. But if it's that simple, why do these kids struggle so much to lose weight and maintain it? The answer to that question is also pretty simple: They 'use' food to cope with life. The postings on comfort eating in Chapter 9, stress eating in Chapter 10, and boredom eating in Chapter 11 reveal that these kids use the sensations of food and the action of eating to numb unpleasant feelings and to relieve stress and boredom. The disaster is that they are unable to stop. They overeat to the point that they make their lives miserable.

We don't feel pleasure and pain at the same time. As one researcher put it, "If a behavior eases pain or boredom for only 30 seconds, the behavior will be repeated." [Foster 2006]. Thus, kids may become involuntarily 'hooked' on using food to comfort themselves and to cope with stress. It's likely simple pleasure, to begin with, which causes them to overeat. They eat "because the food is there." But once their brains realize that pain is eased by the pleasure of the food and that stress is relieved by the displacement activity of eating, they may be driven to continue the behavior, even though they become distressingly overweight as a result. These kids hate being fat, yet they struggle to resist cravings for pleasurable foods, e.g. 'junk food,' knowing full well that eating those foods will result in additional weight gain and further damage to their lives. Many openly post that their eating is out of control. This is highly suggestive of an addictive quality, or 'psychological food dependence.'

The common expression by the kids on the boards of feeling 'out of control' with eating is confirmed by the poll results below. Most of the 145 kids responding feel that their eating is out of control. (http://www.blubberbuster.com/cgi/poll_new_56.cgi)

Do you feel that your eating is out of control?

YES: 96 votes (66%)

NO: 49 votes (34%)

---

145 Kids voted

Below are some comments from kids responding to this poll:

Age 15, female, 5 foot 4, 295 lbs - I know that Im obese but **I cant stop myself eating** fatty foods. **Its comforting to eat even though I know it will just make me even fatter.** Ive tried to lose weight before but it always fails and I just end up at least as fat as I was before, **so I get depressed and eat more which ends up making me fatter.** Its so annoying to never be able to lose weight

Age 15, female, 5'5, 156 lbs - **I love the way junk food tastes and I have so much trouble avoiding it because of that. Also, if I eat just one chip or have the smallest amount of candy or ice cream, I want more.** I end up eating like 3 candybars instead of part of one, or ice cream, a few cookies and some candy, or the whole bag of chips.

Age 12, female, 5"8, 280 lbs - **i only eat when i am bored or depressed which is all the time lol**

The overeating addictive quality and apparent psychological food dependence of kids posting on the bulletin boards is disturbingly similar to tobacco, alcohol, and drug dependence. Many kids have posted that they feel "addicted" to certain types of food, particularly 'junk food' and 'fast food' (see Chapter 9), as the post below relates:

Age 14, female, 5', 178 lb.: its so hard cuz **its like an addiction.** . i mean **its not like crack or anything but its almost as hard to quit** and it can kill u just as sure, slowly. ;.that's wat i think about when i want **junk food or fast food.**

We asked kids what they thought about junk food and addiction in a poll (http://www.blubberbuster.com/cgi/poll_new_62.cgi):

Do you think that high pleasure food (junk food) is addicting, like drugs or cigarettes?

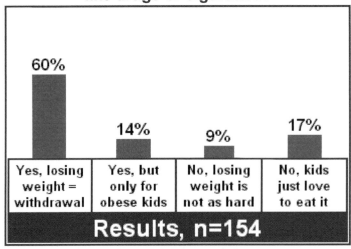

154 kids voted

Most kids voting feel that junk food is addicting like drugs and cigarettes and that losing weight is similar to the 'withdrawal' of quitting smoking or getting off drugs or alcohol. It's noteworthy that only a small percentage of the kids feel that losing weight is not as hard as quitting smoking or getting off drugs. Furthermore, most of the kids feel that they are addicted to junk food, per the results below.

Do you feel that you are addicted to junk food?

YES: 104 votes (68%)

NO: 50 votes (32%)

154 kids voted

Probably very few overweight kids know the scientific definition of "addiction." Nevertheless, they do know that something very powerful is driving them to consume large amounts of pleasurable foods, in spite of the dreadful effects of inevitable weight gain.

From sonnie, Age 16 - 02/24/09
Ht. 5'6", Start: 240 lb, Current: 230 lb, Goal: 140 lb - does anybody have an info on **how to resis the urge 2 eat, knowing that later on you'll regret**..i need help bad!!

*The scientific definition of 'addiction' is actually just that: being driven to a behavior, even though the individual knows that the action will later result in significant problems. An overwhelming need to ease pain or an unpleasant emotion outweighs the delayed consequences. The word "addiction" may seem too severe to apply to kids and uncontrollable eating, conjures up ghastly images, and may be offensive to some individuals. Nonetheless, acknowledged addictive behaviors include shopping, gambling, sex, sports, TV, workaholism, and many others. Furthermore, some overweight kids on our boards literally say that they use food "**like a drug**," as shared below:*

From elle, Age 14, female - 10/25/08
I weigh fifty seven kilos (125 lb.) and am 166cm (5'6") tall. **I lost about 35kg (77 lb.) maybe more** in just one year. ..I used to eat not only a lot of junk food but also large portions and just binge even when i wasn't hungry. **Food was like a drug for me**...

Withdrawal period?

What these kids say suggests that in order to break their dependence on certain foods, they must go through a 'withdrawal' period of bad cravings, antsiness, irritability, even depression - similar to coming off tobacco, alcohol, or a drug. Withdrawal is what happens when a substance or behavior, which eases pain, is suddenly stopped. It is the brain's way of reacting to the jolt. The emotional discomfort of withdrawal may be worse than the emotional pain that started the addictive behavior in the first place. This is perhaps why many kids quickly give up on weight loss and start overeating again. Gastric bypass/banding probably accomplishes 'enforced withdrawal' during that period.

Fortunately, kids say that this withdrawal discomfort seems to get a lot better within 10-14 days (see Success Stories, Chapter 14), again an experience similar to coming off tobacco, alcohol, or a drug.

From randi, Age 15 - 8/17/07 -
Ht. 5'10", Start: 211 lb, Current: 209 lb, Goal: 150 lb
- **if u can have enough self control and stay off the sugar for two weeks you stop craving sugar completly** and some sugar free sweets that you might not have liked before taste really good

It's unclear whether stopping displacement activity eating (stress eating, binge eating) results in these withdrawal-type symptoms. Antsiness certainly occurs when trying to stop stress eating, similar to trying to stop nail biting, but the antsiness may not improve in 10-14 days, as it seems to do when kids stop comfort eating.

Vicious Cycles

Once kids become hooked on using food to cope with their lives, they frequently become caught in vicious cycles, as described in Chapter 13, where they eat more and more to numb the shame, stress, and depression of being overweight in itself. In addition, the more they engage in the addictive-type behavior, the worse the withdrawal cravings when trying to give it up, which tends to keep them hooked, again like a vicious cycle. Even worse, they lose none-food coping skills, which makes it even harder to give up the addictive-type behavior. Plus, the more they fail at attempting to get through withdrawal, the worse the pain and need for the addictive numbing of food, as described below:

From Carissa, Age 16 - 08/01/09
Ht. 5'5", Start: 260 lb, Current: 254 lb, Goal: 140 lb - ... have struggled with my weight ever since I was about 5 yrs old... In fifth grade my mom took me to weight watchers with her... **I failed.** After that My weight kept balloning... **I felt lyk a failure which caused me to gain more weight.**

What is it that kids actually are hooked on?

Although the kids' postings imply an addictive quality (i.e. psychological dependence) to their overeating, this may be an entirely new form of psychological dependence, very different from chemical dependence (drugs, alcohol, and tobacco). It appears to be the action of eating (biting, chewing, swallowing) and the immediate sensations of food in the mouth (taste, texture) that these kids are hooked on (see post below), rather than a central chemical response, as with a drug. Also, bulimic kids, who vomit up the food they eat, still get comfort or stress relief from overeating and continue the behavior.

Reply from Jennifer, Age 16 - 07/28/09
.. drinking much water helps to feel full, but **i miss the taste... of food... could it be that I'm addicted to food?** It's hard NOT to eat...

From Jessica, Age 13 - 06/24/08
Ht. 5'3", Start: 362 lb, Current: 384 lb, Goal: 120 lb - ...I just love to eat. ... **I know it's bad for my health, but I don't even care.** Ever since my dad left things have been down hill, but **eating fixes that if just for a little while**... I always eat until i feel like I'm about to pop, and even then I don't stop because **it tastes so good** and **feels good** too

Displacement activity, eating to relieve stress (see Chapter 10), seems to be a significant component of overeating in kids' postings on the boards, possibly as significant as emotional numbing by the pleasure of food (comfort eating). Does displacement activity eating, binge eating for example, have an addictive quality? It certainly causes severe problems in kids' lives and can make them feel 'out of control.' However, unlike comfort eating and other addictive behaviors, displacement activity eating just gets rid of nervous energy or distracts from life, but does not numb pain, as addictive behaviors generally do. Nevertheless, certain addictive behaviors (e.g. gambling, shopping. sex) may include significant displacement activity and stress relief.

Note: Kids don't get hooked on just any food. They don't get hooked on broccoli or dry toast. They get hooked on high pleasure, high action foods. 'Junk foods' seem to be the most problematic foods, according to the kids who post on our site.

Where did satiety go?

Pleasure, comfort, and stress relief from certain foods seems to override the fullness or 'satisfied' feeling, which normally stops kids from overeating. Many overweight kids say they eat until they feel "stuffed," which is uncomfortable, so then they finally stop. Stomach stapling surgery and stomach banding cause weight loss because the stomach is made much smaller. As a result, the uncomfortable, 'stuffed' feeling occurs after only small amounts of food are consumed, which causes the person to stop eating much earlier. Some kids, however, say they like feeling stuffed, as explained below:

From Aaron, Age 13 - 09/10/01
Hi. I have a tendency to eat whole lot! I eat all kinds of junk food and overeat at regular meals. I notice when I'm full, but I just keep eating and eating. I know this is not healthy, and I really should stop, but **it is just such a good felling to be stuffed to your gill**...

Might this possibly be a feeling of relief that (for a brief time) the child is not compelled to eat?

Has food become so pleasurable that kids hardly recognize the satisfied feeling anymore? If so, kids need to consciously think about what amount of food their bodies need and stop when they have eaten that amount. Putting just the needed amount of food on their plates is also a good idea.

Boredom Eating

Overeating from boredom appears to be a major problem for overweight kids, as described in the many postings and chatroom conversations in Chapter 11. However, when kids say that they are "bored", they actually may be depressed, anxious, or stressed. Many posts mention being 'bored' in the same sentence with being 'sad' or 'depressed,' as described below. Being bored is more socially acceptable than being depressed.

From Madi, Age 17 - 04/27/09
Ht. 5'6", Start: 286 lb, Current: 286 lb, Goal: 180 lb -... I don't know what to do anymore... Im extremly over weight and I was just diagnosed with type 2 Diabetes... **I have a eating problem and go to food when im sad or bored or stressed.** Im so lost and dont know what to do.

Boredom eating may be due to a lack of distractions that numb or avoid emotional discomfort. Pleasurable food and eating is an effective numbing distraction. Boredom has also been defined as a feeling of powerlessness. Because of this kids may detach from life. As noted in Chapter 13, a boredom vicious cycle may result. The cure for boredom eating thus seems to be for kids to take action, to take on their problems and fears head on. It may help for kids to write down their problems and fears in a notebook with a plan (see pp. 287).

Pacifier effect

We've all seen screaming infants calmed by inserting a rubber pacifier in their mouths. The sucking activity soothes the infant, without their tasting or swallowing anything. Kids probably never completely outgrow the pacifier effect, as illustrated by sucking on a lollipop, a straw, or a popsicle. Could overeating by kids to relieve stress and unhappiness be partly due to the persisting pacifier effect? If so, non-calorie pacifiers, like carrots or celery, and distracting activities like hobbies and sports may help.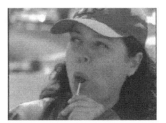

When does it start?

When does getting hooked on the pleasure of food or displacement activity of eating seem to start? Does it start with the baby getting a bottle every time she cries or M&M's every time he throws a toddler fit? The rate of obesity in infants and toddlers is rising faster than in any other age group. Someone else is feeding them. Infants whose parents frequently soothe them with food have higher rates of obesity as children [Agras 2004]. Parents should find ways to soothe their infants other than food, especially if the infant is not due to be fed, for example rocking the infant or using a teddy bear that emits the sound of a mother's heartbeat.

Denial

Kids may not accept that they are psychologically hooked on eating and the pleasure of food. They may be unable to identify emotions or connect them with eating. They may say, "I don't use food to cope with life, I just love to eat." Yet they are unable to stop. They continue to overeat, knowing that being overweight harms their social life and their health. At the same time they may ask for help with weight loss. What is likely occurring here is that they are psychologically hooked on certain foods (e.g. junk food), but it is unconscious. Or, they may simply be in denial. The below story illustrates this, as the teen asks for help:

This is DANIELLE's story:
Hi lucy, its me Danielle, Im a **13 year old** girl(about to be 14 july 27) and **i weigh 190 pounds**... it seems as if im getting bigger at the momment. i do eat alot, **i dont eat it out of depression or anything but i eat beacuaes the food is there and its good**, i **need some help**... i wanna weigh 150 at the most, so i can look great for school, so **please help me so i can be healthy**. Thank You!

Why now?

If kids truly are hooked on the comfort and stress relief of certain foods, comparable to an addiction, and they become overweight and obese because of this, why is this happening now? Pleasurable food has long existed. Why is the childhood obesity epidemic occurring today?

A Perfect Storm

Several extraordinary factors, which alone would not produce the childhood obesity epidemic, appear to have come together at the same time to produce the epidemic, in the same manner as unusual weather conditions occurring together produce a 'Perfect Storm.'

There appear to be five key factors contributing to the childhood obesity epidemic: 1) high technology junk food and fast food production; 2) junk food and fast food availability to kids; 3) increased stress in kids; 4) comfort food science and marketing; and 5) kids are less active.

1) Industrialization of junk food and fast food

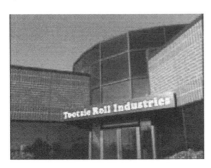

The History Channel "Modern Marvels" TV series has released several impressive documentaries on the technology of high pleasure food production in the U.S., most notably, "Snack Food Tech" and "Fast Food Tech," which are available on DVD. The level of technology and industrial production of snack food and fast food is mind-boggling: "Fryers that cook thousands of pounds of sizzling potato chips an hour, machines that wrap candy faster than the eye can see, plants that chill millions of gallons of ice cream a year." Industrialized mass-production has brought high pleasure food to an unprecedented level: "The output of the Chicago Tootsie Roll factory (above left) is staggering – they make 83 million Tootsie Rolls a day, 16 million Mason dots, and about 20 million lollipops!!!" [Snack Food Tech 2007]. Cheap, high pleasure food is now available to everyone, including kids.

2) Junk food and fast food availability to kids

Junk food

Many schools in the U.S. are attempting to rid themselves of soda and junk food in their cafeterias and vending machines. Nevertheless, kids still have major exposure and ready access to junk food outside of school. The photo on the following page is an inside shot of one of the large U.S. drug chain stores. As one enters the store, he/she is immediately confronted with center isle shelves full of candy. The store is open 24/7. The shelves extend down to floor level, so that even a toddler walking by with a parent could easily grab a candy item.

Convenience stores, such as 7-Eleven, are also a 24/7 source of junk food for kids, as well as many supermarkets. And of course vending machines are everywhere.

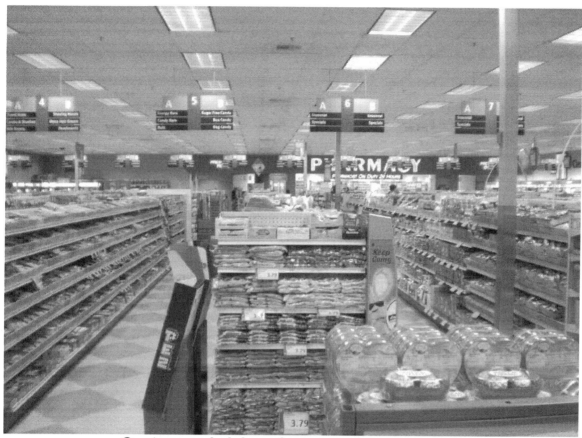

Center candy isles of a large pharmacy chain store

Fast food

Below is a graph of the number of fast food restaurants in the U.S. from 1980 to 2000. On the following page a second graph depicts the percentage of obese kids over the same time period. Do the two graphs seem to be increasing at the same rate? Could there be a connection between the number of fast food restaurants and the number of obese kids?

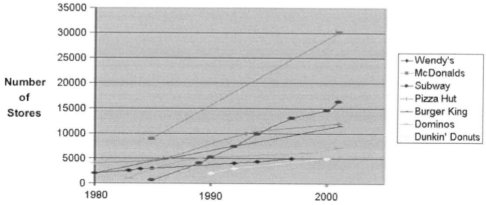

Number of fast food restaurants in the U.S. from 1980 to 2000
(Source: adapted from an image on www.stillwell.com)

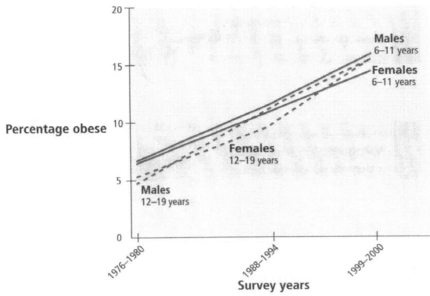

Percentage of obese kids in the U.S. from 1980 to 2000
(Source: U.S. Center for Disease Control and Prevention)

3) Increased stress in kids and using food to cope

As presented in Chapter 10, kids on our site give the impression that they are under more stress today than kids in past times, and in a poll 80% of kids responding say that their stress has increased over the past three years (see pp. 170). They say they use food to cope with this stress. This appears to be 'displacement activity,' similar to nail biting and hangnail picking. Even though kids hate wrecked fingernails and painful, bleeding hangnails, many are unable to stop those behaviors as a way to relieve stress. In the same manner, kids hate being fat yet are unable to stop overeating as a way to cope with stress.

Furthermore, kids become caught in a vicious cycle of overeating to cope with stress, feeling disappointed in themselves resulting in increased stress, more overeating to cope, more weight gain, more stress, and so on. Binge eating appears to be a reaction to sudden severe stress, resulting in a displacement activity of frenzied overeating. Kids on our site frequently report that their eating habits are tied to stressed out parents in their lives. Probably not noticed by the kids is the fact that being a parent is stressful.

In October 2007 the American Psychological Association conducted a study on Stress in America. Forty eight percent of 1848 adults surveyed felt that their stress had increased over the previous five years; 43% overate when under stress. The majority of foods eaten when under stress were high pleasure foods, 'junk food' [Stress In America 2007].

4) Comfort food science and marketing

Comfort food science

Needless to say, food companies would love to get kids hooked on their products, and food companies appear to have developed comfort food to a science. On a recent airplane flight I was given a 'snack,' a small package of assorted chips. WOW!! The flavor and taste were so powerful that it made it very difficult to save the remainder, so that I could later take the photo at right.

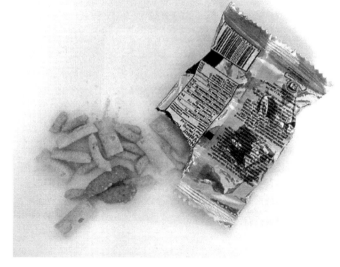

The Modern Marvels TV documentary, "Snack Food Tech", describes how a corn chip manufacturer applies the flavoring as a thin layer to only one side of the chip: "The goal is to have a flavor that peaks quickly in the mouth and quickly fades, forcing the consumer to eat more and more" [Snack Food Tech 2007]. The posts below attest to the success of chip manufacturers' strategies to get kids hooked on their products.

From Jayni, Age 11 - 10/09/08 -
Ht. 4'6", WT: 148 lb - Over the summer vacation i have .. become obese. .. **I just can't stop myself stuffing my face with chips...**

From DancingDamsel, Age 13 - 01/30/09
Ht. 5'2", Start: 175 lb, Current: 175 lb, Goal: 130 lb - Okay, so today I did kinda badly...**I went over-board with the chips.**

From Emily, Age 13 - 06/27/08
Ht. 5'5", Start: 130 lb, Current: 154 lb, Goal: 105 lb - **ugh! i ate an entire bag of chips today!**

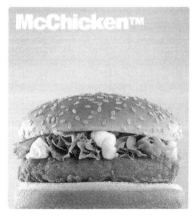

The same appears true for fast food. I recently ate a McDonald's McChicken™ sandwich (left). For several days afterwards I kept remembering its grabbing flavor, which far surpassed that of the last fast food I had eaten several years earlier. It certainly was comfort food, as the highly pleasurable taste made me forget all my troubles for the time it took to eat it.

Kids say that "food today tastes so good," that it's very hard to resist, as described in the post on the following page.

280

Age 14, female, Ht:5*8 ,Wt:140 lbs - it's just to hard to watch what you eat since the food today tastes so good. well that;s my opion

High fructose corn syrup *is a new cheaper, easier to use sugar, which currently is being added to thousands of foods. It's now in soft drinks, candy, ice cream, bread, crackers, salad dressing, jelly, pickles, soup, applesauce, juices, even baby food and some types of baby formula. High fructose corn syrup is probably no unhealthier than table sugar, but it's significantly cheaper to produce and use. It's likely that the many-fold increase in food's total sugar content is contributing to obesity. The sweetness of sugar is very pleasurable and comforting, so people eat more of sweetened foods. Is the food industry trying to sweeten as many foods as possible, so people will buy more of them... and get hooked on them? Are food companies selling pleasure rather than nutrition? Industrial mass production now makes such pleasure affordable and available to everyone, most notably kids. But such pleasure might be addicting and may result in obesity at an early age.*

From sabina, Age 16 - 10/28/06
Ht. 5'6, Wt. 157 - …. i have the worst **addiction** to strawberry icecream. **God i hate that junk food tastes good!!!**

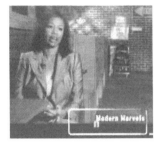

Food companies are very aware that the pleasure of food is comforting. In the Modern Marvels 'Fast Food Tech' TV documentary (left) a fast food magazine editor said, **"It's about taste… part of the reason for the success of fast food is the 'comfort food' level of it."** *[Fast Food Tech 2007].*
[To see video, click on image at left or below link]:
(http://www.blubberbuster.com/school/comfort-food.html)

In other words, food companies are aware that food is comforting when it tastes really good.

Comfort food marketing

Food companies conduct market research on the emotional needs of consumers and advertise with emotional slogans, such as "Help yourself to happiness" (Golden Corral restaurants) and "Pop Tarts: MADE for FUN" (Kellogg Company).

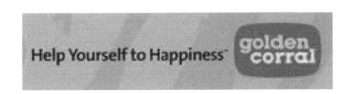

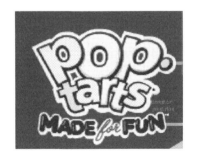

McDonald's Chicken McNuggets are marketed as "Little nuggets of joy."

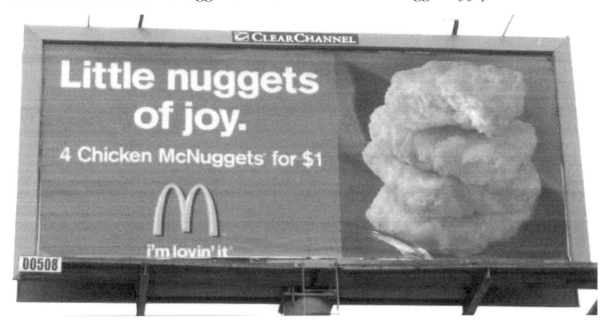

The slogan of MilkyWay is: "Comfort in Every Bar." - www.youtube.com/watch?v=KuoSc67vksc

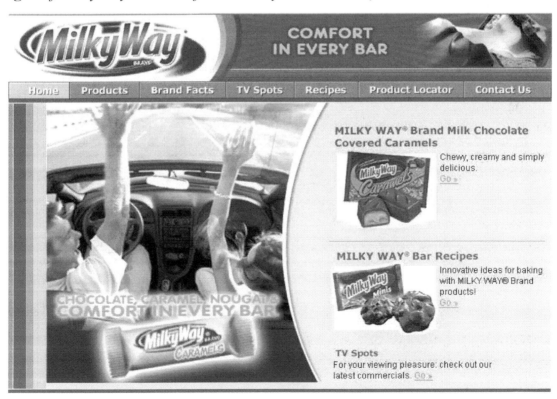

(Source: www.milkywaybar.com, 11/16/2007)

Even 12 year olds understand the power of comfort food:

Age 12, female, 5' 1'', 108 lbs - **Junk food=comfort food. food listens to our problems. its like a therapist**

McDonald's has the "Happy Meal" and "PlayPlaces" for kids. According to the History Channel Modern Marvels TV Series, McDonald's is one of the largest toy distributors in the world.

McDonald's Big Mac was 40 years old in 2008, with the ad, "CURING MAC ATTACKS FOR 40 YEARS." But who, or what, causes Mac Attacks?

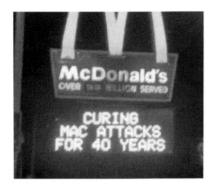 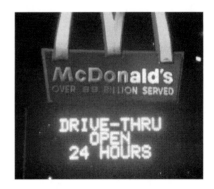

Fast food places may be described as, "Drive through pain treatment." Fast food drive-through windows are now open 24 hours a day, just like an ER.

McDonald's advertises relief to stressed consumers:

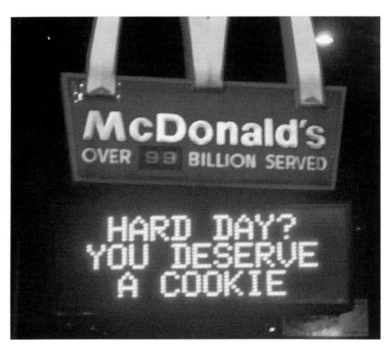

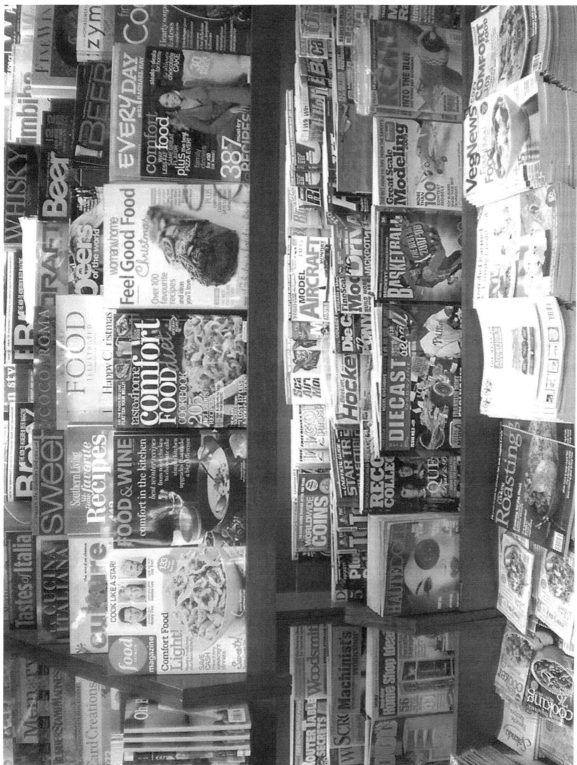

The number of magazines in the cooking section of a Barnes & Noble book store in Feb. 2009 with the words "Comfort Food" or "Feel Good Food" on the front cover is rather striking (there are seven visible here).

5) Kids are less active

Kids today are definitely less active than in the past. There is less outside play, less PE (physical education) at school, and more video games. Physical activity does burn calories, but more importantly, physical activity releases natural chemicals in the body called endorphins, which produce feelings of well being.

Fun activities, especially non-competitive sports, games, and activities with other kids, improve mood and self-esteem and distract from eating for comfort and boredom. Exercise also is a form of displacement activity, relieves stress, and helps to avoid stress eating.

Are food companies 'feeding' psychological food dependence?

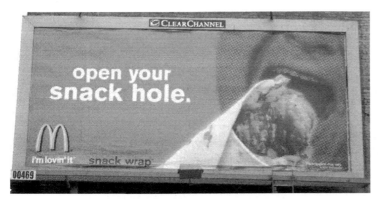

The childhood (as well as the adult?) obesity epidemic may be due to a perfect storm of cheap, highly available comfort food combined with significantly increased stress in kids. Kids describe using the pleasure of food and the displacement activity of eating as coping mechanisms. Food companies are aware of this, design products accordingly, and market to this ('comfort in every bar'). Are food companies fostering and capitalizing on psychological food dependence? According to CNBC's TV documentary, "Big Mac, Inside the McDonald's Empire," McDonald's new Snack Wrap was developed in response to the "grazing" behavior of consumers. Grazing is now thought to be a form of binge eating [Williamson 2008]. McDonald's has the above ad for the snack wrap.

Pillsbury advertises to mothers: "Kids are hungry after school... Totinos Pizza Rolls... Kids can't resist their delicious pizza flavor... It's how kids help themselves." The ads show that kids can easily prepare the food themselves. Arriving home from school is when kids say they overeat the most (poll results, pp. 163), as they're stressed from the day. Many are also alone at that time.
(http://www.blubberbuster.com/cgi/poll_new_86.cgi)

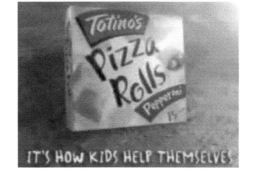

How then do kids lose weight?

If the childhood obesity epidemic is occurring today because of a perfect storm of widely available, high pleasure foods combined with stressed out, depressed kids, who are hooked on the comfort and displacement activity of eating, how then do these kids become unhooked and lose weight?

Withdrawal period

As discussed earlier in this chapter, it appears that successful kids go through a period of withdrawal - extreme cravings, feeling antsy, feeling stressed, even depressed – when they cut down or stop the foods they are hooked on. Plain willpower is rarely enough to get them through withdrawal. The kids need lots and lots of support and distracting fun activities. Kids say in their posts that the discomfort of withdrawal usually gets a lot better within a week or two (see Success Stories, Chapter 14).

It may be that morbidly (severely) obese kids can make it through withdrawal only by gastric bypass surgery or by live-in weight loss centers, such as weight loss camps or boarding schools, where access to food is strictly controlled. Camps and live-in weight loss centers, although expensive, seem a far better solution for kids than gastric bypass, which has lifelong side effects, as well as a small risk of death. However, even if kids can get through withdrawal cravings, once they leave camp or the center, they must then cope with life without seeking comfort or stress relief from food. They may thus still experience unbearable cravings after the withdrawal period, particularly if their food dependence is in part displacement activity (stress eating). At the live-in Insula weight loss center for youth in Berchtesgaden, Germany, I talked with a teen who was about to return home after losing nearly 80 lb. He confided that he greatly feared being unable to handle the temptations of fast food and junk food, once he returned to the uncontrolled environment of his home and school.

Below are strategies and techniques that successful kids have used to make it through the discomfort of withdrawal and become unhooked from their problem foods:

1) They first develop motivation

The kids focus on why they want to lose weight (see Chapter 7). So they won't be teased? So they can attract the opposite sex? So they won't get diseases? So they can move faster in sports? So they can wear clothing in style? They post their reasons on the board. Which is more important: the reasons that they want to lose weight... or being entertained and comforted by food? Also, they post their weight goal and other goals (make the baseball team, etc.).

2) They make a plan

They post their plan:
a) What foods will they cut down or cut out? Junk food, fast food? Portion sizes, second helpings? For example, they could cut everything they usually eat in half and save half for later.
b) What supportive, distracting things will they do when they go through withdrawal, such as take a walk with their dog or a friend, ride their bike, work on a hobby, shoot basketball, go dancing, take a course, decorate their room, or call a friend?
c) How else will they deal with cravings? Having sweet apples, frozen grapes, or baby carrots in the fridge or flavored ice water helps. A little bit of pleasure in their food can also help manage cravings (as noted on pp. 245). Squeezing their hands really tight together helps with cravings or antsy feelings.
d) Their start date.
e) Getting through withdrawal is looked at like a job - a job that they get paid for later.

From anne, Age 16 - 8/22/03
- i read the blubberbuster advice for cravings and it said to **hold your hands together**. i was like yeah right! that is not going to work for me! but last night i watched my boyfriend eat a reeses sunday and i didn't have a single bite. as simple as it sounds- **it works**, hey- if you don't have your hands free then you won't grab and eat stuff.

3) They arrange support persons

Before starting, the child or teen arranges support from a health professional - a doctor, school counselor or nurse - and from friends and family. He/she tells these people about the plan to lose weight, and that he/she needs their support in order to make it through withdrawal. He/she informs them of the start date. They agree to be available by phone or email. This requirement for support persons may be a problem, given the disconnect between many overweight kids and their caregivers (parents, doctors) as revealed in Chapters 5 and 6.

From PRESHUS - 01/28/06
.. I was at my highest wieght of 190 pounds... I lost 15 pouds.. **FIND supportERS TO HELP ENCOURAGE NOT DISCOURAGE YOU...**

4) They eliminate, hide, and stay away from 'hookable' foods

Most of us cannot resist the temptation of having comforting, stress-relieving foods in front of us. So... these kids try to not put these foods where they can see them. They empty the house of junk food. They stock the house with fruits and veggies for snacks. They stay away from fast food restaurants. They go shopping with their parents and buy low-fat, sugar-free foods for comfort and healthy foods like fruits for snacks. They have fun with it... smoothies anyone?

The kids get out of the house. But they don't put themselves in front of a bakery or a Burger King or Wendy's. They go for a walk with the family dog or a friend. They go for a bike ride, or rollerblade, or go on a hike, or visit a museum, or the library, or volunteer at the local animal shelter by caring for lonely pets.

5) They learn ways to cope with life without using food

Even before symptoms of withdrawal fully ease, the real work begins. The kids learn to cope with life - unpleasant feelings, loneliness, stress, and boredom - by substituting other things for the numbing pleasure and comfort of food. Many overweight and obese kids have never learned to cope with life's pains, without seeking comfort and stress relief from food, or they have long ago lost those coping skills. Successful kids find soothing and stress relieving activities, such as non-competitive sports, pets, hobbies, books, musical instruments, volunteer work, counseling - anything they enjoy besides food. Relaxation and deep breathing exercises, like yoga, help relieve stress. They look at life as a 'glorious adventure' and they remember that 'life is too important to be taken seriously.' They write down their problems, 1,2,3, with a plan for each problem, as shown below:

My Problems

#1. My mom always comments about my weight and what I eat. She's pretty and thin.

Plan:
- write a letter to my mom about how I feel and tell her that when she does this, it stresses me out and makes me overeat more.
- find someone (maybe my minister?) to help me deal with my mom.

#2. I hate doing my homework. I eat when I do it cuz I'm stressed. I don't understand math.

Plan:
- do my homework as soon as I get home from school and take a walk when I'm stressed.
- don't watch TV while doing my homework
- get a tutor in math
- do my homework with a friend who can help.

They make a sign like the one below and put in on their wall. And then they do it!

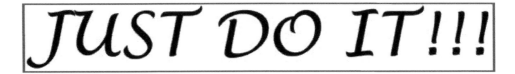

Gradual method that kids use to lose weight (removing the culprit one by one)

Stopping 'cold turkey' all hooked-on foods at once is quite hard. The resulting withdrawal discomfort may be too much to bear. A 'divide and conquer' approach is more achievable.

Here's a method that some kids use for getting unhooked from problem foods, one at a time, make it through withdrawal for each one, and thereby lose weight:

1) Kids pick one food that they have a problem with, like candy, soda, or french fries.
2) They stop eating that one food completely. They stay away from it, if possible.
3) They go through withdrawal for that one food. They expect to feel extreme cravings, antsy, maybe even stressed or depressed.
4) They realize that the withdrawal discomfort will mostly go away in a week or two.
5) They then pick a second food that they are hooked on and stop it completely.
6) They go through withdrawal for that food.
7) They do this for as many foods as they are hooked on.
8) Large portion sizes is also something they stop, but again, they must go through the withdrawal feelings for a couple of weeks.
9) They are careful not to substitute a new high pleasure food for the foods from which they become unhooked.
10) Removing high pleasure additives from food is also a way kids get unhooked, such as breads without added sugar, or low fat milk instead of chocolate milk. Mixing chocolate and low fat milk or regular and low fat milk together is a way to gradually change.

We asked kids in a poll (http://www.blubberbuster.com/cgi/poll_new_87.cgi) about their use of the above method. (Results on following page).

What about losing weight by cutting out just the foods you have the most problem with?

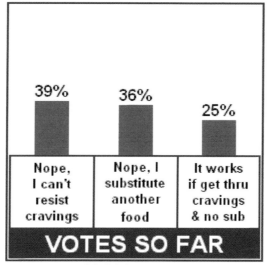

69 kids voted

Of the 69 kids responding, most say that the method doesn't work, because they are not able to resist cravings or because they just substitute another problem food for the problem food they are able to stop. But one fourth of the kids indicate that the method does work, if they can get through the cravings and don't substitute another food. Below are some comments:

The gradual method works

Age 16, female, 5'6, 225 lbs - **this is good** - I mainly have a problem with pastery stuff.

Age 19, female, 5'5", 170 lbs - **I have been in this situation before and I know that it works. The hard part is getting through the cravings.** Unfortunately over the past few years I "relapsed" so to speak and now have to repeat the process. - I don't have a problem with mainly one food.

Age 10, female, 4'7, 89 lbs - **Yes it does work** when you think about the HUGE downside. Medical problems, health issues and so many more and some of it can be stopped by not eating that food. - I mainly have a problem with Chocolate cravings.

Age 14, female, 5'5, 140 lbs - **I really think this would work** because if people push themselfs to do it they could get over there bad habit of eating junk food and move on a good habit to eating healthy food. - I mainly have a problem with pizza.

The gradual method doesn't work

Age 15, female, 5'5, 144 lbs **- this is ridiculous** - I mainly have a problem with anything salty.

Age 12, female, 5"2", 329 lbs **- I just end up quitting cos I cannot resist my cravings of chips and cake.** - I mainly have a problem with chips and cake.

Age 15, female, 5"4', 165 lbs **- When I crave Chocolate or Pepsi, I don't think "Hey..I'll just go drink water or eat a salad"..my mind unconciously thinks..."Okay, find something else that's equally good."--Might work for some people, but not for all. I went off Candy and Soda for an entire year, and to resist it was easy...I just thought "Ew..that looks gross", and it worked...But that's also the year I gained all my weight, because I substituted other foods for candy and soda...Sometimes it just doesn't work.** - I mainly have a problem with Chocolate and Pepsi.

In this same poll we asked the kids if there is mainly one food that they consider a problem. Most said yes.

Do you have a problem with mainly one food?

YES: 43 votes (62%)

NO: 26 votes (38%)

69 kids voted

We further asked the kids to list their one main problem food. Their most common one main problem foods were chocolate, candy, chips, and fast food.

Critics of the gradual substance avoidance approach described on pp. 288, claim that "food is necessary for life... and is not a substance from which children can simply abstain." [Pretlow, R. 2008]. Nonetheless, are chocolate, candy, chips, and fast food necessary for life? Jamie Jeffrey, MD, Director, HealthyKids Weight Management Program says: "No!! Weaning from a patient's particular 'addiction' with replacement of healthy foods and/or healthy habits is what it's all about... the fact that 'food' is so readily available makes treatment, and especially maintenance, even harder."[Jeffrey, J., 2008]

If kids can get unhooked from just a few foods, with which they have the most problems, this may result in significant weight loss. Unfortunately, they may need to stay away from their problem foods essentially forever, or they will relapse, as the post below describes:

From Emily, Age 11 - 06/24/09
Ht. 4'10", Start: 149 lb, Current: 149 lb, Goal: 110 lb - ...I am trying to loose

weight, but what happens when you have one of those school valentine parties, or christmas parties? **I want to eat all the sweets, and junk food, but then I can't stop the next day, and the next day, and the next day! I just completely get thrown out of wack and gane EVERYTHING back!**

Staying away from problem foods forever may seem extreme and unreasonable. Yet, as a comparison, if a child were allergic to a particular food, they would need to avoid that food forever, in order to protect their health. Is avoiding foods, which cause them to be overweight or obese, any different? Protecting their health has the same priority. Even small amounts of problem foods may put the child right back into food dependence mode once more.

Most importantly, successful kids do not substitute other problem foods in place of the foods they are able to stop. The idea is to get through withdrawal and at the same time substitute non-food items or activities for the comfort or stress relief that the problem foods gives to the child or teen. The first step is that kids become AWARE that they are using food to relieve stress or to comfort bad feelings. The next step is that they experiment in the moment with different tools to keep from eating or from eating as much, such as getting out of the house, turning on music and dancing, or calling a friend for support.

From Laura, Age 19 - 4/25/06 -
Ht. 5'6, Wt. 125 - I was once overweight and know exactly how it feels to be the fat person. **I know what it feels like to be emotionally addicted to food; but now food only means something nutritional that I need to put in my body.** I want to give you all the best of luck in making your lives healthier. You have to start somewhere...although it isn't easy... it is worth it in the end. I promise!

*The above described withdrawal method applies mainly to **comfort eating, which has an addictive quality.** It may not apply to displacement activity eating (stress eating, binge eating). Stress eating may respond better to stress management techniques (deep breathing, squeezing one's hands together, fun activities), although successful kids find that avoidance of stress foods does seem to help.*

Withdrawal cycling

All too often kids move back and forth between trying to lose weight and the discomfort of withdrawal, then giving up and going back to overeating again, then back to trying to lose weight and withdrawal again, as the below post illustrates. Because they never get completely through withdrawal, they pretty much have bad cravings and antsy feelings continually, which is agonizing.

From Amanda, Age 19 - 10/08/08
Ht. 5'8", Start: 225 lb, Current: 173 lb, Goal: 150 lb - okay so i pretty much **let**

myself go for like, 2 weeks. big mistake, i went from like 167 to 173. so i gained like 6 pounds... my main concern right now is to get back to where i was a couple weeks ago (between 166-168). i know i can do it. i just really have to stick to my guns this time. i want to be 165 by christmas (i weighed 185 last christmas so i want there to be 20 pounds difference) i think i can do it. anyways good luck everyone. **resist temptation beause once u give in once, ur bound to keep on going (like i did).** byee!

Knowledge about healthy eating is not enough

If a psychological dependence on certain foods is what's causing kids to be overweight and obese, then simply teaching kids about healthy eating is not enough. Most kids responding to a poll on our site say that they are overdosed on healthy eating information (see pp. 5), which they have been taught in school. Instead, they need information on the emotional reasons they overeat and how to resist cravings.

Here are more of those kids' comments about healthy eating information:

Age 14, female, 5 foot 5, 199 lbs - **The info is useless.**

Age 15, male, 5'10", 284 lbs - **I know what foods are healthy. I just actually WANT the things that aren't healthy, cravings are much more of a problem in my eyes.**

Age 15, male, 5 11, 192 lbs - **I usually do the exact opposite of the pyramids message.**

From sara, Age 13 - 06/04/06
Ht. 5'7, Wt. 175 - **i know alot about food and nutrion i just keep binging though ugggggggggggg......;/**

Age 15, female, 5,6, 230 lbs - **this paper is crap it doesnt help anything to lose wieght all you have to do is have will power and cut down your eating alone you dont have to eat healthier or anything you just have to cut down ur meals and exercise**

Age 14, female, 5'4, 150 lbs - **no one really talks to me about healthy eating and when they do they just say don't eat that eat this and this is usually something completely disgustig**

Furthermore, even complete awareness by kids that they are eating emotionally or that their overeating is like an addiction is not enough, as illustrated below:

From Ray Ray or Rach, Age 12 - 11/19/03
Ht: 5'6", Wt: 227 lb. - I really need help! I do really good on my diet at school usually...
but **when I get home I can't stop eating!** I've tried to just not start eating until dinner
becuase once I start I can't stop but that never works and I end up eating anyway and
I've tried like just eating a little bit of something but **for me food is addictive so I jsut
keep eating more of it.** Please help me!

 *Ray*Ray* 14 in 8!!!
I do have emtional eating problems...any suggestions on what to do for that? I'll
try the goal thing - thanks.

*The above 14 year old has apparently been aware of her emotional eating for at least three
years, which she describes as addictive (see also her below reply at age 11 to another child).*

Reply from Ray Ray, Age 11 - 11/11/02
r u really starving or just bored or sad or mad
sumtimes people eat because they r one of the things above

*Yet even with that knowledge, three years later at age 14 (above) she has been unable to stop
her emotional eating.*

*Another teen expresses her frustration in the post below, and a teen has an epiphany in the
post below that:*

From ann, Age 17 - 11/02/04
does any 1 else notice how desperate we r to find out how to lose weight and **ask how and
then dnt follow it. we all no how to lose weight.** anywayz bye

From Ellie, Age 13 - 05/10/09 -
Ht. 5'5", Start: 163 lb, Current: 142 lb, Goal: 125 lb - You know what I figured out?
It might sound stupid, but **it's the closest i've ever come to an epiphany.** Ok, here it is;
I was thinking to myself, wow, i'm really fat. I can't even fit into the shorts I just got.
That's really actually very depressing. Then, I had the sudden urge to go get a fudgsicle,
even though we had just had lunch 10 minutes ago and I was really full. Right after I
thought that, it hit me. I wasn't hungry. **That was my epiphany. Eating isn't supposed to
be meant the way that overweight and obese people use it. It's not some kind of
coping mechanism, it's a way of keeping your body ALIVE.** Not your solution to
boredom or like me, being fat. So, I've been thinking lately before I pick up a piece
of food, Am I hungry? Do I really need this, or am I just bored or upset? It usually
works :) Like I said, might sound crazy but It's working for me. **BTW can you please
help me with this?**

Ellie in the post on the previous page has realized that she uses food to cope, but she still asks for help with this.

Even when kids are aware that they eat emotionally and use food for comfort, the previous posts show that it is difficult to stop with that knowledge and sheer willpower alone. Successful kids say that they distract themselves with fun activities, ideally with other kids, like non-competitive sports, cheerleading, volunteer work, hobbies, books, or learning to play a musical instrument.

Keeping a food-feeling diary also helps. Kids write down everything they eat and what they feel before, during, and after they eat it. This helps them see what foods they overeat and whether they are using food to cope with emotions, as illustrated by our online food/emotion diary below:

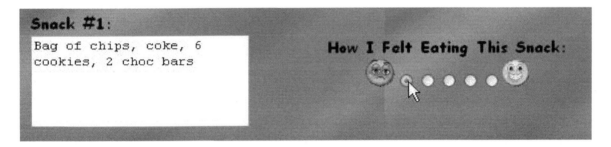

Tolerance

Many kids say that they eat progressively more as they become more overweight, as noted in the posts and poll in Chapter 9. Chapter 9 further describes 'tolerance' as where an individual must use more and more of a substance or behavior to obtain the same pleasurable effect, which is a characteristic of addictive-type behaviors. If the childhood obesity epidemic is indeed due to psychological dependence on at least certain types of food (addiction?), then tolerance might be a factor that is worsening the epidemic and contributing to development of severe and morbid obesity in some kids. Severe and morbid obesity in children and adolescents has tripled in the past 25 years [Skelton et al. 2009]. The comment below from a 14 year old girl speaks powerfully to this tolerance idea:

> Age 14, female, 5' 2", 201 lbs - **It's like a drug. What used to satisfy you before now has no effect. I feel like i've become immune to the foods that used to comfort me. And like drugs you keep moving on to bigger, worse things in order to get the same feeling as when you started out.**

If kids need more and more food to achieve the same comfort effect, this would certainly worsen the childhood obesity epidemic.

Public Policy

If psychological food dependence (addiction?) is in reality a major cause of the obesity epidemic in children and teens, what might be done about this on a public basis, in view of what kids say? Here are some possibilities:

1) Evaluate limiting exposure and access by kids to junk food and fast food

This involves removal of junk food from schools, taxing junk food and fast food, eliminating government subsidies to industries that produce ingredients commonly used in junk food products, such as high fructose corn syrup, and restricting marketing to kids. But would this actually help? On the one hand, motivated kids say that banning junk food would help them to control their weight (out of sight out of mind – see below comments from kids). And limiting exposure and access by kids might possibly help prevent them from getting hooked at the outset. On the other hand, kids who do not want to avoid such foods will still find a way to obtain them (i.e. a black market – see below poll). And parents would still bring junk food home and take kids to fast food outlets. Furthermore, limiting soda availability in schools has not been found to influence student soda consumption [Blum et al, 2008]. We asked kids what they thought about removal of junk food from school (http://www.blubberbuster.com/cgi/poll_new_55.cgi):

Would removal of junk food from your school help kids be a healthy weight?

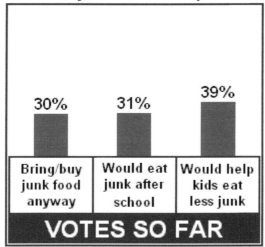

124 kids voted

Less than half of the 124 kids voting feel that removal of junk food from their school would help kids be a healthy weight. More than half feel that kids would either bring junk food to school or obtain it after school.

> **Has your school removed vending machine or cafeteria junk food?**
>
> **YES:** 33 votes (27%)
>
> **NO:** 91 votes (73%)
>
> **Are kids selling junk food in your school?**
>
> **YES:** 48 votes (39%)
>
> **NO:** 76 votes (61%)

Slightly more than a fourth of the kids' schools have removed junk food, but nearly 40% of kids voting say that kids are selling junk food in their schools.

Here's what kids say about limiting their exposure to junk food (http://www.blubberbuster.com/poll/comments_72.htm and http://www.blubberbuster.com/poll/comments_62.htm):

Age 13, female, 5'1, 128 lbs - **If we don't have junk food, we won't eat it!**

Age 10, female, 4''11, 91 lbs - **i think bad foods that kids are addicted to my not stock the food in markets or stores so kids or teens can be healthier and live a longer life.**

Age 17, female, 5'4", 121 lbs - Although I am not personally addicted to junk food, I have seen more and more teenagers my age who do seem to display signs of being addicted to junk food. As for the whole "McDonalds" issue, I believe that fast-food corporations, while they should be able to make money, are corrupt when they add addictive sweeteners and hook children with gags like "Happy Meals" and a skinny clown (Ronald Mc D, who appears to have never eaten the food in any of the commercials he appears in.) While an individual does have some responsibility to control their own diet, greedy CEOs have no right to addict children with seeteners to make $$$. This is just like how cigarette companies add honey to sweeten the otherwise vulgar, nasty nicotine tast of cigarettes and thus appeal to teenagers - very immoral to profit off

Age 16, female, 5'6", 185 lbs - **If they didn't put addicting sugers in them they wouldn't be**

Age 11, female, 5'0, 140 lbs - **i belive that the kinds of stores that make junk food are to blame because nowdays what ever kind of junk food is set in front of a kid they are going to eat it**

Age 16, female, 5'8, 178 lbs - **IT WILL HELP THEM A LOT, BUT THEY WILL REALLY SUFFER, FOOD IS EERY FAT KID, FRIEND, AND LOVE**

Age 14, female, 5ft 4in, 153 lbs - **I think that its our fault that we eat this "junk food" but the companys need to see what there products are doing and stop making the junk food so accsesible!**

Restricting exposure of kids to highly abused foods may seem extreme. But if kids were catching an infectious disease from such foods, wouldn't we want to limit their exposure? Why is obesity different?

Here's what kids say about blocking access to junk food:
(http://www.blubberbuster.com/poll/comments_42.htm)

Age 13, female, 5 foot , 128 lbs - **OMG THIS WOULD HELP SO MUCH!!** i find myself at the deli buying candy behind my moms back ugh. **if that happened i think alot more people wouldnt be overweight**

Age 13, female, 5'5'', 133 lbs - I think that by blocking access to unhealthy food, it won't stop the adults from buying that stuff, for themselves, and **since these parents are irresposible obviously they would give it to their kids.**

Age 13, female, 5'6'', 160 lbs - I think that they (whoever) should **block off all reach to junkfood. that way, we wont be tempted to eat it.**

Age 13, female, 5ft.4", 177 lbs - **duh! it would help alot of people**

Age 17, female, 5'2", 110 lbs - most people r aware of how junk foods hurt u but how can you expect anyone to not eat them? **theyre always there!**

Age 15, female, 165 cm, 154 lbs ... I used to be a very obese teenager. I used to weigh about **210** pounds and **lost 56** pounds. Anyways, I believe that **it's very easy for teenagers to obtain junk food.**

Age 12, female, 5'3, 186 lbs I think that **if we had more healthy food places and less places like Taco Bell then kids would be skinner and wouldnt be over weight.** I hope you show this to other people

From James, Age 14 - 05/04/06
Ht. 5'1", Wt. 178 - Hey I come from a **school where everyday for lunch we have something from either burger king mcdonalds** etc.. I don't think theres one kid of normal weight in the school. ...O by the way, **we cant bring a lunch because it could be a bomb** (public skool)

Age 17, female, 5'7, 240 lbs - **I do believe the out of sight out of mind thing because I'm tempted everyday to go to the snack bar**. But kids would still bring things from home, just a smaller number of them will.

Hence, kids who are trying to lose weight say that restricting access to junk food and fast food would help them. Nonetheless, kids who are not trying to lose weight would rebel at this, as shown below:

Age 13, female, 5'5, 125 lb. - **this is gay**

Age 14, male, 6,0, 230 lb. - **i love to eat junk food**

Even though less access may deter kids somewhat, one teen notes" **its stupid. dose the beer probation act ring a bell?"** *As revealed in the poll on pp. 296, when schools remove junk food, entrepreneur kids sell junk food on a black market at school. How about a junk food tax? At the 2008 National Childhood Obesity Congress I asked acting U.S. Surgeon General, Steven K. Galson, if a tax on junk food was feasible. He felt that taxing junk food was unrealistic, as consumers and food companies would strongly resist such. Even so, taxing junk food, for example a sugar tax, is unlike prohibition. A black market would seem less likely, and the higher cost might curtail consumption of soda and junk food by kids. An added benefit might be less tooth decay, which occurs commonly in overweight kids [McDougal2009].*

2) Focus on the reasons kids overeat

Restricting access by kids to junk food and fast food may seem to be a direct way of impacting the childhood obesity epidemic. Nevertheless, what is really needed is a cultural shift so that overeating is 'not cool' and so that junk food is 'yuck.' It may be helpful to define what a 'food' is, versus simply a pleasurable substance which may be consumed by kids. Imagine if a new junk food were developed, which was so pleasurable that no one could resist it, the 'ultimate junk food.' Would we want to give that to kids? How close are we to the ultimate junk food?

Proposing to ban junk food and fast food in kids parallels the recent proposal to ban cigarettes in the military. This has generated an outcry that soldiers need cigarettes to cope with the stress of training, war, etc., even though they become addicted to smoking in the process. Similarly, kids say they use junk food and fast food to cope with stress, depression, and boredom, even though they become overweight in the process. Shouldn't we address the reasons that soldiers need cigarettes, and similarly, the reasons that kids need the comfort and stress relief of junk food and fast food? Why are kids so stressed and depressed today and what can be done about this? For example, something as simple as giving a kid a hug, a pat on the shoulder, or even a smile might do wonders to break overeating vicious cycles, as the post below suggests:

From renee, Age 13, female - 1/31/02
... i have **lost 18 pounds** ... i weighed **207 now i am 189**.... **this doc is great .. she is like my biggest cheerleader**. last time i **lost 9 ponds in one month and she hugged me!!!!** she **always asks about how i feel about the weight loss and she really cares**... i think the biggest thing is support from people who care about you!

Unfortunately, such "touchy, feely" approaches tend to be uncomfortable for clinicians and policy makers and raise liability issues for those who deal with kids, e.g. teachers, school nurses, PE teachers, counselors, YMCA leaders, etc. If kids can't get warmth and comfort at home, they usually can't get it elsewhere either.

Age 12, female, 5'3, 186 lbs - ... **If parents took the time to actually listen to their kids I think less kids would be depressed and less kids would go to the fridge when they were depressed.**

In a poll on our site, arriving home from school is the most common time that kids say they overeat (see pp. 163), (http://www.blubberbuster.com/cgi/poll_new_86.cgi). Communities might offer fun activities after school, on weekends, and during holidays, which would combat stress, loneliness, and boredom in kids. Counseling could be available for kids who need it. Schedules of schools, busing, and parents could be adjusted to allow for these activities. Hobbies, books, and musical instruments could be included, along with non-competitive sports, to cater to kids of all weights. Most overweight kids have low self-esteem, and raising their self-esteem is essential for motivation to lose weight. 'Charm' and fashion classes for girls and body-building classes for boys are ways to build self-esteem and reverse the low self-esteem vicious cycle. Federal, state, and local resources could be allotted for these activities.

3) Address the reasons for the adult obesity epidemic

In a poll asking what kids think would help the most to reverse the childhood obesity epidemic, more than two thirds of 110 kids voting say that parents being healthy role models would have the most effect (http://www.blubberbuster.com/cgi/poll_new_63_percent.cgi). In a second poll only one fourth of 201 kids responding say that their parents help them with weight loss (http://www.blubberbuster.com/cgi/poll_new_13_percent.cgi). Two thirds of their parents are overweight, which is the main reason the kids say that their parents don't help. Most of the kids say that they keep weight loss a secret from their parents (http://www.blubberbuster.com/cgi/poll_new_48_percent.cgi), and most say that they can lose weight without help from parents (http://www.blubberbuster.com/cgi/poll_new_59.cgi).

However, the kids add that if parents frequently bring home junk food and take the family to fast food restaurants, this makes it much harder for the kids to be a healthy weight.

Personal health risks appear to be not as motivating to adults as risks to the health of their children, although studies have shown that many parents of overweight kids are in denial that their kids are overweight. Health risks from obesity in children may prove to be the catalyst which reverses the adult obesity epidemic and its effects on children. The realization that kids will live shorter lives than their parents is a wakeup call that we must do something about the reasons for obesity in adults, which are very likely the same as in kids, i.e. stress eating and comfort eating, and which result in availability of hookable foods to kids. Again, probably not noticed is the fact that being a parent is stressful. A study comparing obesity rates of parents who have children in the home vs. adults of the same age who are child-less might shed some light on a possible link between parental stress and adult obesity. Might kids and parents both be stressing each other and overeating to cope?

4) Design weight loss programs to be more like substance dependence programs (addiction medicine).

As described earlier, in order to lose weight, the kids seem to have to go through unpleasant 'withdrawal' symptoms, similar to coming off alcohol or a drug. Hence, camps and live-in weight loss centers are needed for the most obese kids to help them through withdrawal. Weight loss centers and programs must recognize that once through withdrawal, kids need help to find alternative ways to comfort them and deal with stress and boredom, other than food. As many overweight kids have never learned how to cope with bad feelings, other than eating them away, it's thus an educational process on how to cope with life.

Furthermore, the self esteem of most obese kids is so low, that in order to motivate them to give up the comfort of food, instilling self-pride and caring about their bodies is first necessary.

There are many worthwhile childhood obesity initiatives, such as healthy lifestyle programs. But perhaps these programs should be examined through a psychological food dependence/addiction lens (right). Do such programs help psychological food dependence? If not, kids may become discouraged when such programs fail to help them lose weight or maintain their weight. Discouraged kids may comfort eat more and seek help less, another vicious cycle.

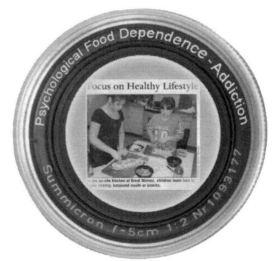

Psychological Food Dependence Lens

Out of the Mouths of Babes

Age 15, female, Ht: 5'4, Wt: 196 lbs - I've **lost 117 pounds**, and I've gone down 10 pant sizes. **I used to weigh 313,** I was huge... **I think it's awful that we as teens and kids are one of the first generations to have a lower life expectancy than our parents and even grandparents, it's so sad with the society we live in today.**

From Katraena, Age 9 - 06/17/06

....It really was hard for me to resiste foods,... I was **130lbs and only 4'11"** I was a big ol 9 year old. .. what I had been eatting when I lived with my mother ... **Did you know hot pockets and corn dogs are bad for you? THEN Y DO THEY MAKE EM? GRRRR** I was eatting about 6 hot pockets a day or 4 corn dogs a day ...

*A teen on the TV show, 'The Secret Life of an American Teenager,' remarked to an overweight classmate, "I don't hate you because you're fat; you're fat because I hate you." There's profound truth in that statement. Kids are hurting, and they're overeating because of it, which results in their hurting more. Compelling evidence points to overeating as a form of substance dependence, an emotional, psychological dependence on certain foods, appallingly similar to dependence on tobacco, alcohol, and drugs. Overweight and obesity in kids appears to be a psychological problem, **not** a nutritional problem. When kids ask, "How do I lose weight?" it appears that they are really asking, "How do I get through withdrawal?" and "How do I cope with life without using food?"*

Childhood obesity is at epidemic levels worldwide. Adequate treatment and prevention is just not happening. The health profession seems to be unaware of the psychological dependence (addiction?) of kids on food or is resistant to the idea. Kids understand it, as do food companies, so why doesn't everyone else?

You may say, "Okay, so overeating and overweight is like tobacco or alcohol abuse - it's just another vice... big deal." But we are talking about kids here, plus the enormous health costs! We need a dose of truth. Isn't the major difference between drugs of abuse, alcohol, tobacco, and high pleasure food simply that high pleasure food is given to children? Recall that cocaine was frequently given to children to soothe them in the early 1900's. And candy cigarettes were commonly given to kids as late as the 1950's.

> A 16 year old girl eloquently summed it all up:
>
> "A teen who does drugs or smokes would get in trouble if their parents found out. But no one's going to ground you for eating, which can be equally as damaging, and is equally as difficult to stop."

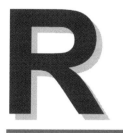

References

1. Adams,K., Lindell, K., Kohlmeier, M., and Zeisel, S., **Status of nutrition education in medical schools**, Am J Clin Nutr. 2006 April; 83(4): 941S–944S.

2. Agras, S., **Risk factors for childhood overweight: a prospective study from birth to 9.5 years,** J. Pediatr. 2004 Jul;145(1):20-5

3. Alexander, H., **"Pennsylvania: Designing Services to Treat Overweight and Obese Medical Assistance Children.",** NICHQ Q-Call **"Pay Now or Pay Later – Financing Childhood Obesity Prevention and Treatment,"** Dec. 2008

4. Austin SB, Field AE, Wiecha J, Peterson KE, Gortmaker SL., **School-based overweight preventive intervention lowers incidence of disordered weight-control behaviors in early adolescent girls**, Arch Pediatr Adolesc Med. 2005 Mar;159(3):225-30.).

5. Bennett, W., and Gurin, J., **The Dieter's Dilemm**a, Basic Books, 1982

6. Black J. and Macinko, J., **Neighborhoods and obesity,** J.Nutr Rev. 2008 Jan;66(1):2-20.

7. Blum J, Davee A, Beaudoin C, Jenkins P, Kaley L, Wigand D., **Reduced availability of sugar-sweetened beverages and diet soda has a limited impact on beverage consumption patterns in Maine high school youth**, J Nutr Educ Behav. 2008 Nov-Dec;40(6):341-7

8. Davis B and Carpenter C, **Proximity of fast-food restaurants to schools and adolescent obesity**, Am J Public Health. 2009 Mar;99(3):505-10.

9. Drewnowski A, Darmon N., **The economics of obesity: dietary energy density and energy cost.,** Am J Clin Nutr. 2005 Jul;82(1 Suppl):265S-273S

10. **Fast Food Tech**, Modern Marvels series, HistoryChannel.com, 2007.

11. Fennoy, I., **Treating and Evaluating Pediatric Obesity and Its Complications**, American Academy of Pediactrics NCE, San Francisco, October 2007.

12. Foster, G., Session on **"Cognitive Behavioral Treatment,"** Obesity Society Meeting, Boston, 2006.

304

13. Hambly, C., Adams, A., Fustin, J, Rance, K, Bünger, L., and Speakman, J., **Mice with Low Metabolic Rates Are Not Susceptible to Weight Gain When Fed a High-Fat Diet**, *Obesity Research (2005) 13, 556–566; doi: 10.1038/oby.2005.59 (http://www.nature.com/oby/journal/v13/n3/full/oby200559a.html)*

14. Hetherington M, **Chewing Gum May Help Reduce Cravings and Control Appetite** *Obesity Society Annual Meeting poster, New Orleans, 2007. (http://www.newswise.com/articles/view/534512/?sc=mwtn)*

15. Hill, J., Q&A and discussion following **Update on the National Weight Control Registry**, *Obesity Society Annual Meeting, Boston, October 2006.*

16. Jeffrey, J., Director, HealthyKids Weight Management Program, Children's Medicine Center, Charleston, WV, email **personal communication**, 2008.

17. Kalich K, Chomitz V , Peterson K , McGowan R, Houser R, and Must A, **Comfort and utility of school-based weight screening: the student perspective**, *BMC Pediatrics 2008, 8:9, March 2008.*

18. Koch FS; Sepa A; Ludvigsson J, **"Psychological stress and obesity"**, *The Journal of Pediatrics, Volume 153, Issue 6, December, 2008.*

19. Kubik MY, Fulkerson JA, Story M, Rieland G., **Parents of elementary school students weigh in on height, weight, and body mass index screening at school**, *J Sch Health. 2006 Dec;76(10):496-501.*

20. Landhuis C, Poulton R, Welch D, and Hancox R, **Childhood Sleep Time and Long-Term Risk for Obesity: A 32-Year Prospective Birth Cohort Study**, *Pediatrics, Vol. 122 No. 5 November 2008, pp. 955-960.*

21. Leatherdale ST, Wong SL, **Modifiable characteristics associated with sedentary behaviours among youth**, *Int J Pediatr Obes. 2008;3(2):93-101*

22. Martin, C., **Assessment and Intervention for Food Cravings**, *Obesity Society Annual Conference, Phoenix, 2008.*

23. McDougal S, Certo M, Tran J, and Bernat J, **Overweight Kids More Prone To Cavities**, *International Association of Dental Research meeting Buffalo, 2006.*

24. Neel JV., **Diabetes mellitus: a "thrifty" genotype rendered detrimental by "progress"?** *Am J Hum Genet 1962;14:353-62.*

25. NICHQ, National Initiative for Children's Healthcare Quality annual conference, **Childhood Obesity Forum**, *Miami, 2008.*

26. Nihiser AJ, Lee SM, Wechsler H, McKenna M, Odom E, Reinold C, Thompson D, Grummer-Strawn L. , **Body mass index measurement in schools.**, *J Sch Health. 2007 Dec;77(10):651-71; quiz 722-4.*

27. O'Malley, G., Trinity College, Dublin, Ireland, **personal communication**.

28. Pretlow, R., **Overweight and Obesity in Childhood**, *Letter to the Editor, Pediatrics, Vol. 122, No. 2, August 2008, pp. 476.*

29. Schwimmer JB, Burwinkle TM, and Varni J., **Health-related quality of life of severely obese children and adolescents**, *JAMA. 2003 Apr 9;289(14):1813-9.*

30. Selye, H., **"A Syndrome Produced by Diverse Nocuous Agents"**, *J Neuropsychiatry Clin Neurosci, reprinted in Nature, vol. 138, July 4, 1936, p. 32.*

31. **Snack Food Tech**, *Modern Marvels series, HistoryChannel.com, 2007.*

32. Skelton JA, Cook SR, Auinger P, Klein JD, Barlow SE, **Prevalence and Trends of Severe Obesity Among US Children and Adolescents**, *Acad Pediatr. 2009 Jun 26.*

33. Spangle, L., **Life is Hard, Food is Easy**, *Lifeline Press, Washington, DC, 2003.*

34. Stice E, Killen JD, Hayward C, Taylor CB, **Age of onset for binge eating and purging during late adolescence: a 4-year survival analysis**, *.J Abnorm Psychol. 1998 Nov;107(4):671-5.*

35. **Stress in America**, *American Psychological Association Report, October 2007 (http://apahelpcenter.mediaroom.com/file.php/138/Stress+in+America+REPORT+FINAL.doc)*

36. Striegel-Moore RH, Dohn F, Kraemer HC, Taylor CB, Daniels S, Crawford P. **Eating disorders in black and white women.**, *Am J Psychiatry.2003; 160 (7):1326 –1331(Binge eating onset).*

37. Swinburn B, **Obesity prevention in children and adolescents**, *Child Adolesc Psychiatr Clin N Am. 2009 Jan;18(1):209-23*

38. Nicklas T, Baranowski T, Cullen K, and Berenson, G, **Eating Patterns, Dietary Quality and Obesity,** *Journal of the American College of Nutrition, Vol. 20, No. 6, 599-608 (2001)*

39. Torres SJ, Nowson CA, **Relationship between stress, eating behavior, and obesity**, *Nutrition. 2007 Nov-Dec;23(11-12):887-94. Epub 2007 Sep 17.*

40. Washington, R., **Childhood Obesity Difficult Cases**, *Contemporary Forums Obesity Prevention & Treatment, San Francisco, May 2008.*

306

41. Williamson, D., *Assessment and Treatment of Binge Eating Disorders*, Obesity Society Annual Meeting, Phoenix, 2008.